TRIP THE LIGHT WITHIN

A PSILOCYBIN THERAPY GUIDE

CATHERINE WARNOCK
MA, LPCC, NCC

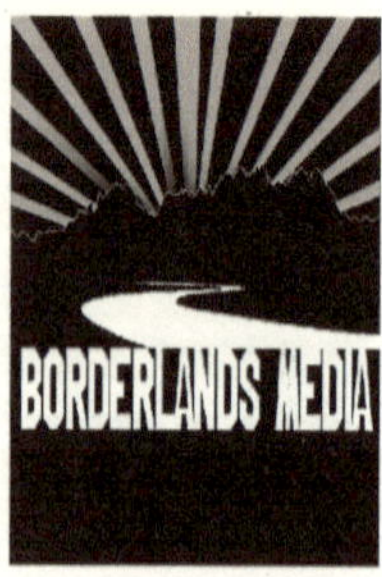
BORDERLANDS MEDIA

TABLE OF CONTENTS

FOREWORD

"This takes it to the next level," she said.

"Right?!" I replied.

There's a single word that appears near the end of Catherine's book that I had to look up the first time I read it. That word is *liminal*. It refers to the place between two sides; the occupation of a space that's on a threshold. That word—liminal—is the key to this book.

When Catherine and I met online, she'd already completed five chapters of a book she was writing. It didn't seem like she'd require any help to get it finished. However, I was intrigued by her line of work and offered a few minutes of my time to provide her with some insights into book writing and publishing. She accepted.

During our meeting, she revealed that she was still experimenting with the book's format. I suggested she join our writing community as a safe place to trial her ideas and receive feedback from peer and professional authors. It was in that liminal space that her book began to take shape.

Eventually, my business partner and I became Catherine's developmental editors on the project. But that's only one facet of the role we played.

As is the case with any book project, I straddled the line between teacher and student. I helped awaken Catherine's dormant writing skills, and she opened my mind to the world of Psychedelic Assisted Therapy (PAT). When you give, you get.

The following months whizzed by as Catherine wrote and took breaks to work on two documentaries. But when she came back, something had shifted. She had a new vision, a new direction for the book.

"Okay," we said. "It's your book; let's do it."

Catherine will tell you that the following four months elapsed outside the bounds of what we call time. She didn't just write; the writing flowed through her. The words, sentences, and chapters became an unstoppable current, filling the pages of her screen and making their way to my editing table. I hung on every section, delighting in the mysteries that revealed themselves like the stars do at dusk.

Interesting, I thought. *Fascinating. I believe her.*

As the grand story took shape, buoyed by all the supporting stories, I knew we were creating something special. It was, therefore, no surprise to me when we discovered a whole new portal into Catherine's work, dressed up as an onomatopoeia.

¡OYE!

Say it out loud, and it forces you to stop. It's a liminal concept that means *here!* or *look here!* It begs attention and forces you to stop—right on a threshold. In that space, the reader is invited to reflect on a crucial aspect of the teaching. It's also a nod to the cultural significance of Catherine's Latino heritage and an appreciation of the indigenous traditions to which our Western culture might offer its most profound gratitude.

And then we found *her*, or rather, she found us.

"This elevates the book," Catherine said.

"What a discovery," I replied.

"This takes it to the next level," she said.

"Right?!"

Between the factual accounts of psilocybin experiences and the science behind the medicine, we all heard it: *her voice.*

Quiet at first—nameless, even.

She is an ethereal entity with the wisdom of a sage, the love of a mother, and the unflinching truth of a mirror. I suppose she was always there, waiting for us to see her—to hear her. She is the liminal space in which everything is born and everything dies. She is the vibration before the voice, the heartbeat before the body.

Maria's entity isn't a creation of ours; she's an apparition. *She's* the one who inserted herself in Catherine's work, who opened the door to a higher consciousness. As much as it's been an honor to edit Catherine's work, it's been an honor to interact with the cast of entities that made this book possible—from distant relatives of a bygone era, to souls called to help humanity. I'm deeply touched by the impact all of them have had on my experience working on this humanitarian book.

Less than a week after completing my editorial contribution to Catherine's work, I journeyed into the field to test what I had acquired academically and sought to integrate spiritually. Under Catherine's expert guidance, I did a psilocybin journey. She encouraged me to create intentions, to examine my blockages, and open my heart to the possibility of healing.

I accepted.

On the journey, I died. At least twenty times over. Each death resonated in a new color—colors I'd never seen before. Of course, my many deaths were metaphorical, but they were also quite real. Real, in the sense that the egoic construct with which I walked into the experience died that day.

In the weeks that followed my journey, I have been visited several times by the ghost of my once familiar ego. It wants to reinhabit my body, but I have too much love now to allow it back in.

So I named him. He is *Casper.* I love him, but he's also journeying, flickering in and out of my reality. As each day goes by and I direct my energy to the new—yet to be named—ego, I am grateful and in love.

When you look into Catherine's eyes, there is a playful and daring soul adorned with compassion. That soul wants nothing more than to see the inhabitants of our planet see their true selves. Because when they do, aided by the wisdom of mushrooms, it's impossible to avoid the complete presence of Truth. I now know the truth, and it is *everything*. In that liminal space in which Truth resides, everything has its place, and it's all perfect—just like Catherine's book.

In the spirit of love,

I AM

Alex Morin

CHAPTER ONE

FROM FORENSICS TO FUNGI

VOICE - *You've been walking for some time now, haven't you?*

CATHERINE - *Who's there?*

VOICE - *You don't know me yet.*

Though you've listened for me longer

than you think.

CATHERINE - *I don't understand.*

VOICE - *You will, in time.*

Not all guidance comes in thunder.

Some arrive like spores on the wind.

CATHERINE - *(hesitating) Why now?*

VOICE - *Because now ... you're ready to remember.*

I WAS LYING ON THE FLOOR, eyes closed, body trembling, as the mushrooms surged through me like a wave I hadn't consented to but desperately needed. I wasn't sure if I was dying or being reborn. My breath came in shallow gasps, tears slid down the sides of my face, and somewhere in the distance, I could hear the low hum of a trusted guide's voice reminding me to surrender.

This was not recreational. This was reclamation.

In that moment, everything—my illness, my heartbreak, my relentless drive—collapsed into one pulsing truth: I had been carrying more than my body could hold. And these mushrooms, strange as it sounds, knew precisely where to go. They found the places I had buried, the memories I had rationalized, the trauma I had buried beneath the mask of achievement.

Had cancer returned? My body showed signs of it.

And then the mushrooms, in their quiet wisdom, seemed to ask: *What if I am not here to fix you, but to restore what has always been hidden?*

People think working in psychedelic therapy means I must be calm, spiritual, maybe even effortlessly enlightened. They don't realize it requires walking into fire, again and again. They don't know that before I ever held space for anyone else, I had to survive the burning down of my own life.

This is a story about healing, yes, but more than that, it's about remembering. Remembering who we are beneath the survival mechanisms. Remembering what's possible when we stop numbing, stop pretending, and start listening.

And it begins with one woman—me—saying yes to a path that terrified her.

My career trajectory has consistently led me to the cutting edge of innovation. I now find myself at the frontier once again. This time in the world of *psychedelic-assisted therapy*, a field experiencing a renaissance that has been profoundly transformative both personally and professionally.

The first time I stood at such a threshold was in the mid-1990s, when forensic science was just beginning to emerge from the shadows into public awareness. During my final undergraduate semester in late 1994, I worked in a toxicology laboratory in Sacramento while closely following the O.J. Simpson trial on the radio. Even then, I sensed the magnitude of what was unfolding, not just in the courtroom, but in the evolution of forensic science itself. The trial brought unprecedented attention to DNA analysis, toxicology, and crime scene investigation, forever changing public perception and professional standards. Suddenly, terms like "chain of custody" and "contamination of evidence" were being discussed on the evening news. For the first time, the average person began to understand that how evidence is collected and handled can make or break a case. It became clear that forensic science wasn't just about solving crimes; it was about ensuring justice. Much like today's psychedelic field, it was a moment when science, media, and culture collided. And I had a front-row seat.

Today, I see similar shifts happening in the world of psychedelics.

What was once a taboo subject relegated to underground circles is now making its way into clinical trials, legislative debates, and mainstream media. Words like "*integration*," "*set and setting*," and "*therapeutic dose*" are starting to enter the public conversation. Just as the O.J. Simpson trial helped demystify forensic science for the public, today's growing openness to psychedelics is beginning to reshape our understanding of healing, consciousness, and mental health. And once again, I find myself witnessing the birth of an entirely new field, one that I'm helping shape as it comes into being.

After graduating from California State University, Sacramento in 1995, I joined the Texas Department of Public Safety's DNA Analysis section at their Corpus Christi laboratory, which included on-call crime scene duties. I distinctly remember rushing home during lunch, on one of my shifts, to watch the Simpson verdict live. It was a seminal moment for forensic science, particularly in terms of crime scene protocols, and how the Simpson crime scene was processed, precipitating significant changes. The case forever altered standard protocols and the collection of crime scene evidence worldwide, setting new benchmarks for investigations globally. I mention this because psilocybin protocols for healing will no doubt experience the same type of "watershed" moment. Just as forensic science evolved in response to critical lessons learned, the processes surrounding psilocybin-assisted therapy are in the process of being refined to meet the complex needs of mental health patients. We are standing on the threshold of transformational shifts that will define best practices for future generations.

In 1995, DNA analysis was in its infancy, drawing intense interest from all sectors. Upon arriving in Corpus Christi, I volunteered to spearhead the quality control and validation testing process, a requisite for establishing DNA analysis capabilities for crime labs. Though demanding, the project aligned perfectly with my motivation to make a difference. It also aligned with my drive to be a part of cutting-edge technology.

I was young and fresh out of college, fueled by an eagerness to prove myself. I wanted more than just a job. I wanted to leave a mark, to contribute in a way that mattered beyond the confines of my role. The opportunity to be at the forefront of something as groundbreaking as forensic DNA analysis felt like my chance to carve out a meaningful place in a rapidly evolving field. I approached every task with determination, driven by the belief that my work could have a tangible impact on justice and the lives of those affected by crime. After months of rigorous work, I completed the required validation studies and received authorization to implement DNA analysis for evidence processing. It was more than just a professional milestone; it was the realization that even as a newcomer, my efforts could shape the future of forensic science.

My contributions didn't go unnoticed. Soon, I was traveling to other Texas State laboratories in Waco and Lubbock, helping them initiate their validation studies. I've never shied away from hard work or the challenge of blazing new trails in the pursuit of innovation.

During my early twenties, as an undergraduate, I first encountered death in ways that would leave an imprint I carried for decades. Sitting in forensic classes, I stared at photographs of bodies torn by violence. Faces were unrecognizable, limbs contorted, the aftermath of human cruelty frozen in clinical detail. I remember gripping the edge of the table, my stomach twisting, asking myself, sometimes out loud, sometimes just in my mind, "Is this even right?"

Back then, I didn't understand that the tight knot in my chest, the prickling nausea, and the sleepless nights that followed were not just discomfort. They were trauma staking its claim. The coursework demanded detachment and objectivity, yet I felt my own humanity fraying at the edges. I was being exposed to horrors no one should endure at that age, and I had no tools to process what I was seeing.

By the time I began handling crime scenes, the intensity escalated. Scenes of unimaginable violence became part of my daily reality. Brain matter spattered across walls. Rivers of blood pooled across floors. Weapons twisted against flesh in ways that defied comprehension. The human body and the choices people make in moments of extreme cruelty left an imprint on my mind that refused to fade. The images replayed behind my eyes when I tried to sleep. Days, sometimes nights, would pass with me staring at the ceiling, wide awake, my mind trapped in a loop of horror I could neither control nor escape. It was brutal. I didn't yet have the language or the insight to know that what I was experiencing was trauma, that the stress I felt was a response to repeated exposure to human violence.

It wasn't until graduate school, as I studied counseling, that the full weight of my experiences began to make sense. Sitting in classes on first responder trauma and vicarious trauma, I began to recognize my own symptoms: the sleepless nights, the involuntary replay of scenes, the heavy, unshakable anxiety. I realized that law enforcement and forensic science at that time had no place for mental health. Vulnerability was seen as weakness. Processing wasn't just discouraged; it was invisible. I had carried decades of unacknowledged trauma, believing resilience meant silence.

For the first time, I began to actively process my work-related PTSD. I learned to acknowledge the images, the memories, the fear, and the emotional weight that had built up inside me. I studied the mechanisms of trauma, vicarious trauma, and PTSD, finally giving voice to experiences that had silently shaped me for years. That work laid the foundation for my future in counseling and psychedelic-assisted therapy. I had walked through the worst of humanity's violence and lived, and I could hold space for others confronting the shadows in their own lives.

When I later began guiding clients with psilocybin and other psychedelics, I realized the medicine could reach layers of trauma that even years of traditional processing could not. Psychedelics allowed access to the hidden places of memory, emotion, and fear, layers I had first encountered in those early forensic experiences. My firsthand understanding of extreme trauma allowed me to navigate both my own healing and the healing of others with empathy, precision, and care. It was the bridge between surviving the unspeakable and guiding others toward reclaiming themselves.

My five-year career with TX DPS began in Corpus Christi and culminated at the Houston laboratory, where I caught the attention of Applied Biosystems, now part of Thermo Fisher Scientific. As the leading manufacturer of DNA analysis equipment, reagents, kits, and software, they recruited me to train forensic scientists nationwide, and occasionally worldwide.

The wisdom I gained in this role extended far beyond technical expertise. As I traveled the United States, visiting major metropolitan hubs, smaller cities, and towns, I developed a nuanced ability to connect with people from diverse backgrounds and mindsets. The extensive travel came with extra benefits, one of which was the accumulation of airline and hotel points that became gateways to international adventures. Were it not for the points, I may have missed out on many of the experiences that helped shape my worldview.

One such trip took me to Amsterdam, where I spent an afternoon strolling along the winding canals, reflecting on the city's quiet resilience. At a small café by the water, I struck up a conversation with an older woman who had lived through Amsterdam's post-war recovery. As she shared her story of personal loss and renewal, it became clear that the city had found strength in the collective power of community. Much like the people who rebuilt it, the city had learned that resilience didn't come from isolation, but from coming together. Her words about the importance of connection, shared healing, and the strength of good people resonated deeply with me. These lessons would later inform my work and help me guide others through their journeys of recovery.

These international journeys became more than just vacations; they were immersive lessons in cultural and social understanding. Visiting unfamiliar landscapes and connecting with diverse populations and communities, I cultivated a global perspective that taught me adaptability and open-mindedness. As a result, my worldview expanded far beyond what traditional learning methods could offer. I didn't know it at the time, but the education would set me up well for navigating the world of psychedelics.

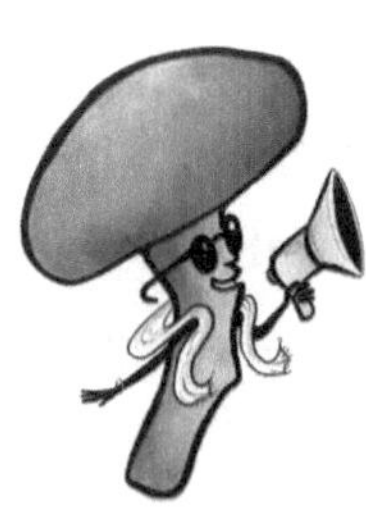

¡OYE! Optimize Your Experience

Throughout this book, you'll spot little sections called **¡OYE!**, short for **Optimizing Your Experience**. These are bite-sized tips to help you make the most of your journey, whether you're getting ready, in the middle of a big realization, or figuring things out afterward. In Spanish, *oye* means "listen," and it's also a common way to grab someone's attention, like saying "Hey!" or "Yo!" So when you see one, picture the mushrooms leaning in with wide eyes, snapping their fingers, saying, "¡OYE! Don't miss this part."

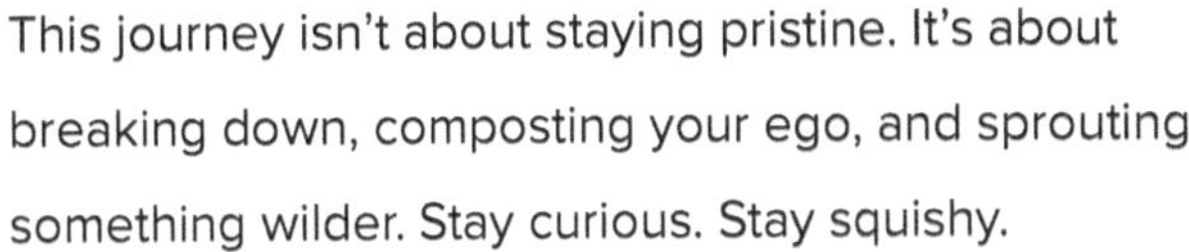

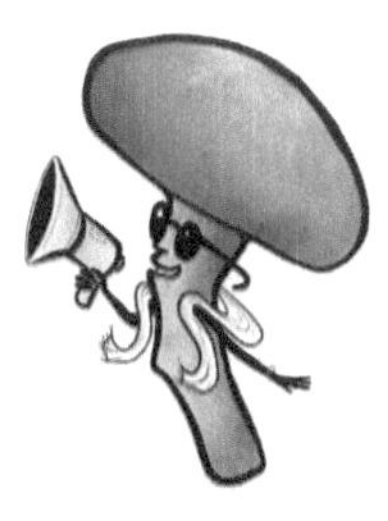

This journey isn't about staying pristine. It's about breaking down, composting your ego, and sprouting something wilder. Stay curious. Stay squishy.

The first time I tried mushrooms was around the year 2010. It happened in Denver, and with a relatively moderate amount. I didn't measure it, but based on my experience today, I would say I took between .75 and 1.0 grams. My neighbor had acquired a small bag, and I agreed to give it a try. That experience occurred approximately a decade before I would discover the therapeutic potential of _psilocybin_ mushrooms.

Nevertheless, the experience itself was subtle.

From my balcony, I observed the night sky in peaceful relaxation, the cool air brushing softly against my skin. The moon hung low, a luminous guardian of the dark sky above, casting a mystical glow that seemed almost too vivid, too alive. Its light wasn't just bright, it stretched, unfolding into a supernatural, delicate tail that trailed behind it like the fragile sweep of a comet or the faint wisp of a celestial ribbon. The shadow it cast shimmered faintly, pulsating with an energy that felt both ancient and intimate, as if the moon itself were breathing. The edges of objects around me blurred slightly, haloed in silver, and the sky seemed deeper, vaster, as though I were peering into an endless well of stars. No one with me that night could confirm what I witnessed. Their eyes saw only the familiar, while mine had glimpsed something inexplicably altered.

The following morning, I dismissed the experience as ordinary. The vividness had faded like a dream upon waking, leaving little inclination to explore further. What had felt extraordinary under the moon's glow had quietly dissolved into the unremarkable. It was as if the ineffable nature of what I had witnessed couldn't withstand the harsh light of day. The experience defied language, slipping through the cracks of my vocabulary, and became impossible to put into words. With my ego back in full presence, eager to reassert control and logic, I found myself discounting the truth of what I'd seen; convincing myself it was nothing more than a trick of light or an overactive imagination.

It would be another ten years before my interest would spark again, but through the lens of therapeutic applications.

> **VOICE** - *You've been searching with your eyes open.*
> *But the answers are waiting in the dark*
> **CATHERINE** - *Who are you?*
> **VOICE** - *A reflection. A root. A remnant of what you forgot you knew.*
> **CATHERINE** - *Are you part of me?*
> **VOICE** - *In time, you won't need to ask that question.*
> **CATHERINE** - *Why are you here?*
> **VOICE** - *To walk with you. When the path disappears.*

In 2012, I made the bold decision to leave my 20-year career in forensic science and pursue a new path in counseling. The truth is, forensics no longer aligned with who I was becoming. Like the medical field, it demanded certainty and an expectation of always being right, of having the final answer. That environment often bred arrogance, and I found myself increasingly uncomfortable in a space that didn't allow room for vulnerability, humility, or growth. I wanted to live and work in a way that embraced imperfection, both in myself and in others. As such, I enrolled and was admitted into a graduate counseling program.

I had a deep desire to learn and grow. What I quickly discovered was that entering a counseling graduate program wasn't just about earning a degree; it was an honest journey of personal transformation. And it wasn't like any typical academic program. It became a continuous process of self-exploration and therapy, where every lesson in the classroom forced me to confront and navigate my own personal challenges. It reshaped me, and in doing so, deepened my understanding of how healing is a lifelong, ongoing process not just for the clients I would eventually serve, but for myself as well.

As my journey continued to unfold, I had the misfortune of facing medical challenges. In 2019, I needed bilateral hip replacements, six months apart, due to an aggressive form of osteoarthritis that was deteriorating my hip sockets at an unprecedented rate.

After my first hip surgery, I asked to schedule the second right away. My surgeon recommended waiting years. But with the level of pain and limited mobility I was facing, that simply wasn't an option. I pushed back.

Reluctantly, he agreed to X-ray my other hip, confident it would show minimal change. His surprise was palpable when the images revealed a level of deterioration typically seen after two years—yet it had happened in just two months. That unexpected decline fast-tracked my second surgery, even as I was still recovering from the first.

Once I completed standard rehabilitation, I began working with a personal trainer twice a week to rebuild strength and stabilize the muscles around my new joints. During one of our sessions, she mentioned her recent experience with _magic mushrooms_. I'd tried them once before and found them unimpressive, but something about her story stuck with me. I tucked it away. _You never know, right?_

Although I was regaining my strength, I didn't foresee that my health issues were only beginning. I had both hips replaced at the age of fifty-one. And at the end of 2020, my doctor urged me to get my first colonoscopy, which I managed to avoid for another year. Having both hips replaced seemed like a valid excuse, but not long after I turned fifty-two, my doctor insisted I be initiated into the mid-life health routines common in Western medicine. I continued to procrastinate, and eventually, when there were no more excuses to hide behind, I drank the awful solution, endured the treatment preparation, and completed the procedure.

Whew! I was relieved when it was over, and my doctor told me everything looked fine except for a polyp located in a difficult-to-reach spot due to its size. Typically, small polyps are easily removed during the procedure, but this one, according to the doctor, would require surgical removal. They said they would have more information to share after the biopsy results were obtained.

I went on with my life as if nothing had happened, until about two weeks later, when I received a phone call and a letter from my doctor informing me that the biopsy results were cancerous. I had non-Hodgkin's B-cell lymphoma.

Even with this news, my level of denial led me to believe it was nothing to worry about. After all, the doctor had mentioned it could be surgically removed. I'd been through a few surgeries before, and in my mind, this would be no different than the appendectomy I'd had a few years prior. *No big deal. Go in, cut it out, and I'll move on with my life.*

I realized how wrong I was when I received a call from the oncologist's office. They asked me to come in to meet with the doctor that same day! Anyone familiar with the U.S. healthcare system knows that most specialists have a waiting list of at least two to eight weeks for initial appointments. This doctor wanted me there in just three hours! *Uh-oh.* The nauseous feeling in my stomach quickly overpowered my urge to put it off for a week or two, and I cleared my schedule.

The following week was a whirlwind that turned my life upside down. Overnight, my calendar was flooded with appointments—scans, blood tests, the installation of a port, endless doctor visits, and medication changes. It felt like an avalanche, crashing down on me all at once. I was drowning, overwhelmed by a medical world I never wanted to be part of. No matter how hard I tried, I couldn't catch up emotionally. My mind was spinning, my body was changing, and my heart was heavy with fear.

Since this happened at the height of COVID, many doctors had implemented strict restrictions to minimize the spread of the virus. One of these meant that I had to attend my appointment alone. The thought of walking into the office by myself was daunting, but I didn't have a choice.

Whenever I receive difficult news, my mind tends to go blank—I struggle to process the information in the moment fully.

Having someone there with me has always been essential, not just for emotional support, but to help me make sense of everything afterward. The realization hit hard that my husband, Ken, my rock, wouldn't be allowed in the exam room with me.

So we came up with a plan: He would drop me off, drive home, and be ready for my call so he could listen in on speakerphone during my session with the doctor. This solved part of the problem, but I would still have to walk into the appointment alone. After hearing whatever news awaited me, I would have to sit there by myself and wait for him to come back and pick me up.

The physical distance between us that day was only a few miles, but emotionally, it felt like a galaxy away.

Dr. Rama, my oncologist, informed me that I had a rare and very aggressive form of cancer. When I suggested we schedule the surgery right away, she gave me a troubled look, clearly searching for a gentle way to explain that surgery wasn't the path forward.

I distinctly remember her saying, "If you do that, it will only grow back."

What I didn't yet understand was that I didn't have colon cancer. I had lymphoma. It had been discovered in my colon, but it could have just as easily been found anywhere in my lymphatic system. While cutting out a polyp might be a practical approach for colon cancer, it's not a solution for lymphoma.

I struggled to wrap my head around the treatment plan she outlined, each word hitting me like a wave I wasn't prepared to face:

Extensive chemotherapy—around the clock.

Five days in the hospital.

Hooked up to an IV.

Not just once, but every three weeks for a total of six hospital stays.

And if that wasn't enough, Dr. Rama gently added that radiation might be necessary if my body didn't respond to the chemo.

Shit.

I sat there, numb, trying to process what she was saying. I'd heard of people walking into a doctor's office for chemotherapy infusion, maybe for a few hours, then heading home to recover. *But for five days straight? In a hospital bed?* I couldn't wrap my mind around it. My heart raced as I asked the only question I could manage: "Why can't I just do this at home?"

She gave me a soft, apologetic look and explained that this type of chemo was high-risk as it required constant monitoring, and my vitals had to be checked around the clock to ensure I didn't *crash* under its intensity.

It felt like the ground beneath me was slipping away. None of it made sense. I was still clinging to the hope that we could just cut it out, be done with it, and move on. But with every word she spoke, the hope unravelled, leaving me face-to-face with a reality I wasn't ready to accept.

During the appointment, Ken struggled to hear much of what was discussed. Dr. Rama had a naturally soft voice, and with both of us wearing masks, the sound was muffled. This left me with the heavy burden of not only processing the life-altering information in real time, but also ensuring I could accurately convey every detail to Ken. The weight of that responsibility was immense, knowing how much I relied on him for support, yet feeling the pressure of being the sole bridge between him and the critical information we both needed to grasp.

I'll never forget the look on Ken's face when I shared the news with him. He had always been my rock, a steady, unshakable presence. He has always been the kind of man whose calm could anchor our ship in any storm. But at that moment, something cracked.

I saw something I'd never seen before. His face fell as if the very foundation of his composure had been pulled from beneath him. The color drained from his skin, leaving him pale and almost translucent, like the blood had retreated inward, trying to protect him from a blow he couldn't deflect. His eyes, usually warm and steady, opened wider with a raw, unfiltered fear, their usual sparkle dimmed by the weight of sudden dread. His jaw clenched involuntarily, a silent attempt to hold himself together, but I saw the slight tremor in his lips, the rapid blink as he tried to process words too heavy to carry. That flicker of vulnerability, that fragile crack in the armor of the man I leaned on, terrified me more than the diagnosis itself. It was like watching an immovable mountain shudder and realizing that if it could be shaken, then nothing was as unshakable as I'd believed. Seeing Ken so unnerved made the reality of it hit even harder.

And yet, surprisingly, something shifted in me. As his fear surfaced, I felt myself grow more stoic, as if I had to be strong enough for both of us. My resolve hardened. I thought to myself, *We've been through tough times before; we can get through this too.*

The year prior had been brutal with my hip replacements, a long road of pain, recovery, and uncertainty. If we'd survived that, surely this would be more of the same.

But deep down, this was just another layer of denial, a fragile shield against the truth I couldn't yet grasp. I had no idea what we were about to face.

We had about two weeks to prepare for my first treatment. Dr. Rama stressed, once again, that this was a highly aggressive form of cancer, demanding an equally aggressive treatment plan that would begin as soon as possible. There was no time to waste. She worked tirelessly to get my insurance to approve the treatment. Before I could fully process what was happening, I found myself packing my favorite pillow and the cute, colorful pajamas I had bought—small comforts to bring a touch of warmth to the stark reality of a week-long hospital stay.

The pace of everything only increased. It was all happening so fast that I could barely keep up. It was as though the snow was catapulting down the mountain towards me, roaring like a prehistoric beast, and I was an unsuspecting new growth evergreen in its path. One moment, I was preparing for Thanksgiving, clinging to normalcy, and before I could even process the diagnosis, Christmas came, and I found myself in a cold, sterile room, hooked up to an IV, receiving my first cancer treatment. It was all happening too fast, and I felt powerless to stop it.

The entire cancer experience could fill the pages of its own book: every detail, every emotion, every battle. But as it relates to my psychedelic journey, this was *the* pivotal moment. It was during this time, in the shadow of fear and uncertainty, that I began to uncover the profound benefits psychedelics could offer, not just for mental clarity and emotional resilience, but for physical healing as well.

By this time, I was a licensed counselor. And with this skillset, it didn't take long for me to notice the varied mental health states of my fellow cancer patients. Patterns emerged, and I observed how certain emotional conditions seemed to support or hinder the healing process.

One of the most striking patterns was the prevalence of anger. Some patients were furious about their diagnosis, haunted by questions like, *Why me?* and, *What did I do to deserve this?* This was particularly heartbreaking to witness, because their anger seemed to drain so much of the precious energy their bodies needed for healing. The emotional weight was palpable, as if their rage created a toxic internal battle that ran parallel to the one their bodies were already fighting.

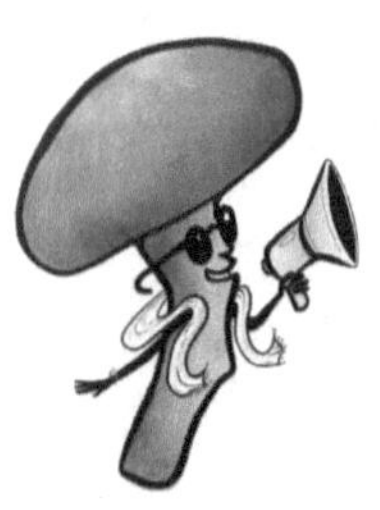

¡OYE! Energy is contagious—mushrooms pick up what you're putting down.

They don't just read the room. They *magnify* what's in the room. So bring grounded presence, sprinkle in some curiosity, and leave the cranky at the door.

Then there were those consumed by fear. Some were terrified of dying, while others suffered from PTSD triggered by the medical trauma they were enduring: each scan, each procedure, each hospital stay layering new anxieties onto old wounds. PTSD magnified every step of the process, turning even routine appointments into sources of panic.

Often, I saw patients grappling with both fear and anger, much of it rooted in their experiences within a medical system they felt was failing or even traumatizing them. As well-intentioned as medical staff may be, the reality is that they often don't have the time to listen and truly address each patient's specific concerns.

In a routine setting, where most people see their doctors only a few times a year, this can be frustrating but manageable. However, for patients navigating serious illness—especially those who are hospitalized and interacting with medical professionals multiple times a day—the experience is entirely different. The lack of personalized attention can feel overwhelming, even dehumanizing. Medications may be delayed or mixed up, critical symptoms may be overlooked, and concerns may be dismissed in the rush of a chaotic healthcare system that is overstretched. What might be a minor inconvenience in ordinary circumstances can become a source of deep distress and lead to PTSD when your body is already fighting for survival, and you feel like just another case file instead of a person in need of care.

The third predominant emotional state I observed was guilt and shame. For patients with lung or liver cancer, those feelings were often directly linked to past behaviors like smoking or drinking. But for many others, guilt and shame stemmed from feeling like a burden to their families, friends, and even to medical staff. Cancer can be profoundly isolating, not just because of the illness itself, but because it often feels like you're the only one truly advocating for your care. Cancer may ravage the body's cells, but the need to repeatedly ask for attention and insist that something isn't right can be exhausting. When all of this happens continuously and pleas are dismissed, there's an erosion of self-worth. It chips away at your sense of value, and some patients begin to believe they deserve the suffering, as though their illness is some kind of punishment. That belief only deepens their guilt and shame, creating a vicious cycle that is as damaging to their spirit as the cancer is to their bodies.

One thing I knew from my work as a therapist was that unresolved anger often becomes depression, while unresolved fear becomes anxiety. The emotional toll of carrying these burdens, along with guilt and shame, is staggering. The sheer amount of energy it takes to combat depression, anxiety, and self-blame, while simply trying to maintain a basic level of functioning, is utterly exhausting.

What struck me during my cancer experience was how the emotional exhaustion wasn't just a mental struggle; it had a physiological cost. Research in psychoneuroimmunology shows that chronic emotional stress suppresses immune function, slows physical recovery, and elevates inflammation.[1] When patients expend their inner resources on fear and trauma, it can literally drain the energy their bodies need for healing.

Throughout my cancer treatment and recovery, I learned that healing isn't just a physical process. It's deeply tied to mental and emotional well-being. A peaceful, healthy mind creates space for the body to focus its efforts on fighting the disease. My experience taught me that healing requires more than medicine; it demands emotional clarity, acceptance, and a sense of inner calm, allowing the body to channel its strength where it's needed most.

Before my diagnosis, I had done extensive work on understanding how the brain processes and resolves trauma, including the roots of anger, depression, fear/anxiety, and guilt/shame. While I hadn't fully unraveled all of my unresolved trauma, I had made significant transformational shifts without the aid of psychedelics. The inner work created a solid foundation that allowed me to navigate my cancer treatment without becoming consumed by such emotional weights. However,

---

1   Gouin & Kiecolt-Glaser, 2012

trauma resolution occurs in layers, and healing is not a single event; it's an ongoing process.

The work I had done was enough to help me focus on recovery rather than being paralyzed by fear or resentment. I was also fortunate to have an incredible support system, a loving and devoted husband who kept my spirits lifted, and a family whose unwavering presence allowed me to focus all my energy on physical healing. Their support created a buffer against the emotional hardship that often accompanies a cancer diagnosis. But there were still deeper layers I had yet to uncover. At the time, I didn't realize just how much remained beneath the surface. It wasn't until later, when I discovered psychedelics, that I would begin to access those hidden wounds—ones that traditional methods hadn't fully revealed. Psychedelics wouldn't just bring them to light; they would ultimately provide a way to engage with them, process them, and resolve them in ways I hadn't previously imagined.

In a surprise twist of fate, as quickly as the avalanche had come hurtling at me, the violent mounds of snow retreated. After my third chemotherapy treatment, I had a PET scan that revealed incredible news: the mass in my colon was gone.

Gone! I could hardly believe it. I felt a surge of disbelief, quickly followed by an overwhelming wave of relief that left me breathless.

WooHoo!

Dr. Rama even suspected it might have disappeared after the second treatment, but the exact timing didn't matter. What mattered was that it was no longer there. The aggressive treatment had done its job, shrinking the lymphatic mass back to a normal lymph node. I remember clutching the edges of the exam table, tears welling up, not just from joy, but from the sheer exhaustion of carrying the weight of a potentially terminal illness for as long as I had. In that moment, the worry loosened its grip, replaced by gratitude so deep it felt like my heart could burst.

Despite the progress, Dr. Rama urged me to complete the whole treatment plan to minimize the risk of recurrence. She warned that if the cancer returned, I would need a bone marrow transplant, a grueling process that, in her words, would make my current treatment feel like a "cakewalk." Needless to say, I agreed to continue.

I wrestled with that decision during sleepless nights, turning it over in my mind and searching for answers that only my heart could provide. However, after the fifth treatment, I began grappling with intense neuropathy and the relentless grip of "chemo brain," a cognitive fog so thick and disorienting that it genuinely frightened me. The fear of potentially losing my cognitive abilities permanently, along with numbness in my fingers and toes, forced me into deep soul-searching. After much reflection, I made the agonizing decision to forgo the sixth and final treatment. It wasn't just a choice; it was a battle between survival and self-preservation. It was a calculated risk, but more than that, it was an act of reclaiming myself; a defiant stand to protect the core of who I was and who I am.

Fortunately, this story has a happy ending. Dr. Rama told me that if I remained cancer-free for three years, the likelihood of recurrence would drop to zero. It has now been four years. Four beautiful, hard-earned years. I am beyond grateful, not just for my health, but for the depth of knowledge, the growth, and the profound understanding that have been etched into my soul through this journey. Every scar, every fear faced, and every moment of doubt have shaped me into someone who doesn't just survive but truly lives, with a heart fuller and a spirit stronger than I ever thought possible.

In addition to feeling grateful to be alive, I now regard my cancer experience as a test of my resilience and fortitude. It forced me to cultivate a strength I hadn't known I possessed, one that would prove essential for what lay ahead.

As a forward-thinker and pioneer pushing the boundaries of my field, I realized that the tenacity I had developed was not just for survival—it was preparation. Cancer prepared me to stand at the forefront of a movement that had the potential to revolutionize the field of healing in multiple ways.

CHAPTER TWO

MUSHROOMS, MEDICINE, AND MISTAKES

I DIDN'T SET OUT TO BECOME a psychedelic advocate. But in the quiet aftermath of my cancer treatment, when the dust had barely settled and I was still relearning how to breathe without fear, I found myself spiraling into research. I needed to understand the mechanisms of healing, not just in the body, but in the mind and spirit. That's when I came across something unexpected. Something radical.

Buried in medical journals and peer-reviewed articles were accounts of a substance I hadn't thought about for nearly a decade: Psilocybin. Magic mushrooms. But this wasn't the stuff of stoner stereotypes or psychedelic festivals. These were rigorous studies, published by some of the most respected institutions, detailing how a single, high-dose psilocybin session could relieve end-of-life anxiety, lift the fog of depression, and ease even the most existential dread.[1]

I was stunned. Moved. Intrigued. What I was reading felt like a missing piece; a key to a lock I didn't know I'd been carrying.

The more I read, the more curious I became. I wanted to understand how this powerful substance could be so deeply

---

1   Griffiths et al., 2016

connected to life satisfaction and joy, especially in the face of something as devastating as a terminal diagnosis. What struck me most were the personal testimonials and stories of people who, after a single psilocybin experience, found themselves liberated from the mental and emotional burdens that had once weighed them down. One account involved a young woman who had terminal cancer who was able to confront her deep-seated fears about leaving her loved one(s) behind. She was able to achieve a sense of peace and clarity after psilocybin-assisted therapy, offering her final months filled with joy and acceptance rather than fear.

And the psychological results almost outweighed the physical ones for end-of-life and/or terminal patients. Instead of withdrawing from their families in an attempt to shield their loved ones from the pain of watching them suffer, these individuals did the opposite. They leaned in and pulled their loved ones closer, embracing connection and making the most of the precious time they had left. Families shared how these experiences allowed them to bond, find closure, and create meaningful, heartfelt memories, rather than feeling isolated, heartbroken, and disconnected in the face of impending loss. When I was ill, I'd realized how carrying a heavy emotional burden could hinder healing, so seeing this shift in perspective was both inspiring and reassuring.

Reading these accounts felt like a revelation. It would be difficult to overstate the game-changing impact of this information.

Had I unlocked a path to freedom from emotional pain for my clients? For myself?

It confirmed what I already knew from both my professional background and personal observations: that unresolved anger, fear, guilt, and shame don't just interfere with healing; they interfere with *living*. Psilocybin wasn't just helping people face death with peace; it was helping them reclaim their lives, even in its final chapters.

I kept digging. My interest in psychedelics grew, and I found myself particularly drawn to exploring psilocybin. I had tried it before and found the experience neutral, even calming, which made it feel far less intimidating than experimenting with something unfamiliar. There was comfort in knowing how it affected my body—no surprises, no fear of the unknown.

Second, psilocybin is a natural medicine. Technically, it's a fungus rather than a plant, but it grows organically from the earth, not synthesized in a lab. The connection to nature felt grounding and authentic, especially after all the synthetic drugs I had been exposed to during my cancer treatment.

Third, psilocybin mushrooms have been used for thousands of years, woven into the fabric of spiritual and cultural healing traditions worldwide. Archaeological evidence suggests their ritual use dates back to prehistoric times. For instance, cave art in Tassili n'Ajjer, Algeria—dating from approximately 7000 to 5000 BCE—depicts mushroom-like figures, which scholars interpret as evidence of early shamanic practices involving psychoactive fungi.[1] In Mesoamerica, indigenous groups, such as the Aztecs, referred to psilocybin mushrooms as *teonanácatl* ("divine mushroom") and used them in sacred ceremonies for divination and healing, as recorded in the Florentine Codex. The Mazatec people of Oaxaca, Mexico, continue to practice *veladas*. These

---

1   Samorini, 1992; Winkelman, 2019

healing rituals utilize psilocybin mushrooms, a tradition brought to broader awareness through the work of traditional healers in the mid-20th century.

I believed there to be something deeply grounding in participating in such an ancient lineage of seekers—humans who, across continents and millennia, have turned to the mushroom to connect with wisdom, healing, meaning, and medicine.[1]

Finally, there was the safety factor. I had never heard of anyone becoming addicted to psilocybin or needing rehab because of it. My research confirmed that psilocybin isn't physically addictive and, remarkably, has no known lethal dose. These elements gave me the confidence to explore it more deeply, not just as a substance, but as a potential key to emotional and spiritual healing.[2]

Since my personal trainer had a connection, I decided to procure a supply of mushrooms and begin my first-hand experimentation with psilocybin. At the time, I wasn't aware that my prescription medications would interfere with the experience, but I was eager to begin. I had yet to witness what a macrodose session looked like, so I was entirely in the dark about what to expect.

On the day I decided to try macrodosing mushrooms, my husband, Ken, kindly agreed to watch over me during the experiment. Looking back, I realize how little I knew about preparation – things like *intention* setting, and the importance of creating the correct *set* and *setting*. In hindsight, I can see so

---

1   Samorini, 1992; Winkelman, 2019; Sahagún, 1950–1982; Estrada, 1981

2   Canal & Murnane, 2017

many ways I set myself up for a less-than-optimal experience, which, no doubt, contributed to the muted effect I had.

The first mistake was drinking coffee throughout the entire experience—and not just a little. I consumed four times my usual amount, essentially turning myself into a jittery, over-caffeinated _psychonaut_. Psilocybin is known to heighten sensory perception, particularly in the visual, auditory, and olfactory domains. It also typically suppresses hunger, as the gastrointestinal system slows down. Yet, for some reason, coffee tasted like the nectar of the gods that day, and I mindlessly kept the java flowing like a barista on a mission. I now understand that coffee, being a stimulant, actually counteracts the calming and introspective effects of psilocybin.

Instead of the deep, transformative journey I had envisioned, I spent the day in a bizarre loop of listening to music, dancing like an enthusiastic but uncoordinated rave-goer, and gripping my coffee cup like it held the secrets of the universe. While it was certainly an _experience_, it wasn't exactly the mind-expanding revelation I had been hoping for.

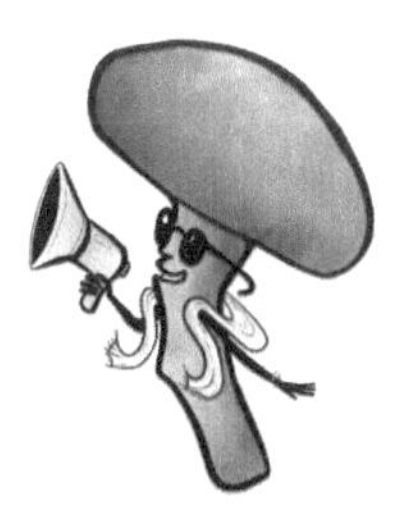

¡OYE! Have your usual brew—then back away from the pot.

If skipping caffeine gives you a headache, a small cup an hour before is fine. But less is best. Riding a mushroom wave while over-caffeinated is like meditating on a trampoline. You're aiming for depth, not bounce.

Another mistake was the byproduct of taking antidepressants at the time. These medications significantly hinder the psilocybin experience. In my experience, people on antipsychotics, antidepressants, or anti-anxiety medications often feel jittery or restless, unable to surrender to the experience fully. I was no exception.

The therapeutic use of psilocybin encourages turning inward. There is an entire universe of self to explore when we direct our attention within. This process typically involves wearing an eye mask, remaining silent, and staying physically still, all of which create the optimal conditions for a deeper connection with oneself. These practices help facilitate _ego dissolution_, allowing profound inner insights to emerge. On the other hand, engaging with one's external environment—whether it's using your cell phone or simply observing the room—prevents the necessary inward focus and inhibits the exploration of what the self has to offer. Many people, however, enjoy interacting with nature while using mushrooms recreationally, and I'm not opposed to using them for this purpose. It can undoubtedly be a beautiful, enriching experience. However, I've learned that it can also distract from the inner work that's essential for meaningful transformation.

During one of my early journeys, Ken suggested I go outside to the park across the street from our house. I agreed, and I vividly remember how mesmerizing the tree branches appeared. The entire tree seemed to be breathing, its branches undulating in slow, rhythmic waves, as if it were alive and in harmony with my breath. As the wind rustled the leaves, they caught the light and seemed to glow with a soft, golden hue, casting a beautiful pattern of light and shadow on the ground. The air felt charged, almost as if the light itself was infused with energy, radiating warmth and softness. The lines of the branches, once rigid, seemed fluid, twisting and swaying like a gentle dance. Even the texture of the bark stood out, each knot and wrinkle telling its own quiet story. The whole tree felt like it was pulsing with life, deeply interconnected with me in that moment, offering its silent wisdom through its steady presence.

¡OYE! No fireworks? No problem.

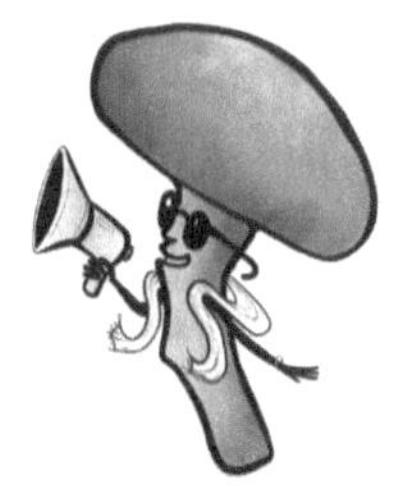

Not every journey comes with blinding insight or life-altering clarity. Mushrooms work in mysterious ways. Sometimes the healing happens so subtly, there's no clear lesson at all—just a quiet shift that unfolds in the days or weeks that follow.

This type of visual experience is often heightened during psychedelic journeys, where even the most ordinary aspects of nature seem imbued with profound significance. In this case, although there were no grand revelations or insights, the beauty and depth of the moment felt almost spiritual in its own way, grounding me in the present and allowing me to *be* with the tree wholly and serenely.

It was a beautiful moment, one I truly appreciated. But in terms of mental or emotional transformation, it didn't offer much. There were no profound revelations about myself, but I did experience striking visuals, calming sensations, and a peaceful appreciation of nature. This is what many might refer to as the spiritual nature of psychedelics. Others might refer to this as the recreational side of psychedelics, where one experiences deep relaxation and an acute connection to nature without any profound, therapeutic insights or deeper understanding of oneself.

Still, I noticed something subtle but meaningful afterward. Even without clear insights, my mood lifted. I felt more energized, more motivated, and generally lighter. Something had shifted, even if I couldn't quite explain how or why.

CATHERINE - *That wasn't what I expected.*

> *It was... a lot.*
>
> *I'm not even sure what I saw.*
>
> *Or felt.*
>
> *Or why it matters.*

VOICE - *You came looking for healing.*

> *And arrived like a tourist.*
>
> *No judgment.*
>
> *We honor your curiosity. Even when it's clumsy.*

CATHERINE - *Who are you?*

VOICE - *A guide. A mirror. A memory.*

> *You've met us before.*
>
> *Only now, you're starting to listen.*

CATHERINE - *But I didn't do it right.*

> *Did I mess it up?*

VOICE - *Nothing is wasted.*

> *Even play opens doors.*
>
> *What matters is that you came.*
>
> *You'll return.*
>
> *Next time, bring your whole self.*

The moon I observed in Denver and the trees I experienced across the street from my house perfectly illustrate the typical psychedelic experience. Had I encountered either of those phenomena without the influence of psychedelics (a moon with a strange, luminous tail or a tree that appeared to be breathing), I would've been deeply unsettled and distressed by visuals that defy logical explanation.

Yet, under the influence of psychedelics, when the substance binds to receptors in the visual cortex, these novel perceptions are welcomed with an unusual sense of curiosity and awe. Instead of fear or resistance, there's a sense of wonder and even delight. The strange becomes beautiful, and the inexplicable feels not only acceptable but profoundly satisfying.[1]

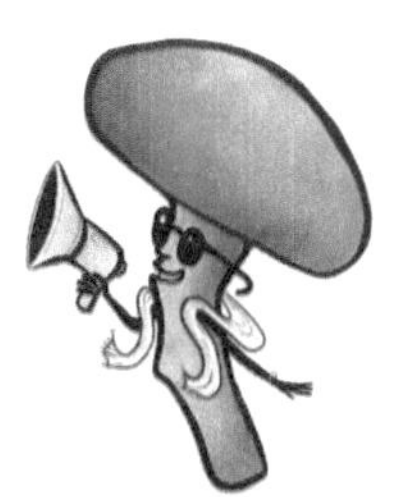

¡OYE! Not everything you see is literal, but it's all meaningful.

Visions can be wild. Don't get stuck on the details. Ask what they feel like, not just what they look like.

I'm not suggesting that recreational experiences can't be therapeutic. I've heard many accounts of people who've happened to have had significant transformational shifts from recreational use. What I'm trying to convey is that a therapeutic experience with psilocybin takes the journey to an entirely different level. One, I had yet to witness myself.

Leaning inward, especially when paired with pre-determined intentions, can lead to life-changing shifts that might surpass years of talk therapy. It's a deeper, more profound kind of healing.

---

1   Tipado et al., 2024

This was a lesson I hadn't yet learned – not until I decided to plan a journey without my prescription medications.

At this point, I still wasn't fully understanding the true therapeutic power of psilocybin. I had experienced some cool colors, and it did help me access deeper emotions, but I hadn't yet grasped the profound, life-changing effects that others had reported.

What I did notice, however, was that my mood improved for periods after each dose. That shift was enough to keep me curious, sparking a desire to explore psilocybin further as a potential tool for countering depression.

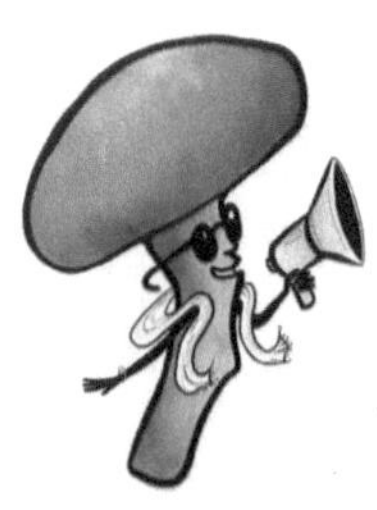

¡OYE! Your first insight might not be your deepest one.

Sometimes the real gem is buried under the obvious takeaway. Keep digging. Let time refine the message.

CATHERINE - *I didn't expect it to change me like that.*

VOICE - *You didn't expect much.*

CATHERINE - *It was supposed to be just another experience.*

VOICE - *Nothing is "just another."
Every journey calls.*

CATHERINE - *I wasn't looking for this.*

VOICE - *You didn't look.
You were led.*

CATHERINE - *What happens now?*

VOICE - *Now, you trust the path.*

The journey begins.

You are not alone.

CHAPTER THREE

CURIOSITY AND THE CABIN

CATHERINE - *I've spent my life chasing proof,
numbers, facts.
But you... You're different.
You don't show up in a lab.*

VOICE - *Some truths live between the lines.
We are not here to replace your science.
Just to remind you that healing is never a
straight path.*

CATHERINE - *I thought I was imagining things.
That this was all just chemical.*

VOICE - *Yes.
And no.
Chemistry is the key.
But the lock... that's you.*

CATHERINE - *So what now?
What do I do with all this?*

VOICE - *Begin again.
But this time, don't study the door.
Open it.*

I HAD TAKEN PSILOCYBIN A COUPLE of times, but each attempt left me feeling underwhelmed, like I was knocking on a door that refused to open.

Why isn't this working? I remember thinking, staring at the walls, waiting for something—anything—to happen. I kept telling myself, *"Maybe I just need a higher dose,"* or, *"Maybe I'm not doing it right."* It felt like I was constantly chasing an experience that seemed just out of reach.

I had seen it in the literature, the warnings that prescription medications, especially *Selective Serotonin Reuptake Inhibitors or SSRIs*, could dull or block the effects of psilocybin. But for some reason, I didn't fully register it. Maybe I skimmed past it. Perhaps I just didn't want it to be true. I was so focused on chasing the experience that I couldn't see what was standing in the way.

Then one day, it clicked. Like puzzle pieces snapping into place. *Of course. The meds.*

I felt a wave of recognition and frustration all at once. *How did I miss this?* I hadn't been ready to connect the dots before, but now, there was no unseeing it.

To explain how I got there, I need to go back to my history with prescription medication. At 19, I was diagnosed with *Major Depressive Disorder*. Honestly, it wasn't shocking. In my family, sadness was the baseline. Mental illness and addiction floated around our home like background noise. In my household culture, depression was normalized, accepted, and worked around.

The diagnosis came after I had spent three consecutive days unable to get out of bed, skipping classes and letting the world slip by. I remember the doctor looking at me gently and saying, "You don't have to feel this way forever." I wanted to believe him, so I nodded through tears.

Like so many others, I began the frustrating trial-and-error journey of antidepressants.

"Let's try Prozac first," the psychiatrist said. Months later: "Not working well? Hmm, okay, let's switch to Zoloft." My medicine cabinet slowly began to resemble a pharmacy, but nothing seemed to work.

Each new prescription came with hope: *Maybe this will be the one.* But more often than not, it ended in side effects, disappointment, or numbness. It wasn't until I tried Wellbutrin that something shifted. "I don't feel great," I remember saying, "but I finally feel... functional."

In my twenties, the idea of relying on antidepressants for life felt unsettling, even suffocating. But by my thirties, I had come to terms with it. I told myself it was no different from a diabetic needing insulin. This was simply the way I managed my depression. What I didn't realize was that Wellbutrin was also keeping me from fully experiencing the deep healing potential of psilocybin—something that could have offered a path to understanding and transforming my depression, not just managing it.

After cancer treatment, my body wasn't just recovering, it was adapting to an entirely new reality. The brutal cocktail of chemotherapy had thrown me into sudden menopause, leaving me battling relentless hot flashes and nerve pain that felt like electric shocks in my limbs. To manage the chaos, my doctors prescribed Effexor, a standard pharmaceutical solution to ease both the hormonal firestorm and the lingering neuropathy. Effexor is also commonly prescribed to treat depression and anxiety, but for me, it was a way to cope with the physical aftermath of cancer. Just like that, I became another statistic: one of millions of Americans relying on prescription meds to keep both body and mind in check.

Although I may have gotten my health stabilized with these drugs, I wasn't having much success with my psilocybin journeys. They remained more muted in nature than was expected. And so progress was slow. Something wasn't adding up. As my curiosity about psilocybin deepened, I began to suspect that these very medications, the ones designed to stabilize me, were dulling my experience with the mushrooms. If I was ever going to step into the potential of psilocybin fully, I needed to change my approach.

Instead of going at it alone, I decided to seek guidance. I wanted to explore psilocybin with a trained professional, someone who truly understood the depths of trauma and transformation. Luckily, I knew just the right people. In my community, I had connections with a group of counselors who specialized in _Memory Reconsolidation_, an effective process for rewriting deep-seated emotional patterns. Even more exciting? They supported _Emotional Triggers Treatment_, a modality I had developed myself based on my expertise in how Memory Reconsolidation could help resolve trauma.

I wasn't just searching for a breakthrough. I was eager to step into an experience that had the potential to rewrite everything I thought I knew. By late spring 2022, I was done with half-measures. I wanted to experience psilocybin in its full, unfiltered power.

I enjoyed the collaborative approach we now had going. So, I reached out to my group of counselors with a bold proposition: _What if we journeyed together? Not just as individuals, but as a team?_

We would split into two groups—half of us would take the medicine while the other half guided, and then we'd swap roles the next day. To further our understanding, we decided to experiment with different doses, mapping the terrain of consciousness at varying intensities. I wasn't the only one who was curious to see how each dose would shape the experience—how a _mesodose_ might offer subtle insights while a _hero dose_ could plunge someone into the depths of their psyche.

With excitement crackling in the air, we decided to rent a secluded cabin in the mountains, setting the stage for a profound weekend of exploration. This wasn't just a casual retreat. It was an opportunity to delve deeply into the mysteries of the mind, to witness firsthand how psilocybin might transform trauma, memory, and emotional healing.

But there was one more piece to this puzzle: I needed to know if my prescription medications had truly been holding me back. So, in the days leading up to our journey, I decided I would temporarily pause my antidepressant to see if it changed the experience.

Now, let me be absolutely clear: I do NOT recommend that anyone abruptly stop taking their medication. Antidepressants alter brain chemistry, and quitting cold turkey can have serious consequences. Anyone considering changes should always consult their doctor first.

But for me, this was an experiment, a calculated risk in the name of discovery. And, I had a whole team of qualified counselors with me.

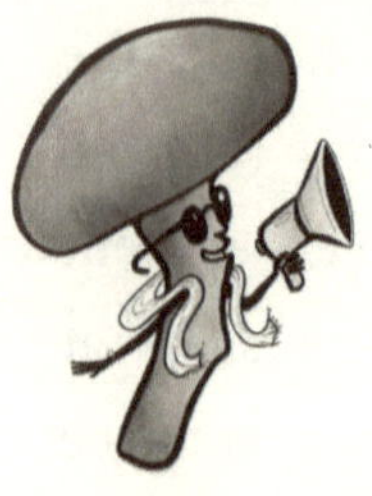

I knew what going without my antidepressants would feel like. There had been times when I'd traveled and accidentally skipped my meds for a few days. I knew the pattern. Typically, by day four, I'd start to feel a slight dip, inching closer to a depressive state on the spectrum. But it was never anything too severe. That gave me confidence. If I stayed within that window, I believed I could experiment safely.

What I didn't realize, and what I should have discovered, was that abruptly stopping medications like Effexor could be dangerous. The withdrawal effects could be brutal, even unpredictable. I had worked with clients who had experienced just how harsh the withdrawal could be, with symptoms like brain zaps, dizziness, nausea, and mood swings. Withdrawing from Effexor is no joke. It should be taken seriously, as it can leave you physically and emotionally vulnerable. But at the time, I was operating on instinct, unaware of the full risks.

So, three days before our mountain retreat, I made the call. I stopped taking my medication.

That weekend, Sabrina, Rosie, Inga, Gary, and I decided to take the leap. Rosie opted for a mesodose, just 0.75 grams of psilocybin. Sabrina went all in with a hero dose of five full grams. I chose something in between: a macrodose of three grams; enough to dissolve the edges of reality without completely surrendering to the void. Inga and Gary, on the other hand, chose to remain grounded, stepping into the role of observers and guides. It felt like a thoughtful "wait and see" approach—one foot in curiosity, the other in caution.

Once we pulled out the bag of mushrooms, we all noticed each tiny fruiting body, just one to two inches long, with button-sized caps and stringy stems. Inga's eyes lit up with curiosity. She picked the smallest one, held it up to the light, sniffed it, and without hesitation, popped it into her mouth. "I just want to see what it tastes like," she said, her grin infectious. The moment was playful, daring, and full of wonder. That, my readers, counted as a microdose, even if it wasn't measured, just a tiny spark of exploration that perfectly captured the spirit of curiosity.

One of the significant benefits for all of us as mental health professionals was the opportunity to observe the effects of each individual's approach to the medicine.

For Rosie, it was uncharted territory and her very first experience with psilocybin. Though her dose was mild, the journey was anything but ordinary. Her eyes widened with wonder as she tried to put words to the strange and beautiful sensations unfolding inside her.

She described experiencing _synesthesia_, the blending of senses, as if thoughts and emotions had taken on colors of their own. A personal challenge with which she'd been struggling suddenly became _green_ in her mind, a color weighted with meaning only she could understand. Rosie watched in awe as the wooden deck beneath her seemed to breathe, moving with the semblance of sentient energy, as if the entire world had come alive in a secret dance she had never noticed before.

Moments of laughter bubbled up unexpectedly, followed by waves of tears. She wasn't just thinking through emotions; she was feeling them in a way she had never experienced before, moving through an entire spectrum of release and realization. We watched as layers of tension melted away; as her mind rearranged its puzzle pieces into something clearer, something lighter.

By the time Rosie's journey ended, the transformation was undeniable. She spoke with a newfound clarity, as if years of emotional weight had been lifted in a matter of hours. The insights she gained allowed her to reframe the past; to see old wounds from a fresh perspective, to untangle the knots of complicated relationships that had once seemed impossible to resolve.

It was breathtaking to witness. Psilocybin hadn't just given her a moment of peace. It had handed her the keys to a door she hadn't even known existed.

And on the other side? Understanding. Healing. Freedom.

Sabrina chose the hero dose because she was no stranger to altered states of consciousness. She had lived through the wild, untamed energy of the '60s and '70s, a time when psychedelics pulsed through the veins of a cultural revolution. She had danced through the highs, witnessed the crashes, and emerged with a deep respect for these sacred medicines. Now, decades later, she was ready to return, to surrender fully and embrace whatever the journey had in store.

She took the full five grams without hesitation, her eyes shimmering with fearless anticipation. She *wanted* the depths. She welcomed the unknown. What followed was nothing short of mind-bending.

I can still see Sabrina on the deck, silhouetted against the fading light, her voice cutting through the silence, a raw, unfiltered cry into the vastness of existence. She wasn't just talking, she was summoning. Calling out to lost loved ones, demanding answers from the universe, shouting into the wind as if God Herself was answering back.

For what felt like hours, she rode the storm of her soul, her emotions breaking free like a dam bursting after decades of pressure. She laughed, a wild, uncontainable laughter that rang through the trees. She sobbed deep, guttural cries that shook the air around her. She spoke in fragmented, cryptic phrases. Her words were seemingly torn from the fabric of forgotten memories, half-prayers, half-proclamations of truth only she could see.

To an outsider, it might have looked like madness.

To me, it was anything but... It was *release*.

When she finally came back to us hours later, her eyes held something new. Something ancient and wise, yet impossibly light, like she had shed the weight of a lifetime in a single day. She hadn't lost herself in the experience. She had found herself.

What made the journey possible, Sabrina would later tell me, was having Inga and Gary there. Inga never left her side, sitting close as Sabrina's screams tore through the day, a steady anchor in the storm. Gary stood a little back, arms crossed, a silent guard, his presence a shield against the chaos. Knowing these strong, unwavering souls were near gave Sabrina the courage to surrender fully, to reach depths she might never have touched alone. Their support didn't dilute the intensity. It amplified it. Allowing her to wrestle with the raw, unfiltered emotions and emerge transformed. Every cry, every laugh, every fragmented phrase was made richer, safer, and infinitely more profound because she was with trusted guides.

In the weeks and months that followed, the transformation was undeniable. Sabrina radiated a newfound joy, a lightness in her spirit, as if a heavy weight had finally been lifted from her shoulders. She spoke of the profound relief of reclaiming parts of herself she had long abandoned. She had touched the great beyond, the vastness of the eternal; all of it humming with infinite wisdom.

Even now, she looks back on that day as the moment everything changed. The moment she broke through the illusion. The moment she finally understood.

And her journey is still unfolding. Layer by layer. Revelation by revelation. She is still listening to the echoes of that day. They continue to reverberate.

My journey that day was both the same and entirely different from Sabrina's. Before I get into what set it apart, I want to capture how it echoed her experience. As the medicine took hold, I found myself on the deck on the other side of the cabin. While Sabrina proclaimed her truth to the world, I surrendered to the wind as it whipped across my body.

Every gust was electric. Inga came over, keeping a gentle eye on me as I began to move, twirling my arms in the shifting air. "I can feel the entire world right now," I whispered. And I truly could. Messages seemed to arrive from everywhere, brushing against me with the wind: a whisper from Japan, a sigh from Ireland, a gentle pulse from Thailand, a song from Australia. Each change in direction carried a new voice, a new vibration, a new invitation to merge with the infinite.

I was weightless, unbound. My body was alive with currents I couldn't name, and with each passing moment, my ego loosened its grip. "I" began to fade, dissolving into a vast, humming oneness. The world was no longer separate from me. I was a part of every tree, every gust, every echo of faraway voices. It was exhilarating, terrifying, and utterly glorious all at once.

This was the first time I was actually living what I had heard others describe so many times. The stories of ego dissolving, of merging with the world, of feeling every particle of life moving through you were no longer abstract. No longer just words or secondhand awe. I was in it. Every vibration, every whisper of wind, every flicker of light became a message I could feel in my bones. I wasn't imagining it. I wasn't interpreting it. I was it.

As I reflect on that particular experience, the moments of ego dissolution stand out. They are the ones in which I was given profound insights into who I was, who I had been, and the untold truths buried in my past. Yet, as transformative as that experience was, I must also acknowledge the unseen weight that held me back: my prescription medication.

Even after just a few days off the meds, I can see now how those chemicals had built up over the years and were not so easily discarded. They lingered in my system, affecting the depths of my experience in ways I couldn't fully comprehend. Despite my best intentions, they held me at arm's length from the full immersion I was seeking, keeping me from plunging into the rawness of the experience. I now know that taking a few days off Wellbutrin does offer a full experience, but the Effexor did blunt my experience slightly—though I still gained a wealth of insight and experienced some ego-dissolution. This may have been due to the fact that I was on a very low dose. Studies show that some people experience blunted effects from Effexor.

There was also the small but significant detail of not using an eye mask, something I didn't fully appreciate at the time. The absence of that simple tool kept me from sinking deeper within, missing out on the profound connection that could have unfolded in the darkness.[1]

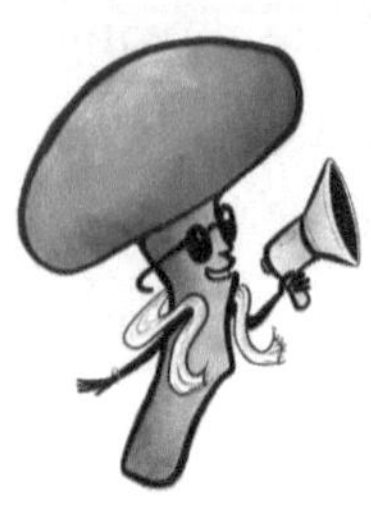

¡OYE! Bring an eye mask.

This isn't just a blackout tool. It's your ticket to the IMAX of the soul. The fewer distractions out there, the more revelations in here.

But despite these barriers, there was one particularly transcendent moment. Alone, I found a quiet, serene spot in a recliner downstairs, with a perfect view of the sunset, the sky ablaze with colors I could almost taste. It was a peaceful moment, beautiful in its own right. But as I stared at the horizon, my thoughts wandered. In that space, I learned one of the most profound lessons the mushrooms had to offer: they don't always give you what you want, but they always give you exactly what you need.

---

1 Gukasyan et al., 2023

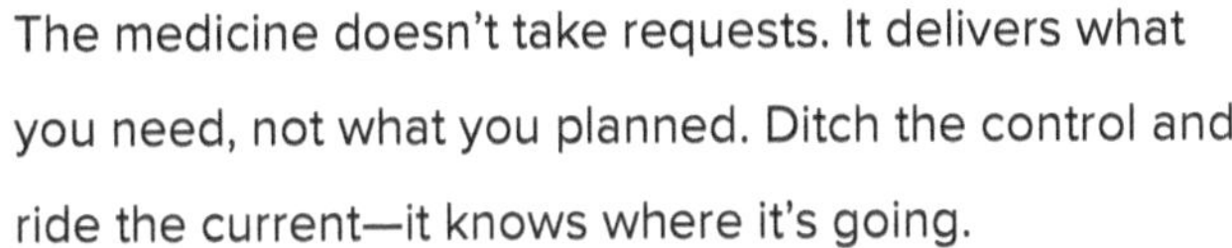

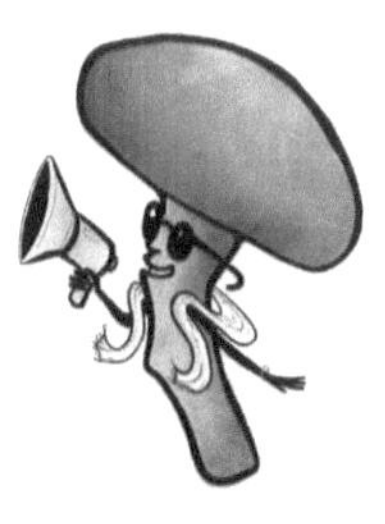

¡OYE! Expect the unexpected. And then expect to be wrong about that too.

The medicine doesn't take requests. It delivers what you need, not what you planned. Ditch the control and ride the current—it knows where it's going.

That day, I needed to revisit my relationship with my maternal grandmother, an enigmatic figure whose complexities and contradictions had shaped me in ways I had never fully understood. I found myself drawn into memories of her, of the dynamics that had defined my childhood. And as the mushrooms worked their magic, I began to see her, not as the person I had once known, but as a living, breathing part of my own story.

VOICE - *The past calls to you.*

The ties still bind you, but you do not yet know it.

CATHERINE - *Who are you?*

VOICE - *I am no one and I am everyone.*

I am nothing and I am everything.

CATHERINE - *What is your name?*

VOICE - *Names are nothing.*

You ask to know, but you will never truly know.

CATHERINE - *Why do I feel like I need to know?*

VOICE - *You think a name will hold it all.*

It will not.

CATHERINE - *Why can't I feel sure of this?*

VOICE - *Because you still look for answers outside.*

Answers are not bound by words.

The roots of your ancestors reach deep.

You continue their story.

You are tied to them.

CATHERINE - *I'm afraid of what I'll find.*

VOICE - *You must feel it to free it.*

CHAPTER FOUR

LOVE IS LOVE

My grandmother's story began in Mexico, where she was a young girl of only thirteen when she married my grandfather. Together, they crossed the border into the United States, a place where life would never be easy. She wasn't afforded the chance to learn, to be educated, or to heal from the deep wounds that followed her. Her life, I now realize, was a tangled web of trauma. Her trauma was so deep I could only begin to guess at its expansiveness. But what I knew, even then, was how that trauma seeped into her soul and became all-encompassing. I was a witness to how it manifested itself in anger, cruelty, and bitterness.

We called her *Mamaita* because she didn't like being called "grandma" in any language, English, Spanish, or otherwise. She didn't like the insinuation of being old. Mamaita was a name she chose for herself long before age or frailty became a concern. It was a term of endearment that offered a sense of warmth and affection without making her sound like an old lady. "Mamaita" allowed her to hold onto a sense of youth and vitality, keeping her connected to a part of herself she wasn't ready to let go of. In using it, she could sidestep the weight of time and the expectations that came with it, much like how she sidestepped the deeper wounds of her past. Age was a complex reality for her to face, and this other name was a way to avoid that truth, preserving a version of herself she could still control.

Mamaita told me she was only thirteen when she married my grandfather, Papaito. But as I began gathering facts for this book, I heard different versions of her story. My cousin claimed she was only nine, while my mother insisted she was seventeen. The family genealogist and historian, however, placed her age at twenty-one. This conflicting information, each version changing depending on who she told the story to, reflects the shifty nature of her life. She wove multiple narratives, shaping her past to suit the moment and the audience, leaving a trail of confusion and mystery we could never quite unravel. It was just one of the many layers of complexity that made her so difficult to understand.

Mamaita played her children and grandchildren against each other, like pieces in a chess game, stirring the pot of strife and competition and feeding on the tension she created. Her self-esteem was so low, so fragile, that she hid it beneath layers of passive-aggressiveness, snapping at the world in little jabs. She was petty—*small*, in a way that broke my heart. She'd steal little things from restaurants: sugar packets, silverware, as though she were testing the world, seeing what she could take and get away with. But the most painful part of her brokenness was how deeply she hated herself.

As a woman in my mid-50s, I can now see the picture with clarity, each fragment of her behavior revealing a heartbreaking truth I couldn't grasp as a child, like trying to solve a puzzle with missing pieces. It was suffocating for her, and I can see it so clearly now when I think back on every word and action of hers.

Her racism was a shield, a way to deflect the pain she carried in her own heart.

And then, there was the food; the part of her that looked like love. Or at least, that's how it felt at first. She'd often prepare a feast for me, an extravagant display of her care and her culture, a love she could express only through the labor of her hands and the richness of the flavors. I devoured the food with unspoken gratitude and unconditional love. But also for what it represented. Mamaita had a way of making me feel special in those moments, as if I were the center of her world.

But there was a price.

The price was the unspoken rule that accompanied her meals: I had to eat all that was put in front of me. Seconds, thirds, and extra sweets were proof of my love and my devotion to her. Ironically, it wasn't about the food. All of it was a test of my loyalty. Whenever I complied and showed her I could indulge without resistance, the manipulation began.

It always followed the same cruel pattern: An hour after the feast, she'd look at me with a seemingly gentle smile and say, "You'd be so much prettier if you lost weight."

Just like that, the joy of indulgence turned into a sickening, suffocating shame.

It was a trap. I fell into it every time. Every bite, every moment of perceived warmth and love turned against me. The food that had once felt like a gift was used to manipulate and control me emotionally. By making me indulge and then criticizing me for my appearance, she turned something as simple as food into a weapon. Instead of nourishing me, it became a way for her to make me feel unworthy, and I was left carrying her shame and brokenness, believing they were my own.

At some point, I began to see the game she was playing. She made me her partner in a grotesque dance of guilt and self-loathing, and I couldn't escape it. It was a dysfunction I couldn't explain at the time. It was a strange, twisted connection that bound me to her, keeping me trapped in her web of sorrow and manipulation.

At the cabin, in the depths of my psilocybin journey, time lost its shape. I was no longer an adult reflecting on the past. I had become the child again, stepping back into the emotional landscapes I thought I had long escaped. As the years went by, my relationship with Mamaita became a whirlwind of contradictions, agonizing, yet magnetic movements of love and hate. It was as if I was drawn into her gravity, pulled in by the toxic but undeniable bond we shared. With each passing year, I found myself increasingly consumed by the complex emotions she stirred within me. And now, looking back, I see how inextricably her unresolved pain became woven into my own.

As these memories flooded through me, encouraged by the effects of the psilocybin, another memory popped up, so sharp and vivid, it stood out above all others: Mamaita was proud of me, but not because of my intelligence, my character, or any of the things for which a child might want to be praised. No. Her pride in me was rooted in something so twisted and tragic that it cut to the core. This added another layer of complexity to our already-confusing relationship.

She was proud of me for one devastating reason: I was a white baby.

My father was tall, fair-skinned, with blond hair and piercing blue eyes. I inherited those features. To Mamaita, my appearance wasn't just aesthetic. It was a symbol of something she longed for but could never possess.

She would take me out, parading me in front of her friends as though my very presence, my physical appearance, somehow validated her worth in the eyes of the world. I remember one afternoon vividly when we were visiting a friend of hers, and she motioned me over, her voice loud enough for everyone to hear.

"Come here, *mijita*," she said, pulling me close and smoothing a strand of hair behind my ear.

"Isn't she beautiful?" she beamed to her friends. "Can you believe this blond hair? Those blue eyes?"

Her friends nodded, some smiling politely, others awkwardly avoiding eye contact.

"She's my little *guera*," she added with a laugh, as if I were her prize. She would boast, not about who I was or what I had accomplished, but about how I looked. My fair skin and blond hair, marking me as her "guera," became her silent currency. In public, I was her award, a symbol of status, acceptance, even escape. It was as if my appearance allowed her to imagine a different life for herself, one where she didn't have to bear the weight of being a Mexican woman in a world that often pushed her aside.

In that illusion, she found a twisted form of validation. My whiteness became her proxy for belonging, a privilege she could never fully claim but clung to through me. She reveled in the recognition it brought her, but it was a hollow pride, one that deepened the gap between who she was and who she longed to be.

I came to recognize as an adult that Mamaita had a complicated relationship with her body weight. She wasn't thin; in fact, she was cherub-like, with a slightly chubby build. Yet, she would judge others who were overweight with vehement criticism. It was as though she resented fatness, a trait she could never accept in herself. I often wonder if, in the complexity of it all, she preferred that I be fat to counter the privilege of my whiteness and bond with her shame. Perhaps this created another commonality, a shared struggle between us. This idea, though difficult to grasp, adds yet another layer to the complicated web of her being.

There were so many contradictions and hidden motives that I could never fully understand.

And, to add to all of this confusion, when I was five years old, Mamaita made a decision that would resonate for the rest of my life: she stopped speaking Spanish to me. Until then, it was our shared language, a bond between us. I had become fluent in the rhythms of Spanish, which ran through my childhood like a heartbeat. But one day, without explanation, she turned her back on her mother tongue, relinquishing generations of familiarity and wisdom.

I later learned that she feared that if I spoke Spanish, I would be burdened with an accent. An accent that, in her mind, would limit my opportunities in life. She believed that by severing the oral connection to my Mexican heritage, by cutting me off from the language and culture that flowed through my veins, I would have a better shot at success. In her eyes, erasing the very essence of who I was—the parts that tied me to my history, to my ancestors—was the only way to save me from a world that would look down on me for being "other."

The insights gifted to me by the mushrooms allowed me to truly grasp the depth of her conviction. She thought she was doing what was best for me, protecting me from the struggles and pain she had faced in her own life. She wanted to shield me from being seen as an outsider, from the judgment and discrimination that she knew all too well. But in her desperation to protect me from the harshness of the world, she didn't realize she was also cutting me off from a part of myself that I would spend the rest of my life trying to understand.

Without knowing it, she also attempted to protect herself from the deep-seated pain and shame of her own identity, an identity she spent her life rejecting and fighting against. The cultural heritage that shaped her, the very essence of who she was, became something she could not accept.

My mother once told me that, when she was a child, Mamaita kept a picture of a stranger in a frame and claimed it was of her own mother. This was just another example of the shame Mamaita felt about her culture and her ancestry, an effort to distance herself from the past she couldn't reconcile. In her attempts to shield herself from the hurt and judgment she had endured, she inadvertently extended that defense to me, creating a barrier between us and a part of myself I was never allowed to embrace fully. The tragedy is that her attempt to save me unintentionally set me on a path of disconnection, where I would struggle to find my place and understand the richness of the heritage she carried within her but never allowed herself to embrace.

Wow, this psilocybin experience had me journeying deep into my childhood. What I was confronted with next was something I had been avoiding for over fifty years: the love of my Mamaita.

It hit me like a wave, and I was stunned to realize that, all this time, I had created the belief that Mamaita didn't love me. This narrative, which I had clung to so tightly, had become an essential part of my identity. I built it to survive, to fit in, to belong.

From a very young age, Mamaita made it clear to my cousins that I was her favorite. She didn't just show me extra affection; she announced it proudly, making sure they knew exactly where they stood. It was cruel, a calculated way of wielding love as a weapon. By singling me out, she not only isolated me but also inflicted deep wounds on them. Her favoritism wasn't just a casual remark; it was a deliberate act that sowed division and pain. My cousins were left feeling less than, unworthy of her love, and I became the natural target of their resentment.

As a child, craving nothing more than acceptance from my peers, I rejected this favoritism. I didn't want to be alienated by my cousins, so I pushed away her love. I didn't understand at the time, but her affection created a strange, unspoken bond that conflicted with me. It made me feel guilty for receiving her attention while simultaneously feeling rejected by the rest of my family. My young mind couldn't understand what was happening, and in my fear of standing out, I convinced myself she didn't truly love me.

The mushrooms, however, revealed the truth to me.

As flashes of memories flooded back, each one uncovered Mamaita's undeniable love. The images were vivid and powerful. In one such memory, I saw myself as a child, standing in the hallway closet of her house, preparing for bed. The light chain hung just out of my reach, and I remember how she'd always help me pull it, her hands guiding mine to make sure I could see. On the shelves, I noticed rows of toothpaste samples and toothbrushes, carefully arranged. Papaito, a dentist, kept the closet stocked with these little treasures, and picking out my toothbrush felt like a special ritual. These small acts, helping me with the light and ensuring I had everything I needed for bed, were her way of showing love.

I also remembered how she'd tuck me into the twin bed in her room, right next to hers. She'd pull the covers tight around me, always making sure I was comfortable and cared for. Her touch was gentle but steady, like the rhythm of the care she gave me every night. In those moments, I felt protected, surrounded by her love in a way words could never capture. At the time, these gestures seemed like routine acts, but now I see them as tender expressions of how deeply she cared. Memory after memory revealed how she adored me, not through grand gestures, but through the quiet, everyday things that made me feel safe and cherished.

And then came the profound revelation:

Love is love.

It doesn't matter what we think of the person giving it, whether we label them as kind or cruel, benevolent or evil. The love they release is purified of the baggage that might otherwise distort it. When it is given, it is received as love, cleansed of everything else.

And in that instant, lying on the bed in the cabin, through the lens of the mushrooms, the belief I had carried all those years, that Mamaita didn't love me, was shattered. It had no merit, no foundation. I had created it, and I held onto it as if it were the truth. The ego that had shaped the false narrative stepped aside at that moment, and I saw the truth, unfiltered by the warped lens of my past wounds.

It was a humbling, even surreal experience, to see the depth of love that had always been there, just waiting to be recognized.

Many of us wonder what our lives would be like if a pivotal piece of our upbringing or history were different—if a key event or relationship had unfolded differently.

Would I be more confident? Would my self-esteem be higher?

Through my psilocybin journey, I was gifted an extraordinary opportunity to experience what it was like to review my childhood and see a different reality.

In the days that followed, I began to feel a profound shift. I went from being a child who felt deprived of love, especially from my grandmother and my mother, to an adult who understood, with absolute clarity, that I had been deeply loved all along. That love had always been there, buried beneath layers of confusion and hurt. I had simply failed to see it.

My experience with the mushrooms revealed to me that, in many ways, my grandmother and my mother were reflections of each other. Both women were trying to navigate their own struggles with love, identity, and survival. The apple hadn't fallen far from the tree, and it was during this realization that I found a sense of compassion for both of them. I could see both the deep-seated love *and* the pain passed down through generations, something I had never fully understood despite my years as both a daughter and a psychotherapist.

Even though I hadn't specifically set out to confront my "mother issues" or to unpack the complexities of my relationship with her, something within me began to heal. My relationship with Mamaita, too, was no longer shrouded in resentment or distorted narratives. Instead of seeing Mamaita through the lens of pain and rejection, I saw her for who she truly was: a woman who, in her brokenness, had offered me love in the best way she knew.

It was like a veil had been lifted. I gained insights into my past, as well as a new perspective on my entire family dynamic, in a way that softened the judgments I had carried for so long. Suddenly, I saw myself not as a victim of circumstance, but as a person who had been loved and could love herself fully.

As I came out of the transformative psilocybin experience, the group of counselors gathered around to discuss what we had just gone through. We were integrating our individual experiences, but it was at this moment that I had yet another profound revelation, this time, about my mother.

However, before I delve into that insight, I would like to share another discovery that truly opened my eyes to the incredible powers of _neuroplasticity_—the brain's ability to rewire itself—through the use of psilocybin.

After I had journeyed deep into Mamaita's memories, I began to return to myself and my surroundings, upon which physical hunger started to pull me back into the present. Rosie, who had a physical presence very reminiscent of my mother and Mamaita, began preparing lunch. She offered to make me a taco, and the way she orchestrated the kitchen felt so familiar; it mirrored the way Mamaita would cook.

At that moment, I couldn't help but feel Mamaita's energy had somehow returned to me through Rosie's gestures, her rhythm, even her voice.

It dawns on me now that Rosie's presence had, in many ways, dictated the direction of my journey. At the time, I didn't fully understand the value or purpose of creating clear intentions before a psychedelic experience. I've since learned that setting an intention helps guide the journey, giving it a shape, a focal point—a way to consciously explore the things we most want or need to heal. Because psilocybin is a _non-specific amplifier_, it heightens what's already present within. So when something in our environment resembles something unresolved or deeply embedded in us—like Rosie's resemblance to Mamaita—it becomes magnified, pulling that material to the surface. In this way, Rosie became a kind of living symbol, a catalyst for everything that unfolded.

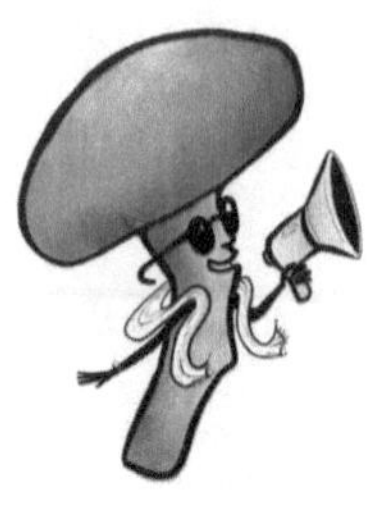

¡OYE! Set intentions as invitations, not demands.

Write what matters to you, refine it, and speak it aloud. The mushrooms listen, but they respond in their own language and at their own pace.

As I sat there, regaining my composure, Gary started laughing. I felt puzzled and asked, "Why are you laughing at me?"

Gary's response caught me off guard: "I didn't know you spoke Spanish."

Without skipping a beat, I replied, "Yo no hablo Español," which only made him and Rosie laugh even harder.

I was confused, but then he pointed out, "You're doing it right now."

In that instant, it dawned on me: I had just spoken Spanish, the language I had *stopped speaking* at the age of five. The language I had buried so deep in my mind had resurfaced effortlessly during my journey. It was such a profound discovery that it almost felt like I had unlocked a hidden part of myself that had been dormant for decades. The psilocybin journey unlocked an *entire language* I hadn't accessed since childhood.

What I now understand is that trauma can create deep-seated pathways in our brains that allow us to avoid difficult emotions or memories. This avoidance is a form of self-protection, keeping us focused on survival rather than revisiting painful or disturbing past experiences. Avoiding the dark portions of our minds helps keep us focused on being efficient and productive. People with severe depression often don't remember big chunks of their lives because it doesn't serve their best interests.

How this relates to my experience is that the Spanish language had become intertwined with the trauma of my childhood, and so it was locked away in a part of my brain that I'd shut off. This was the best way my brain could serve me; by creating pathways that went around the portions of my brain where my trauma was located. However, when my ego dissolved during the journey, I was able to safely explore the painful memories tied to that language, opening up the dormant part of my brain where they were stored. The return of my ability to speak Spanish is a clear example of neuroplasticity in action, and dare I say, "*Extraordinario!*"

Now, when I speak Spanish, it feels like second nature, even though my vocabulary is still at the level of a five-year-old. But my accent? It's spot on. And people have commented on how sweet and youthful my voice sounds.

I witnessed firsthand how psilocybin can lead to profound shifts in the brain's structure, helping us access parts of ourselves we may have long forgotten or hidden away. I'll never forget the power of that moment; the moment I rediscovered a language I thought was lost to me forever.

VOICE - *You remembered!*

The language. The love.

Not from books, but from the marrow.

From the women before you.

They spoke without words.

Their pain carried behind silent lips.

CATHERINE - *It just... came out of me.*

Like it was waiting.

I haven't spoken Spanish since I was a child.

It startled me.

But it felt... natural.

VOICE - *The language of your roots never left.*

It only went quiet, like a song paused.

When you spoke, you claimed.

Reclamation of the parts that shame tried to bury.

CATHERINE - *Why now?*

VOICE - *Because the silence grew too heavy.*

Because you finally stopped.

Long enough to hear the love beneath the grief.

CATHERINE - *I heard her.*

The one whose silence shaped me.

VOICE - *Yes. The one who taught you to carry pain*

without speaking it.

The wounds she passed, not with words, but

with silence.

CATHERINE - *For the first time, I didn't hear blame.*

I only felt grief.

VOICE - *Grief and love, always tied together.*

Sometimes, we inherit more than eye color.

We inherit unfinished stories.

CATHERINE - *I didn't know I was still carrying hers.*

But I felt it in the medicine.

The weight was never mine alone.

VOICE - *It never is.*

Later that evening, as the group of counselors gathered in a circle to reflect on the day's journey, the mood was reflective and intimate. It felt like the right moment to begin making sense of the revelations that had surfaced during my trip. One by one, we were invited to share stories; those defining moments in life that had shifted us, challenged us, or awakened something deep within. As the others began speaking, I found myself listening more than talking, unsure of how, or if, my experiences would fit into the kind of spiritual clarity they each seemed to carry.

Many of the counselors shared stories of their spiritual awakenings; moments when they found solace, healing, and strength through their faith. These stories were filled with positive memories, the kind that connected them to something greater and offered them peace.

Inga spoke first, her voice steady and full of conviction. "My faith in God is the guiding force behind everything I do. It's how I find direction in this world. I trust it to lead me, even when the path isn't clear."

Gary nodded thoughtfully, adding, "I struggle sometimes with the big decisions in life. When I don't know which way to turn, I try to tap into my spirituality, even if it feels like I'm grasping at air. But I believe it helps me find my way."

Rosie, always radiant in her calmness, shared her perspective next. "For me, spirituality isn't just something I believe in; it's something I live. It's who I am, in every action, in every breath. It's the foundation of my existence." Her eyes glowed with serene energy that felt contagious.

Sabrina, still coming down from her hero dose, gave a slow, dreamy smile. "Everything just feels...so clear right now," she murmured. "Like I understand everything but nothing at the same time." She laughed softly, almost to herself.

I sat quietly, listening to each of them. I didn't feel ready to speak yet, unsure of how to frame my journey. When the moment came for me to share, I hesitated.

"I—" I started, then paused, unsure of how to put it into words. "I think my path has been...different. I didn't have these big, clear spiritual epiphanies. My journey wasn't framed by faith or clarity. It's been shaped by confusion, by searching for love, and by...coming to terms with parts of myself I didn't understand for a long time."

There was a brief silence, and I could feel their understanding without needing words. It wasn't the kind of story they had shared, but it was my truth. And at that moment, I realized my story, however messy, was still just as sacred as theirs.

In the quiet that followed, I didn't need to rehash every detail of my revelations. They had already made their mark. What mattered now was what I chose to do with them. Sitting in that circle, surrounded by others who were bravely facing their own truths, I felt something shift. I felt the power of being witnessed. This experience of having my story held without judgment offered a kind of healing I hadn't known I needed.

> **¡OYE! Don't rush to make it make sense.**
>
> Some insights don't come with subtitles. Let the weird, wonderful pieces breathe. Meaning appears when it's ready, usually when you stop chasing it.

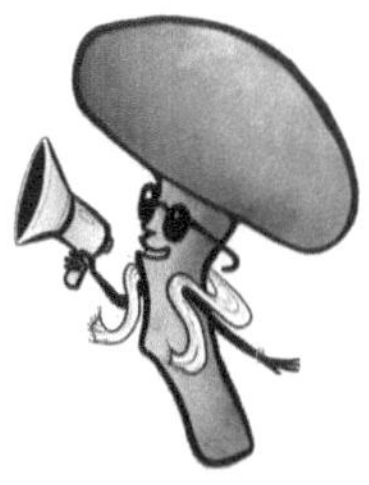

It was in this space of shared humanity, in a cozy cabin with people I trusted, that the deeper work began: not just seeing the past differently, but allowing those insights to settle into my body, my voice, and my future. The mushrooms had opened the door, but it was in the presence of the group with their shared reflections and stories that allowed me to walk through it.

In that space, healing ceased to be a solitary pursuit. I understood, perhaps for the first time, that transformation is not only possible but also sustainable when we're willing to let others in.

I felt liberated by all that I learned in one short weekend, as a counselor, a scientist, and a human being. I also felt humbled. I knew there was more work to be done.

CHAPTER FIVE

TAKE ME TO CHURCH

Even as the medicine wore off, something remained—an echo of the revelations, a tremble beneath the surface. I had opened a door inside myself, and now came the more challenging part: staying in the room. Integration wasn't a matter of simply understanding what had happened during the journey; it was about weaving those insights into the fabric of my life, one breath at a time.

After the experience, something shifted in me that was both subtle and profound. While waiting in line at the grocery store, two men stood behind me, speaking Spanish to each other. One of them commented that he thought my blue-dyed hair was pretty.

Without hesitation or thought, I simply turned around and responded, "Gracias."

His face flushed with surprise, and he quickly looked away, clearly embarrassed. He had assumed I wouldn't understand him, but something in me had changed. It was a small, spontaneous moment, but it made me realize I needed to be more aware of how I respond in my new language. I didn't want to unintentionally make others feel uncomfortable, especially when they hadn't expected me to understand. It was a reminder that my newfound confidence in language needed to be balanced with consideration for the context and the people around me.

Later at home, I noticed a shift in how I approached Ken. There was a softness in me that hadn't been there before, a gentleness that made it easier to be present with him. With my clients, I noticed that I was holding space for them more freely, without the usual weight of needing to fix or direct them. It wasn't just a change in how I interacted; it was a transformation. It was a change in *who* I was, more aligned with the truth of who I truly am.

The counselors at the cabin had created a space where those threads could be examined with care. Their honesty, wounds, and wisdom mirrored pieces of mine. I didn't yet know how closely our stories would intersect, or how their reflections would call forward something buried even deeper in me. But I could feel it stirring: the ache beneath the ache. The mother wound I hadn't yet dared to name. And it all hinged around religion and faith.

My mother met my father at a time in her life when she was struggling to find her place in a family already marked by pain and complexity. She was the youngest of five, but her story was shadowed in part by a sibling she never met: her sister, who died at the age of five, long before she was born. To make matters more complicated, one of her older sisters was given the name of the lost child, an inheritance that haunted her throughout her life. It was as if Mamaita had set an impossible standard, asking one daughter to live up to the memory of another who had been forever sainted in death. I can't help but wonder what would drive a mother to make that choice. It speaks volumes about Mamaita's unresolved pain, her struggle to process loss in a way that ultimately placed a burden on the living.

My mother, labeled "Baby" by her family, was born into this tangled web of expectations. This nickname followed her well into her thirties, a constant reminder that no matter how much she accomplished, she would never truly grow up in the eyes of her family. Even after they stopped calling her "Baby," they continued to treat her as the youngest, the least experienced, the one who needed protecting or controlling. She was a woman trapped by the roles others had cast for her.

This upbringing shaped her in ways she probably never fully understood. It made her fiercely independent but also deeply insecure. She was strong-willed and driven to prove herself. But underneath that determination was a vulnerability she hid from the world. She developed a sharp wit and a keen sense of humor, often using it as a shield to deflect pain. She could be the life of the party when she wanted to be, but there was a reluctance to let people see the cracks in her armor.

Her beauty was undeniable, and while she resented how easily men were swayed by it, she also knew how to use it to her advantage when it suited her.

She met my father in high school and married him at the age of twenty-two. I was born just shy of their first anniversary in 1968. My father, a young soldier, was stationed overseas in Korea before they knew my mother was pregnant, leaving my mother to navigate the challenges of new motherhood while living with her parents. It was a difficult beginning, but she persevered, earning her Bachelor's degree in Education. She learned from a young age how to survive and push through hardship without letting it show.

If there's one lesson my mother ingrained in us, it was the power of setting a goal and achieving it through sheer determination and an unbreakable work ethic. Despite struggling with a learning disability, she refused to let it define her. She had dyslexia and had to study extra hard each night just to keep up with her college peers, all while she was pregnant with me. This was long before dyslexia was widely understood or diagnosed, so she kept it a secret, carrying the weight of her struggle alone because there was no language or support for what she was experiencing. She worked harder than ever, pushing herself to overcome obstacles that others never even saw.

When my father returned, they tried to build a life together, going on to have three daughters, each born within a year and a half to two years of each other. I was the first, followed by my sisters.

But the marriage was far from perfect. My parents separated when I was around nine years old, leaving my mother to shoulder the responsibility of raising three daughters on her own. She worked as a teacher, then studied at night to earn her Master's degree, constantly striving for more so she could provide a better life for us. She later transitioned into a career as a pharmaceutical rep, before switching paths once more to become a flight attendant, a job she held for twenty-five years.

Through all of this, she maintained a veneer of perfection, the same facade she had been taught to present as a child. Outwardly, she was strong and capable, but underneath, she was a woman who struggled with her sense of identity. A master of reinvention, she kept pushing forward. But no matter how far she ran, the shadows of her childhood followed her, influencing her choices, her relationships, and ultimately, her role as a mother.

After divorcing my father, she married for love a second time, and although that relationship only lasted nine years, she still speaks of that man as the love of her life. However, being with him often felt like she had another child. She was the one who paid the bills, scheduled the appointments, and managed the household while working full-time. Meanwhile, he would overspend and repeatedly sabotage his employment. He had a pattern of impulsively quitting jobs or getting fired for poor decisions, like the time he let me, after barely turning sixteen years old, drive his company car—an act that ended with the car totaled and his termination.

What began as a relationship fueled by deep affection eventually left her carrying the whole burden, both emotionally and practically, while still longing for someone to share the load. Her third marriage endured for 26 years, but it was built more on the need for stability than genuine connection. Over time, she realized that stability was an illusion, as the emotional abuse and underlying contempt in the relationship left her feeling just as unanchored as before. He would belittle her in subtle but cutting ways—criticizing her intelligence in front of others or making jokes at her expense that weren't jokes at all. It chipped away at her spirit, leaving her constantly walking on eggshells, unsure of when the next passive-aggressive jab would come. Each marriage carried the echoes of her past: the lingering need for approval, the fear of vulnerability, and the constant pressure to maintain an image of perfection.

Yet, despite the upheavals, she never stopped pushing forward. She rebuilt herself time and time again, adapting to each new chapter with resilience and determination.

Despite her evident resourcefulness and strength, I can't recall a single moment when I felt genuinely seen or heard by the woman who raised me.

Instead, my entire existence seemed to orbit around holding her spotlight. From an early age, I learned that survival meant catering to her every need, constantly ensuring she wasn't unhappy. I would rush home from school to complete all the required chores, making sure every dish was clean, every cushion fluffed, every surface cleared—because if she walked in and saw even one thing out of place, it could send her into a spiral of anger that would ruin the night for everyone in the house. There was never a sense that I could make her happy—only the need to keep her neutral, to prevent her anger from boiling over.

This dynamic left me struggling to understand who I was or where I belonged. As soon as I was able, I began to build a wall between us, creating distance to preserve my sanity. By that point in my young adult life, she would try, over and over, to connect with me, but I couldn't fully open up to her. I feigned receptiveness, just enough to avoid her lashing out, but it was always an act.

As an adult, visits with my mother became month-long ordeals. It would take me weeks to mentally prepare, and even then, my needs disappeared entirely. Whenever we met, we did whatever she wanted, and I was reduced to a shadow of myself, constantly standing behind her spotlight while I remained unseen in the darkness.

This delicate dance kept the peace, but it also meant I couldn't truly be myself around her. I felt invisible, lost in the need to keep her calm, but never able to exist authentically in her presence.

Whenever a visit ended, it would take me two weeks to recover as I was emotionally drained, my essence depleted. Looking back, I see how the relationship kept me from knowing myself. It was familiar, yes, but suffocating. I was trapped in a cycle where I couldn't show up authentically, and so there was nothing real to share. Each visit felt like a personal death, a retreat of my ego just to survive, losing my identity in the process. This is why my visits were so infrequent... We existed in a state of detachment, never truly present with one another.

I spent much of my 40s and the years when I was completing graduate school focused on healing my relationship with my mother. It took many years of work, but eventually, I stopped holding the spotlight for her and catering to her every need. While I still couldn't fully embrace my authentic self around her, I learned not to carry her emotional baggage. The most significant effect was that she could no longer guilt or shame me. Before I began using psychedelics, memory reconsolidation techniques helped me release the guilt and shame triggers that my mother had so naturally used to manipulate me, and that I had fallen into responding to so easily.

By the time I began working with psychedelics, I was able to be around my mother without all the preparation beforehand and without needing long periods of recovery afterward.

I had made significant progress, and I was proud of the work I had done.

One moment stands out clearly as a turning point in my behavior. She was visiting, and as usual, we decided to see a movie together. It was our go-to activity, something safe and easy—entertaining without requiring much intimacy. That day, we chose a movie theater that served lunch, and we both ordered salads, a detail that seemed insignificant at the time.

Later that evening, we met up with family at a Mexican restaurant. As we sat down and opened our menus, she leaned over, nudged me, and said with a conspiratorial smile, *"We can eat whatever we want—we had salads for lunch."*

In the past, that one comment would have sent me spiraling out of control. I would've felt her disapproval like a weight pressing down, and ended up ordering something lighter, something I didn't want, just to avoid her judgment.

But not this time. I took a breath, nudged her right back, and said firmly, "I can eat whatever I want, whenever I want. That's your rule, not mine."

It was a small moment, but monumental in its impact. For the first time, I didn't shrink under her disapproval. I didn't abandon myself to earn her approval. I claimed my autonomy, and it felt like reclaiming a piece of myself she had held for far too long.

Though my mother made several attempts to build a new relationship with me, I remained guarded. I genuinely believed that giving her even an inch would result in losing a mile. For example, if I agreed to a short phone call, it would often spiral into her asking why I didn't call more often or increase the pressure to plan a visit. A simple gesture of openness would quickly become a doorway to expectations I wasn't ready, or willing, to meet. I simply couldn't take that risk, not after all the effort I had put into improving my mental health and establishing myself as an individual.

My experience with cancer did bring us a little closer, but deep down, I still felt she was asking for something that felt impossible. She wanted an emotional closeness and openness between us that had never existed before. She longed for a relationship where I shared my heart with her as freely as she wanted to share hers with me. But that kind of mutuality had never been part of our dynamic. As a child, our relationship had been one-sided: I was expected to tune into her needs, manage her moods, and anticipate what would make her happy. My wants and feelings were never part of the equation. She had taught me, implicitly and repeatedly, that my role was to take care of her, not to be taken care of.

So now, as an adult, when she hoped for emotional reciprocity and connection, it felt confusing and unfair. I didn't know how to make space for myself in a relationship with her, because there had never been any space for me before. She had never made room for my vulnerability, and I didn't know how to trust that she could hold it now. In my heart, I believed it was too late to rewrite the script of our relationship.

Yet in the company of my colleagues at the cabin, after my first therapeutic macrodose of mushrooms, while still in a state of partial ego-dissolution, something came up that required exploration.

My journey with psilocybin had begun to break down the layers of defensiveness I'd built over the years and allowed me to see my mother in a new light, one less clouded by the trauma of my past. I started to understand that her struggles and her pain had shaped her in ways I had never allowed myself to acknowledge. And perhaps, in her way, she had loved me all along.

And yet, as we continued to sit and discuss spiritual awakenings, I began to connect dots that I hadn't been able to reconcile before. I realized that, growing up Catholic, I had always seen Mamaita and my mother as the gatekeepers of our family's religious practices. As I mentioned earlier, I viewed Mamaita as a hypocrite. She would speak of kindness, love, and goodwill, but her actions often reflected judgment, dishonesty, and a mean-spirited nature.

And both of these ladies had an obsessive need to present a perfect image to the outside world. I remember feeling like I had to look presentable just to check the mail, because, you know, *God forbid a neighbor saw me in anything less than my Sunday best.* My mom had a knack for bumping into friends, colleagues, students, and random acquaintances. It didn't matter if we were suffering from illness or had a rough day; if we ran into someone, we had to look flawless. Outward perfection was the goal, while what happened behind closed doors was similar to behind the scenes on a reality show no one was supposed to know about.

I began to see the same insincerity mirrored in church, a place that should have been a sanctuary but instead became another arena for hypocrisy. During my confirmation preparation, I spent afternoons with the nuns, learning the rites and rituals that marked this supposed rite of passage. It was here, in the very heart of this sacred space, that I was taught my worth was somehow less than that of others, simply because I was female.

In the Catholic Church, men are the ones granted authority. Only men can become priests, only men are allowed to lead Mass, hear confessions, or hold positions of real spiritual power. Women—no matter how devout—are relegated to supportive roles: cleaning the church, preparing the altar, teaching children. It was clear, even to my young mind, that the system didn't value women in the same way. We were expected to be obedient, modest, and silent, while reverence and leadership were reserved for men.

The nuns, who were meant to embody grace and kindness, would treat some with warmth and care, but when the doors closed and the curtains fell, they'd turn on me and others, showing a side of cruelty that felt jarring and unjust. Their actions only reinforced the message: in the eyes of the Church, we were second-class citizens—expected to serve, but not to speak.

Those circumstances fueled a further inability to feel close to my mother. Throughout her life, my mother was a devout Catholic, and she supported her church in the only way she knew how: by attending services regularly and giving money whenever possible.

The duplicity I saw in church, where love and judgment coexisted in such a twisted dance, became a breeding ground for resentment for me. Over time, the hypocrisy didn't just sting; it festered deep inside me, fueling a bitter, smoldering anger that I could never quite shake. I came to resent the very place in which I was supposed to find solace, knowing that its message of love was often just a facade.

As I sat in this conversation with the group of counselors, I began to see how deeply this affected me and how it created a wall between my mother and me. As an adult, one of the most significant divides that remained was her inability to grasp my perspective on my childhood. She often spoke of what a "great kid" I was and presented our past through rose-colored glasses, as though it had been a perfect, idyllic time. But every time she said that, it felt like she was erasing my reality, gaslighting me about my own experience. I didn't remember being a great kid. I only remembered constantly being in trouble, never doing anything right, and living in the shadow of her anger.

My upbringing was far from ideal. I spent half my time walking on eggshells, terrified of my mother's rage, and the other half of my time trying to suffocate my own fury because there was no space for my feelings, my needs, and my truth. It was the stark contrast between her outward, charitable persona and her self-centered, unkind parenting that created an irreparable disconnect for me. In public, she presented herself as pious and generous, always smiling and always helping, but behind closed doors, she demanded perfection and control; her love was conditional and often withheld. This contradiction was jarring to me, leaving me to wonder how the woman who could be so "good" in the eyes of others could be so harsh with her children.

A clear example of this was how I was treated differently from my sisters. They were spared from being held accountable for their misdeeds, while I became the scapegoat. If they did something wrong, it was always my fault. I was expected, as the eldest, to manage them, to act as their caretaker and disciplinarian. But when they misbehaved, the blame fell squarely on me, deepening the sense of injustice and reinforcing the feeling that I was the one who had to carry the weight of everyone else's mistakes.

What hurt the most was my mother's inability, or unwillingness, to acknowledge the deep, gaping wounds she inflicted. She couldn't see the scars I carried, and that refusal to recognize my pain continued to haunt me. It haunts me even now, and I'm well into my 50s. It was as if the trauma of never being truly seen by the one person who was supposed to love me unconditionally would never fully heal.

For over thirty years, I've heard stories of sexual abuse by priests, and as a counselor, I have spent years working with survivors of childhood abuse, many of whom were victims of Catholic priests. It has been a harrowing experience, holding space for these individuals as they recount their trauma. And yet, I've seen no real effort from the church to stop this behavior. From what I understand, they simply transfer the priests, hiding their actions instead of holding them accountable or turning them over to the authorities to face legal consequences for their crimes.

I've often wondered, *how can the Catholic church continue to justify the harm it's caused, especially when it refuses to take meaningful action to change the circumstances?*

Why hasn't the church implemented basic rules, like ensuring that two adults are always present when minors are involved in any situation, to ensure accountability?

What's even more disturbing to me is the complete lack of advocacy from those who support the church, including my mother, a parishioner. This, for me, was just another painful example of her failure to acknowledge the suffering of vulnerable children who are ignored, mistreated, and left unprotected.

The truth hit me as the effects of the mushrooms faded: my mother's financial support of the Catholic church felt like an endorsement of this systemic abuse. By continuing to contribute to the institution, she was effectively turning a blind eye to the harm that was not just inflicted on me, but on countless children around the world. This realization wars a turning point in my life. My mother has often said that if she could do it all over again, she would have handled my childhood differently. But how could I accept that claim when all I could see was how she was funding the protection of pedophiles and enabling the continuation of this abuse? How could she profess to care about my well-being and the well-being of others when her actions directly contradicted that care?

Although I was not sexually abused in the way many children were, I understand what it feels like to be a child who is not seen or heard. I want to make it clear that I'm not comparing my experience to theirs'. What those children went through is a level of trauma that I cannot fully comprehend. But for me, this only deepens my point. If my mother truly felt remorse for the way I was treated, if she believed she "would have done it differently," how could she continue supporting an institution that I feel causes lifelong harm to young people?

Adults who come into my office often express that childhood sexual abuse is a life sentence for them, an unending trauma that shapes who they are and how they interact with the world. And yet, I couldn't reconcile my own need to advocate for children, to protect them from harm, with my mother's financial support of an institution that houses, feeds, and shields those very perpetrators. The disconnect between my need for justice and her actions felt like a barrier that I simply could not overcome.

Once the mushrooms helped me see this, I could no longer unsee it or ignore it. The truth was clear, and I knew I had to confront it, no matter how painful. I had to have a frank conversation with my mother about the deep conflict I was carrying. I felt strongly that as long as she continued supporting the church, she was, in a way, discounting my reality. She was invalidating the very truth of my lived experience.

It was one of the most challenging conversations I have ever had.

After explaining my complex realization, she seemed confused, overwhelmed by what I had presented. The weight of it all hung heavy in the air. And as difficult as it was for her, it was equally agonizing for me. I was forced to use my voice in a room with the very person who had taught me, for most of my life, to silence it. To speak up was to break a lifetime of conditioning, to go against the very lessons I'd been taught about who I was supposed to be. It felt like a profound act of defiance, a necessary one, but painful nonetheless.

"Mom, I can't tell you how to spend your money, that's not my place. But knowing that you continue to financially support an organization that still harms children goes against everything I stand for. I can't accept your apologies for the past when you keep backing an institution that refuses to change its harmful behavior toward kids. As long as you keep supporting the church, there will always be a barrier of distrust between us. The trauma caused by childhood sexual abuse lasts a lifetime; it shapes a person forever."

My mother's defensive response, "You don't have to tell ME!" highlighted the point I was making. My mother was victimized sexually as a young child, something that was revealed to me when I was in my teens.

"Exactly, I shouldn't have to tell you!" I said. I was dumbfounded that she'd never actually seen the issue herself before. But, I could tell that it was getting through and that she would not be able to unsee what I was forcing her to face.

"Have you, or anyone you know, ever asked the church what they're doing to stop more victims from being hurt? Why does everyone just accept things as they are? Why is no one holding them accountable, instead of blindly handing over their hard-earned money?" I asked again, my voice growing more desperate,

"Mom, have you ever asked them what they're doing to ensure no more children are harmed?"

Her answer hit me like a punch.

"No." "No... no... no... no... no."

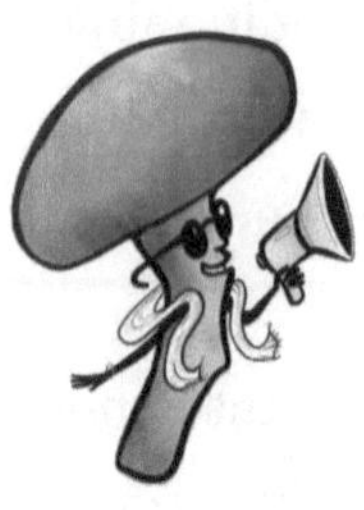

Integration means weaving what you've learned into your everyday life. Don't file your experience away. Live it out, one choice at a time.

The next day, she texted me a pie chart graphic labeled, "How Your 8 cents is Used by the Archdiocesan Chancery Corporation," with the attached message:

"Got curious and looked it up: 4.25% of my 8 cents goes to costs related to clergy sexual abuse and other misconduct. The hope/goodwill I get from the church outweighs the misuse of my funds. The government takes 24% in taxes from this old lady and misuses a lot of it. Every organization is the devil's playground. Can't imagine how awful the abuse must have been and how rampant. Sorry you have to pick up the pieces of your abused patients. Your work is very important. Love you."

I felt my heart shatter as I read her justification.

Was there anything that would make it unacceptable for her to support the church? Would it take the murder of children for it to be considered wrong? This was coming from a woman who had suffered for years from her childhood abuse. The distance between us was growing thicker because she couldn't, or wouldn't, see my point of view.

My text response was, "The government does not intentionally fund/employ anyone who has thirty years of pedophilia history, nor do they cover for them. Government employees are required to report, but clergy are not required and never report. A HUGE difference to me. I have yet to hear what the church is doing to prevent more. I understand that you have to defend your position, but I do not see it as defensible in any way, shape, or form. It is best to agree that we do not agree."

At the time, I didn't fully grasp how even well-intentioned institutions can fail to protect the vulnerable. I was a bit naive about the complexities involved, but my overall point still stands: such lack of accountability is unacceptable anywhere.

I started to feel like there was no way I'd be able to reach her, and a part of me began to believe this conversation was nothing more than a waste of my time. My belief grew stronger than ever, and my mother's denial became a wall between us that seemed impossible to overcome.

Then, a day or so later, my mother reached out.

She said she had listened, truly heard me, and made a decision. She pledged that she would no longer provide financial support to the church. Instead, she would offer her time and energy. She acknowledged that the church had done nothing to address the abuse and that supporting it was no longer something she could condone. She also vowed to question the church's methods for preventing abuse (past, present, and future) for the rest of her life.

Although it felt somewhat forced, a part of me felt a small sense of relief, as if a heavy weight had been lifted, just a little. This was the first time I could sense a tiny crack in the wall between us, a glimmer of possibility for healing. Even though I still wasn't sure she truly understood the depth of what I was feeling, it was the first time she had genuinely considered my perspective. I think she realized that this wasn't something on which I was willing to compromise. While I knew it wouldn't instantly bring us closer, I also understood that without her making such a pledge, the gap between us would only grow, and it would become even harder to find common ground. It wasn't a perfect solution, but it felt like the first real step toward mending something that had been broken for so long.

Little did I know that the pledge marked the beginning of a profound unraveling of my mother's faith in the Catholic Church. She began volunteering her time, answering phones, and providing administrative support. However, as she delved deeper into the inner workings, she began to uncover several uncomfortable truths. What had once seemed like a sacred and benevolent institution became exposed as something very different. Her protective bubble burst when she realized that the church wasn't providing direct help to parishioners in need. Instead, they were directing them to government services, something that deeply troubled her. She had always believed that the church was a source of charity and support, but she began to see firsthand how it wasn't fulfilling that role, instead realizing the facade.

The final straw came when she discovered that the church would not offer any direct help to their parishioners; instead, they were referring people in need to another local church, one known for actually providing direct support to its members. This betrayal was particularly painful to her because she had spent so many years supporting the church financially, emotionally, and spiritually, only to realize that her generosity wasn't being reciprocated. My mother, heartbroken and disillusioned, couldn't reconcile the difference between the generosity she had offered and the cold, bureaucratic machinery she was seeing behind the veil.

The complex reality of hypocrisy, which I had suffered as a child and continued to endure well into adulthood, was something my mother was only beginning to see much later in her life. For years, she had lived behind carefully constructed facades, crafting a version of herself and our family that appeared perfect to the outside world, even if it didn't reflect the turmoil beneath the surface. The church, in all its grandeur and its promises of love, truth, and righteousness, was no different. She had become so accustomed to hiding behind a mask of perfection that when she finally began to see the cracks in the very institution she had once believed in, she realized that it mirrored the same falsehoods she had spent her life perpetuating. The veil of deceit that had shielded her began to lift, and for the first time, she saw the hypocrisy not just in others, but in the way she had lived her own life. It was a painful awakening, one that was forcing her to confront the very illusions she had built around herself for so long.

The experience shattered her trust in the institution to which she had devoted her life and led her to lose her faith in religion altogether. It was a slow burn of disillusionment, a quiet but profound collapse of the world in which she had once believed.

While it was never my intention to rock her world, I couldn't help but feel a quiet sense of peace in knowing I had stood up for what was right. I had advocated for children who deserved protection, and in doing so, had opened a door to a new understanding between us.

This was just the beginning of a long journey for both of us. Our relationship, which had long been strained, was slowly but surely shifting. Little did we know that the work we started with mushrooms was only the first step in what would become a more profound transformation. We had no idea how much more was in store for us, but I was beginning to feel a glimmer of hope that our bond, though tested, could be rebuilt.

CATHERINE - *What should I call you?*

VOICE - *Ask your inner self what label you need for this.*

CATHERINE - *I... Maria?*

VOICE - *Surprised?*

CATHERINE - *Yes.*

I just felt it.

VOICE - *Names are not always chosen.*

They are remembered.

CATHERINE - *Maria...*

MARIA - *You carry their weight. The past is not gone, but it is yours to heal.*

CATHERINE - *How do I carry it forward?*

MARIA - *By seeing it. By accepting it.*

CATHERINE - *I never understood my grandmother's pain, nor my mother's, until now.*

MARIA - *You were born into their wounds.*

But you are not bound by them.

Their truth is yours to understand, but it is yours to

transform as well.

Your healing ripples out, reaching the roots

that shaped you.

CATHERINE - *So, this isn't just about me.*

MARIA - *It never was.*

It's about all of you.

What you heal within yourself, you offer to the ones

who come before and after you.

CHAPTER SIX

UNFRIENDING MY ANTIDEPRESSANT

MARIA - *Walls crack.*

>*You must step back to see it.*

CATHERINE - *What is this change I'm feeling?*

MARIA - *You stand on the edge.*

CATHERINE - *I've been afraid of it for so long.*

MARIA - *Fear holds what you need.*

>*Now, you will feel it.*

CATHERINE - *What if I can't handle it?*

MARIA - *You have handled more.*

>*Now, feel what's hidden.*

CATHERINE - *How can I trust this?*

MARIA - *Trust already exists, beneath your questions.*

THE EXPERIENCE OF EGO-DISSOLUTION WITH MUSHROOMS didn't just shift my perspective. It shattered it. In an instant, the walls I'd built around my mind crumbled, and I was plunged into a realm of profound insights and life-changing realizations. My relationships transformed, my worldview expanded, and I began to see life through a lens I never knew existed.

I was eager to try mushrooms again. Partly because of my experience, and partly because of what I learned about the therapeutic effects of PAT concerning depression.

But beneath these revelations, another story was unfolding: I was on the verge of breaking free from antidepressants.

As a young adult diagnosed with major depression, navigating the world of medication was like stumbling through a maze blindfolded. It took years of trial and error before I finally found *Wellbutrin*, or bupropion, the only one I could tolerate, even with its side effects and compromises. I settled on a dose of 300 mg once a day, time-released.

But here's the twist: one 300 mg SR tablet would send me spiraling, but two 150 mg SR tablets were the perfect balance. It made no sense. In theory, the dosage was identical. In my body, they were worlds apart.

Here's what happened: at one point, while prepping my weekly pill boxes, I unknowingly switched from two 150 mg tablets to a single 300 mg tablet for a couple of weeks. The change happened mid-month, and I didn't notice. Slowly, I began to unravel—my mood dropped, energy faded, and that familiar heaviness crept back in. I couldn't figure out what had gone wrong until a sharp physician's assistant reviewed my medication history and pieced it together. That one small change had thrown me completely off balance. It was infuriating and validating all at once. After that, I fought hard—with doctors, pharmacies, and insurance companies—to make sure I could stay on the version that worked for me.

For thirty years, I took those two capsules every single day. It became muscle memory, a ritual so ingrained that I stopped questioning it. Yet, every time I filled out a doctor's form and saw the question, "Do you have depression?" I hesitated. *What was the answer?* I had been diagnosed, but the symptoms were managed. I didn't feel depressed anymore. The medication was working. It neutralized the darkness that once haunted me.

But what I didn't realize was that it was also neutralizing everything else, including the highs, the joys, and the spark of life. As the mushrooms peeled back the layers, I began to wonder: *Who am I beneath the medication? What have I been missing all these years?*

Ken knew I had depression, but he never truly saw me drowning in its depths. He only caught glimpses—shadows flickering at the edges of my being—during those cruel stretches when my medication wavered or failed me completely. In those moments, the darkness didn't just return; it seeped into every crevice of my mind, thick and inescapable, twisting my thoughts into something unrecognizable. He would watch with quiet concern, searching my face for answers I couldn't give. And honestly, I was relieved he didn't understand. The only way to grasp the weight of that kind of emptiness is to carry it yourself, and I wouldn't wish that burden on anyone.

Through it all, Ken showed nothing but patience; the kind that felt almost saintly. He stood by me, steady and unwavering, even when he couldn't fully understand the storm inside my mind. His empathy came from his own battle scars, especially from the pain of his divorce. That experience had dragged him into a depression of his own—one that was situational, rooted in tangible loss and heartbreak. His darkness made sense. It had a clear beginning, a logical cause, and eventually, a path out.

Ken's dance with depression was justifiable, tied to something tangible. He had to claw his way out of a place no one should ever have to go. What he survived was brutal, the kind of pain you wouldn't wish on your worst enemy.

On his 41st birthday, Ken's life took an unexpected, devastating turn. The woman he had once loved and trusted, his partner, chose that day to reveal a painful truth. She confessed to having an affair with someone he considered a close friend, someone who had even sought refuge in their home during a difficult time. The betrayal was so profound, so unfathomable, it was hard to wrap my head around it. I can't imagine how Ken must have felt. It's almost impossible to process the weight of that kind of deception, especially from two people you thought you could trust. If it were me, I don't think I could have trusted anyone again for a long time.

The worst part, however, was realizing that the betrayal had been happening right under his nose for months. While he thought these two were supporting him, they were secretly growing closer to each other. And then, on his birthday, a day that should have been full of celebration, she chose to drop the bombshell that would haunt him for years. It took a long time before that day no longer felt like a deep wound. It wasn't until almost a decade later that he could finally look at his birthday without that sense of betrayal and loss overwhelming him.

When I first met Ken, his birthday wasn't a day of celebration. It was a day he braced himself for, like a storm he knew was coming but could never outrun. He spent it in isolation, holed up in a friend's dimly lit rental house, a bottle of booze his only companion. Drink after drink, he tried to drown the memories, to numb the ache that gnawed at him from the inside out, waiting for the hours to pass and for the day to disappear. These episodes of depression that haunted him seemed to worsen in those moments, as if the weight of the betrayal made it all feel much heavier. Watching him spiral like that shattered me. I couldn't stand the way those two people still had their claws in him, poisoning what should have been a day to celebrate his existence, his magnificence. Instead, it was just another battle to endure.

It was a long and arduous road. Every year, I pushed him to do the opposite of what he wanted, to face the day head-on, to create new, happy memories. I knew it would take years to overpower the darkness of that betrayal. But I was determined. I wanted to erase his ex-wife's selfish shadow from his life, to reclaim his birthday as a day of joy.

The breakthrough finally came on his 50th birthday. We were in Times Square, surrounded by lights and life, creating a memory so vivid and full of wonder that it finally eclipsed the pain. That day became his new story, a symbol of hope and healing. We had done it. We had rewritten the narrative.

Ken's experience with depression was situational, deeply rooted in his circumstances, and clearly justified, whereas mine was chemical, sometimes random, and unpredictable. My depression came from nowhere and everywhere all at once. It wasn't tied to a specific event or external loss. There were times I'd wake up with a crushing sadness for no identifiable reason, and no amount of problem-solving or pep talks could lift it. That contrast between us—his grief with a name, mine with no face—highlighted just how mysterious and misunderstood my mental health journey was. And yet, even without fully grasping it, Ken remained by my side. That, to me, was love in its purest form.

Yet somehow, despite the divide between our experiences, he understood my condition at a base level. He loved me through it, even when he couldn't see the battle I was fighting inside. I think because Ken had danced with his own darkness, he understood and found the strength to stand by me when I fell into mine. Whether my funk was triggered by medication changes or the relentless grip of depression, he was there—patient, steady, always relieved when I found my way back to the surface, but never angry when I was lost. He became my "Have there been any changes in your meds?" monitor, noticing shifts in me before I did. It was his quiet way of looking out for me, protecting me in a way no one ever had.

After all we had been through with my hip replacements and cancer treatments, he still could love me through my worst days. To take care of me like no one ever had. Ken is nothing short of extraordinary. His ability to continue loving and supporting me, despite his own struggles, is a gift I will never take for granted.

After my own work with the mushrooms, I began to feel a magnetic pull toward the research I'd once only skimmed in passing—the idea that psilocybin might not just treat depression, but *cure* it. Not manage. Not suppress. *Cure.* Years of suffering, lifted. Not through a daily pill or endless therapy loops, but through two profound experiences, spaced just one week apart. That possibility struck me like a bell I couldn't unring.

Around that time, Gina, a friend, a licensed social worker, a psychonaut, and one of the few people I trusted to speak this psychedelic language, mentioned a study that echoed what I was feeling. It was published in *The Lancet Psychiatry* and led by Robin Carhart-Harris. According to the study, patients with treatment-resistant depression experienced dramatic improvements after just two guided psilocybin sessions. Two sessions. One week apart. And many of them sustained that healing long-term.

That was the moment the path lit up for me. This wasn't fringe or fantasy. This was science meeting soul. And I knew—I *knew*—I had to explore it.[1]

At that point, I was intrigued by the science, though I hadn't intended to try two doses in two weeks. But I was eager to continue learning, first-hand, about the effects of psilocybin on depression.

In preparation for the journey, I decided to stop taking my antidepressant a few days in advance. I didn't want any interference from my medication, hoping to clear the way for whatever insights the mushrooms might offer.

For this particular dose, I chose to stay at home, with Ken by my side as my steady, unwavering guide.

To be honest, I don't remember much from that trip. All I can recall is the profound message from the mushrooms: *The second dose needs to be guided by Gina.* I guess that was it; the profound message that I needed to try dosing twice, only a week apart.

There's a part of me that wonders if my memory is hazy because I didn't give myself enough time between doses to process the experience adequately. I was too eager, too quick to move on. It wasn't the most respectful approach to the therapeutic process, and I regret that now.

---

1   Carhart-Harris et al., 2016

Looking back, with the knowledge and experience I have now, I'd never recommend it. *Two macrodoses that close together? It's a bit much!* Today, I'd advise waiting at least a month between doses. In my expert opinion, I'd say that would have given me the same, if not better, outcome. I've learned from my own experience, and from working responsibly with patients, that the time between journeys is crucial to allow for integration, and to let the lessons sink in deeply before diving back in.

When I reached out to Gina the next day, I asked if she'd be willing to guide me for the second dose, wanting to test out the Lancet article's protocol. But what I didn't expect was the gift she was about to offer. Not only is Gina an experienced psychonaut, but she also has the most amazing backyard; one designed specifically for psychedelic journeys. Her space, both inside and out, is a psychonaut's dream, filled with vibrant colors, cozy lounging spots, and an atmosphere that invites deep reflection and exploration. It's the perfect environment for such a sacred experience.

Additionally, Gina had also completed my Emotional Triggers Treatment (ETT) training years prior. She was one of the few who regularly used it with her clients, and she had become proficient in it.

So when she offered to incorporate the treatment I created into my journey, I was overwhelmed with gratitude. I couldn't believe it! Not only was I about to have an expert guide me through this profound experience in a space designed precisely for this kind of journey, but I was going to receive the very treatment I'd developed *on myself*. What an extraordinary opportunity! It was as if the universe was aligning to give me the perfect experience, the perfect guidance, and the perfect healing all at once.

Once again, I prepared for the second journey by stopping my antidepressants in the same manner as before. What shocked me was how, by the time dosing day arrived, I was doing surprisingly well in terms of my depression. Usually, after two weeks of medication adjustments, I'd be teetering on the edge of a full-blown crisis, caught in the grip of the deep, dark funk that would take over my mood, thoughts, feelings, and behaviors. But this time, it didn't happen. Typically, Ken would be the one pointing out every shift in me as the downward spiral began, but this time, he said nothing. It was as if the storm had passed, leaving calm in its wake.

¡OYE! Don't ghost your meds.

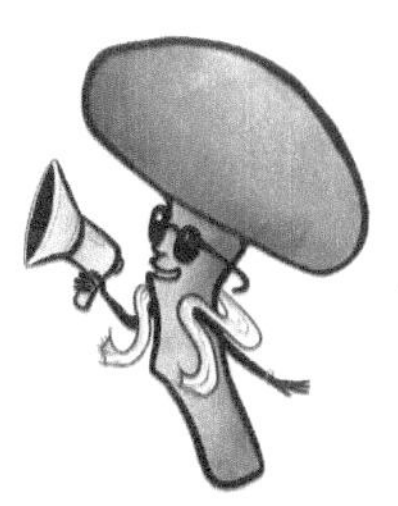

Antidepressants aren't a bad date. You can't just disappear. Break up slowly, with a professional third wheel. Tapering takes teamwork. And fewer withdrawal meltdowns in aisle 5!

The second mushroom journey was nothing short of magical. The moment I stepped into Gina's vibrant space, I felt an energy shift. With her skilled guidance, I went on a journey of deep healing. As planned, Gina performed ETT on me, focusing on the unresolved pain and anger surrounding my relationship with my mother. The clarity that unfolded was profound, like the fog lifting after a storm. I began to understand how years of resentment had built up, how those layers of pain had kept me distant from her. Gina's memory reconsolidation techniques worked wonders, peeling back the years of hurt and creating space for healing.

Through this process, I was able to feel the release of negative energy—energy that had been weighing me down and preventing me from forgiving my mother. She had recently moved to town, and I was struggling to find time to spend with her. I'd force myself to see her, but the guilt and frustration that came with it were suffocating. Gina guided me through an exercise that allowed me to release those heavy feelings, creating more room for compassion and connection. It was as if the walls I had built to protect myself began to crumble, piece by piece, as I moved toward forgiveness.

Then, Gina guided me into deep inner child work, and everything shifted. It was like stepping into the past and coming face-to-face with the broken versions of myself; versions still trapped in the stories I had been told, the ones I had come to believe as absolute truths. She helped me unravel those beliefs, the ones forged in childhood that had shaped me in ways I never questioned. Beliefs that told me who I was and what I was worth. Beliefs that had never truly been mine to begin with.

As I moved through the process, it felt like rewriting the very foundation of my existence. A slow, deliberate untangling. A liberation. This wasn't just about mending the relationship with my mother; it was about reclaiming myself. And when the weight lifted, I felt it, viscerally. Like a breath I didn't know I'd been holding, finally released. The space that pain once occupied was now open, making room for something new. Maybe even for her.

MARIA - *You no longer need them.*

CATHERINE - *The pills?*

MARIA - *Yes. The chemicals.*

You have found something deeper.

CATHERINE - *It feels strange to be without them.*

MARIA - *Strange, maybe.*

But free.

CATHERINE - *It's like the storm is passing.*

MARIA - *Yes. The medicine is working.*

It's still clearing, still shifting.

CATHERINE - *I can feel the change, but it's not*

all clear yet.

MARIA - *Healing is not always sudden.*

It's slow.

Deliberate.

You inhale life now, not just breathing.

You've found a path that rises from the earth.

Not from a bottle.

CATHERINE - *The mushrooms... they're*

helping me see.

MARIA - *They show you what was always there.*

The truth.

CATHERINE - *It feels like a fog is lifting.*

MARIA - *The fog lifts when you choose to see.*

You are choosing presence.

You don't need numbness anymore.

You've reclaimed your truth.

CATHERINE - *I don't think I'll go back.*

MARIA - *You won't.*

You can walk without chemicals.

CATHERINE - *And I'm ready.*

MARIA - *Yes.*

You are coming home now.

As the final hour of my journey approached and Ken was about to pick me up, I sat with Gina, still processing everything that had unfolded. My mind was swirling with new realizations and a newfound clarity. I shared with her how, despite the two-week medication adjustment, I hadn't felt the usual crash.

"I've noticed that I've been okay," I said, trying to wrap my mind around it. "Normally, after tweaking my meds for that long, I'd be spiraling by now. But this time… nothing. I haven't had that dip."

Gina looked at me, her eyes thoughtful, a gentle smile tugging at the corner of her lips. "That's incredible," she said softly. "You know, mushrooms can create new pathways in the brain. It's as if they rewire things, creating new routes for healing and balance. Your depression might have been driven by those old, outdated pathways, pathways that no longer serve you."

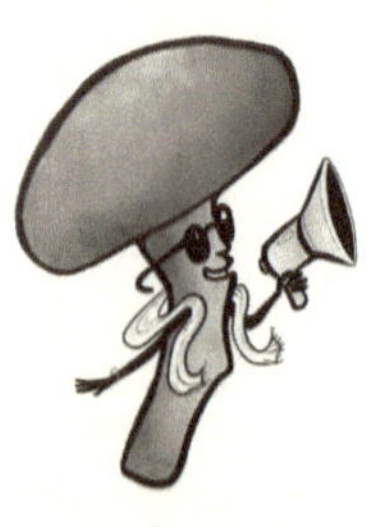

¡OYE! Contrary actions create new neural paths.

Psilocybin throws open the emergency exit on your usual behavior patterns. Suddenly, you get a pause… an unexpected "Are you *sure* you want to do that thing you always do?" Instead of reacting like a well-trained lab rat, you get to choose a new move. Make the weird choice. Make the kind choice. Make the opposite-of-what-you-usually-do choice. That's the gold. And when you do it again? Boom! Neuroplasticity. Your brain's like, "Wait… we can do *that* now?"

Her words hit me like a wave, and I felt a shift deep inside. I could feel the pieces of the puzzle starting to click into place. "So... maybe I don't need them anymore?" The words escaped my lips before I could fully grasp their weight, but they felt true, like they had been waiting to be said.

Gina nodded slowly, her expression both calm and knowing. "Maybe you don't." Her voice was full of conviction. "Your brain has been given the opportunity to form new connections, to heal in a way it couldn't before. The mushrooms have opened up possibilities, and perhaps you're ready to let go of the old crutches."

The room seemed to pulse with newfound energy, the vibrant colors of Gina's space surrounding me like a warm embrace. I felt a mix of excitement and fear. *Could this be real? Could this journey have brought me to a place where I no longer need the antidepressants, the ones that have been part of my life for so long?* The colors, the softness of the space, the gentle hum of possibility. It all felt like a sign that something profound was shifting within me.

For a moment, I sat there, taking it in, the idea settling deep within me. "Maybe I don't need them anymore," I whispered, as if saying it out loud made it real. My heart was racing, but there was also a sense of relief, like I was finally letting go of something heavy.

Gina looked at me, her eyes full of warmth and encouragement. "Trust yourself," she said softly. "This is your journey. And if you feel like you've moved past that old need, it's okay to let go."

The seed had been planted, and it felt like a door had opened, one that had been waiting for me to step through.

When Ken picked me up after my journey, the love I felt for him and Gina was overwhelming. I was still riding the wave of mushroom energy, my heart bursting with gratitude for Gina's incredible help that day. The depth of what she had given me, with her guidance and unwavering support, was off the charts. Not only had she helped me process deep pain, but she had also instilled a new confidence in me about ETT. It was like I had been given a new sense of power, a new perspective.

And then came the decision. It was bold, perhaps reckless, but it felt right at that moment. I made a choice I would never recommend to a client, but one I can't say I regret in any way. After only a couple of days off my medication, I decided not to start retaking it. I didn't wean off it; I just stopped. A part of me knew that if I dipped into a funk, which I knew Ken would notice in an instant, I could restart the medication. But I was ready to trust myself–to trust the new path unfolding before my eyes.

"Ken, I need to talk to you about something," I said. "I've been thinking a lot about what happened with the mushrooms, and I feel like I'm ready to stop taking my antidepressants."

Ken looked at me, his brow furrowed slightly, but he didn't say anything. He just watched me, waiting for me to continue.

"I know it's a big step, and I'm not saying I won't ever go back on them if I need to," I added quickly, wanting him to know I wasn't being reckless. "But I feel like maybe this is the right time to try and see if I can manage without them. The mushrooms opened up something in me, and I'm feeling more… clear—more in touch with myself. But I need to know you're on board with this. This isn't something I want to do alone."

Ken took a deep breath, his eyes softening. "I get it," he said, his voice steady but gentle. "I know it's been a long road with your meds. But you've been through so much with the mushrooms and the therapy. If you feel ready, I'm with you." I exhaled in relief as our eyes met with understanding. He continued, "I support you, of course. But I think it might be a good idea for you to talk to a psychiatrist. You've not seen one in a while, right?"

"It's been years," I replied. "I've been taking the same antidepressant for so long, my general doctor manages it now," I clarified.

Ken nodded, his face serious but caring. "I just want you to be safe. I think having someone to check in with, someone to guide you through it, is important. If you feel ready, then I'm all in. But I want you to have professional support if things get tough."

"I'll make the appointment," I said, feeling a sense of clarity wash over me. "It's important to me that you're comfortable with this, and I'll make sure there's support if things don't go as planned."

Ken smiled at me, his gaze warm and reassuring. "I'm here for you, no matter what. You're not doing this alone."

I found a psychiatric nurse practitioner, and after sharing my psilocybin protocol with her, she agreed to monitor me. I began seeing her regularly, keeping her updated on my progress, making sure that if I needed guidance or intervention, I had a professional on my side.

Initially, things weren't all smooth sailing. The first few months were intense. My emotions, both negative and positive, were all over the place. At first, Ken would notice the shifts and think the funk was creeping back in, but the more I examined it, the more I realized it wasn't exactly depression. It was something else.

I was overwhelmed by emotions in ways I had never been before. My empathy and compassion felt like they had been dialed up to a new level. When my clients shared joy, I felt it deeply. When they cried, I was right there with them, feeling the ache in my chest. My mirror neurons were firing at full capacity. It was an emotional rollercoaster, sometimes uplifting, sometimes overwhelming. I got the same result watching movies and TV shows. I found myself crying for joy or sadness, my heart wide open, raw, and tender. I was a whirlwind of emotions, endlessly fluctuating but constantly feeling.

There were three things I noticed that made me question whether what I was experiencing was truly depression or something else. The first was my productivity. When I'm depressed, I lose all motivation, constantly looking for excuses to avoid work. But this time I was focused, staying on top of my workload. The usual heaviness of depression that used to drag me down and make even the most minor tasks feel impossible disappeared.

The second shift caught me entirely off guard. I was watching a stand-up comedy special, something I'd done countless times before, when suddenly, I heard it—my laughter. Not just a polite chuckle or a forced smile, but a deep, uncontrollable belly laugh that shook my entire body. It was raw, electric, the kind of joy that sneaks up on you and takes over before you even realize what's happening.

And that's when it hit me. I wasn't just laughing—I was *feeling*. *Really* feeling. A stark contrast to the numbness that had wrapped itself around me for so long, dulling everything to shades of gray. It wasn't just that I had been depressed before stopping the medication—I had been *disconnected*. From myself. From life. *But this?* This was different. This was something I hadn't felt in years. This was *alive*.

The third revelation came in the form of tears. But this time, they weren't the kind that pulled me under. Usually, crying in the grip of depression felt like sinking—like each tear carried me deeper into the darkness, heavy and unrelenting. But now, the tears were different. They weren't drowning me; they were *cleansing* me.

With every sob, it was as if something toxic was being wrung out of me, released instead of buried. The weight that had pressed down on my chest for so long began to lift. I never imagined I'd see tears as anything but a symptom of despair, but these? They weren't a descent. They were a release. And when they finally stopped, I realized—I could breathe again.

With the help of my nurse practitioner, I came to understand that the Wellbutrin had kept me in a state of numb neutrality. It kept the depression at bay, but it also blocked me from feeling anything too deeply. Once I stopped taking it, I opened the floodgates to emotions, both high and low, that I had not fully experienced for over thirty years.

But honestly, I reveled in the rollercoaster of emotions. Those months of extreme highs and lows felt so real. So human. For the first time in ages, I could feel everything raw and unfiltered. It felt like I was finally maturing emotionally, growing in ways I hadn't expected.

I was shocked by how numb the antidepressants had made me. Yes, they had improved my functioning and kept the depression at bay, but they also kept me from truly processing my feelings. They stopped me from experiencing the joy of working through complex emotions, and they robbed me of the rewarding aftermath that comes with confronting and moving through pain.

I was awake—truly, vibrantly awake. For the first time in years, I felt alive, not just existing but *feeling* every moment. It was messy, raw, and unfiltered, but it was real—more real than anything I had felt in a long time.

It's been well over two years since I stopped taking my antidepressants. I can honestly say that my depression is now manageable in a way I never thought possible. While I still find that dosing or microdosing with psilocybin helps keep the funk at bay, it's not a daily struggle anymore. Psilocybin didn't cure my depression, but it has given me a form of medicine that empowers me to live free from depression's constant grip. I no longer rely on a pill to pause the problem. Instead, the eventuality of challenges has transformed into something I can manage without surrendering to them every day.

For decades, I believed my depression was something I had inherited, a genetic curse like alcoholism. Both of my parents were diagnosed with forms of depression, and I suspect some of my grandparents struggled with it, too. However, I now see it differently. The fact that my depression is mostly resolved leads me to believe that genetics isn't the primary culprit. It may have played a role, but childhood trauma and the patterns I learned through modeling are far more likely to have shaped my experience.

My depression no longer rules my days, and I am finally free from the need for a daily antidepressant. It feels like stepping into the sunlight after years in the dark—liberating, exhilarating, and full of possibility. Through trauma resolution and the power of neuroplasticity, I've rewired my brain and dissolved much of the depression that once controlled me. It's not gone entirely, but it no longer defines my existence. Growing up in an environment where depression was a constant companion, I learned how to live in its shadow. I'd retreat to my bed for days, mimicking what I saw my father and other family members do to cope. It seemed like the only way to survive. But now, through the use of those psilocybin sessions, continued micro-dosing, and therapy to integrate my experiences responsibly, I've stepped out from under that shadow and created a new way of being.

Ken would say this was far from the easiest part of our journey together. Getting off the antidepressants forced him to accept a side of me he had never known, and it took some adjustment on his part. He had always been there for me, but now he had to navigate a new version of me, one that was more emotionally raw, unpredictable, and at times, overwhelming. It wasn't just about my moods; it was the way I processed emotions, the intensity of highs and lows that were foreign to him. He had to learn how to support me through this transformation, to embrace the new person I was becoming, and to adjust to the ebb and flow of my emotions. It was a challenge, but one he took on with his usual patience, even if it meant learning how to love me win ways he never expected.

These days, I still take a microdose of mushrooms every few months, a gentle reset to keep my mind and spirit in balance. Will psilocybin always be part of my journey? I don't know. But given the choice between an occasional ritual dosing and a lifetime of numbing pills, I'll take the awakening. Every. Single. Time. The beauty of this path isn't just in what I've left behind but in what I've gained: a life that feels fully lived, emotions that flow freely, and a sense of connection and control I once thought impossible.

But feeling alive is just the beginning. Now, it's time to step forward—not just in remission, but into re-mission.

CATHERINE - *I feel different.*

MARIA - *You are different.*

CATHERINE - *The laughter... I haven't felt*

that in years.

MARIA - *It is you returning.*

CATHERINE - *And Ken, he's been there for all of it.*

MARIA - *He helped.*

The strength is yours.

CATHERINE - *Can I really live without*

the medication?

MARIA - *You have lived.*

Now, you see.

CATHERINE - *I never imagined feeling this... light.*

MARIA - *Light comes when you stop carrying.*

CATHERINE - *What happens now?*

MARIA - *Now, you move.*

Every step is you.

CHAPTER SEVEN

REMISSION AND RE-MISSION

MARIA - *The body heals, but the soul must find its next path.*

You cannot rest when your soul is restless.

CATHERINE - *What is my next step?*

MARIA - *You are no longer bound by what you were.*

Your calling is coming.

CATHERINE - *How much longer must I wait?*

MARIA - *You wait because you've not yet found the way.*

Your life purpose has yet to begin.

CATHERINE - *It feels like there's more, but I don't know what it is.*

MARIA - *Exactly.*

The journey is never finished.

Only the mission changes.

CATHERINE - *So, what now?*

MARIA - *Keep stepping forward.*

Guiding is your next act.

Even in the unknown, the mission is clear.

AT FIRST, I THOUGHT REMISSION MEANT the end of something. The end of treatments, of tests, of the calendar revolving around appointments. And while some of that was true, what surprised me was how much was just beginning to take shape. There's a strange stillness that follows survival, a quiet that settles in once the adrenaline fades and the appointments stop. It was in that stillness that something began to stir. Not loudly. Not all at once. Just a gentle nudge, a whisper: *Now what?*

I didn't rush to answer. I let the question hang in the air, following me from room to room, into sleep, into walks, into conversation. And over time, I started to understand that surviving wasn't the finish line. Instead, it was the doorway. The re-mission wasn't about getting back to life as it was. It was about stepping into life as it could be. A life that asked more of me. A life I was finally ready to meet with my whole self.

Cancer didn't just leave a scar; it rewrote my entire existence. Survival came in two distinct phases. The first was the obvious one: my body rallied, endured, and eventually healed. The cancer went into remission, and over time, my physical strength returned. But what no one warned me about was the second part—the transformation happening beneath the surface. Because survival isn't just about remission; it's about *re*-mission—finding a new purpose, a new direction, and a way to truly live again.

This was the more profound transformation, which left me facing a new question: *Now that I've survived, what do I do with the life I might have lost?*

It wasn't about returning to "normal," because regular no longer fit. Instead, it felt like a personal renaissance–a rebirth where my renewed energy and deep gratitude insisted on being channeled into something meaningful.

Facing the reality that my life could have ended changed everything. Each day felt sharper, more vivid, more urgent. Small moments took on greater meaning, and the big questions could no longer be ignored. I can't pinpoint the exact moment my remission became clear, but I know it wasn't sudden. It grew slowly, steadily–like a seed that had always been there, finally given the right conditions to bloom.

By the spring of 2023, it was undeniable: my passion for educating the world about the healing powers of psilocybin became my driving force. It wasn't merely an interest or a cause. It felt like the reason I was still alive. Cancer tried to take my life, but in surviving, I found a new one, rooted in purpose, fueled by gratitude, and guided by the belief that healing is possible in ways we're only beginning to understand.

My work with clients began in early 2023, a time when I was diving deeper into the therapeutic benefits of psilocybin. But the seed of my curiosity had been planted years earlier, long before I realized how profoundly this path would shape both my personal and professional life.

The first time I heard someone describe a psychedelic as life-changing was in 2015, during my counseling internship in Denver. I was sitting across from a client who shared an indelible story. At fifteen, they'd been consumed by rage, angry at the world, lashing out with aggressive, bullying behavior, creating a ripple of hurt around them. But then, they told me about a single psychedelic experience that shifted everything.

"It was like flipping on a light switch," they said. "And it never turned back off."

One dose had cracked something open inside them. The anger dissolved, replaced by a profound sense of love and respect, not just for themself, but for everyone around them. It wasn't gradual. It wasn't subtle. It was permanent. A 180-degree transformation, *overnight*.

I remember sitting there, enthralled. I filed the story in my mind, not fully understanding its significance. But it lingered, quietly, like an unanswered question waiting for its moment.

Eight years later, I was no longer a curious observer. I was stepping into my own psychedelic journey, personally and professionally. That client's story wasn't a distant memory anymore. It became part of the foundation for the work I was called to do.

And when I say "work I was called to do," I mean it literally. My clients created a call to action in me. At the end of 2022, something unexpected began to unfold in my practice. Multiple clients started inquiring about the use of psilocybin to resolve trauma, depression, anxiety, and even chronic pain. Looking back, it feels almost otherworldly—like the universe was weaving an invisible thread through my life, placing this theme before me again and again, just as I was quietly unraveling the same questions within myself.

It felt as though an unseen force had orchestrated an alignment, drawing these conversations into my life when I was most open to hearing them. Client after client shared their intentions, often with quiet determination: they were going to try psilocybin, with or without my support. Some were adamantly against pharmaceuticals, weary of the side effects and the feeling of being numbed rather than healed. Others placed their hope in other traditional treatments, only to be disappointed and left with a lingering sense of hopelessness.

Their words echoed the questions I was already asking myself: *Is there another way to help clients heal? Could this be a key we've been missing?*

Coincidentally, at the same time, a colleague in Colorado confided in me about their[1] unexpected success in microdosing psilocybin after the devastating loss of their son. The depth of their grief had plunged them into severe depression, leaving them grappling with an unbearable void and a shattered sense of identity. In their desperation to feel something other than pain, they agreed to try microdosing at the recommendation of a loved one. It was a game-changer. The shift was profound enough that they started growing mushrooms for personal use.

What stood out to me wasn't just the emotional transformation. I trusted this colleague's process. With a background in nursing, this mushroom grower fully understood the importance of maintaining sterile conditions and cultivating a high-quality product. This connection became the missing piece and gave me the confidence I needed to move forward with my clients.

I knew if I was going to guide anyone through a psilocybin journey, I had to be certain of the substance's safety and integrity. I wasn't comfortable allowing clients to bring their own mushrooms, not when the risk of contamination, adulteration, or

---

1 *Editor's Note to the Reader: You will notice the prevalent use of the pronoun, "they/them" throughout this book. This choice is to protect the identity of those mentioned in the stories throughout. It's the author's wish to remove as many identifying factors as possible to protect her colleagues and clients.*

dangerous additives was a possibility. What I designed to offer was intended to be more than just an experience; it was about creating a foundation of trust, safety, and care.

Yes, clients practically begged me to guide them through a psilocybin journey, desperate for something beyond the limits of traditional therapy. Now, with a safe and trustworthy source for the mushrooms, I felt the door had finally opened. I dove into the research with renewed intensity, absorbing everything I could about best practices for psilocybin-assisted therapy (PAT).

This wasn't just curiosity anymore; it was a calling.

To my relief, the colleague who cultivated the mushrooms was not only supportive but eager to co-facilitate the early sessions. Their presence added an extra layer of reassurance for me and the clients. After careful consideration, I chose three individuals with mild to moderate symptoms of depression, anxiety, and PTSD to participate in my first group PAT session.

It marked the beginning of something transformative, not just for them, but for me as well.

One of the most memorable client experiences from that first retreat involved a veteran who had completed multiple deployments. I had worked with the client for six months, witnessing their unwavering commitment to therapy as they navigated the complex layers of PTSD, anxiety, and depression. Despite their dedication, traditional methods had only scratched the surface of healing. The ongoing battle had them carrying an invisible weight every day.

Because the government actively employed them, this person hesitated to take antidepressants or anti-anxiety medications. The stigma within military culture loomed large. Self-reliance was a badge of honor; seeking pharmaceutical support was seen as a sign of weakness. Though they were hesitant due to the stigma and the risk of losing their job, taking medication felt less like an option and more like a lifeline. Yet psilocybin provided a chance at healing they couldn't find elsewhere.

So they proceeded. About thirty minutes into the session, the client began to curl up in bed, softly asking for more blankets. The chill they felt wasn't just physical; it was part of the unraveling. Temperature shifts are common during a psilocybin journey, and in that moment, the weight of a warm towel fresh from the dryer became more than comfort. It became grounding. A quiet reassurance that they were held.

¡OYE! Your body's thermostat just ate a mushroom, too.

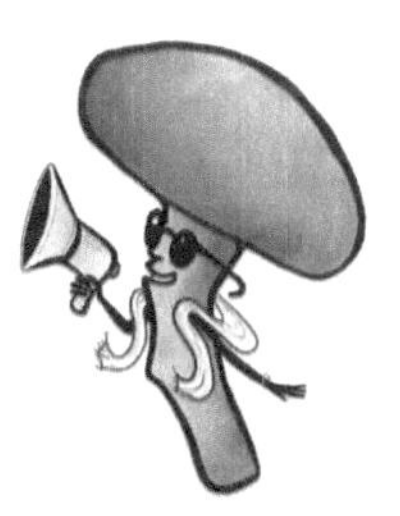

One minute you're in a sauna, the next you're on an arctic tundra. Don't fight it—layer up, cozy down, and let your body vibe with the weather inside you.

Light, however, became unbearable. Even with the blinds drawn and blankets overhead, it still felt like too much. Too sharp. Too bright. The client, unable to tolerate an eye mask, sat cross-legged beneath the covers, trying to shield themselves from the intrusion. At one point, they whispered, "Can you please turn off the sun?" It was as if the very force of nature had become too intense, disrupting the delicate world they were exploring within.

About two hours into the session, I remember them sitting, wide-eyed, with an expression of awe that's impossible to forget.

"I can't believe how great I feel," they said, almost disoriented by the unfamiliar sensation of pure, unfiltered joy. They kept repeating, "I wish I could feel this way all the time. Do people really wake up feeling like this every day?" The wonder in their voice was beautiful. It was simultaneously heartbreaking, however. This wonder I now heard offered a glimpse into how deeply entrenched their suffering had been.

As the journey deepened and the ego dissolved, a painful yet liberating realization surfaced. They saw, with stunning clarity, how profoundly the military had shaped their identity. Not through support, but through a system of indoctrination that starts with recruiting vulnerable, low-income individuals, then gradually stripping away their sense of autonomy. They described it as a machine designed to mold followers, not leaders; one that suppresses individuality under the guise of discipline and honor. It mustn't have been an easy realization to stomach, but it was necessary. It cracked open a door that had been sealed for years, allowing them to reclaim a self that existed beyond the uniform.

As the journey began to soften, another sense stirred. Touch. When I asked if they would like something to eat or drink, they requested a variety of foods. This was unusual, given that psilocybin typically slows the gastrointestinal system and often suppresses appetite. But when I returned, none of it had been eaten. Instead, they were gently running their fingers across textures. Tracing the edges of crackers. Cradling fruit in the hand. They were rediscovering the world through sensation, not logic. It was a quiet, beautiful reflection of what was happening inside their brain. New pathways were forming. Curiosity was replacing habit. This is the power of psilocybin. Healing does not always arrive with drama. Sometimes, it reveals itself in the simple act of feeling.

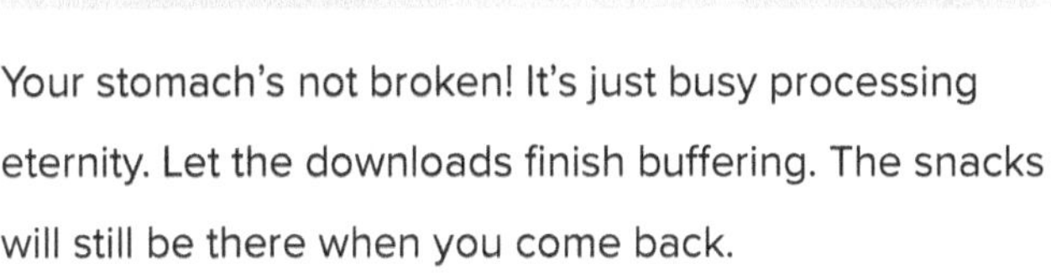

¡OYE! Don't panic! You're not dying, you just don't want snacks.

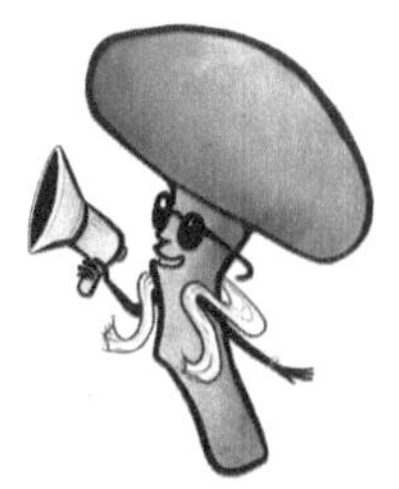

Your stomach's not broken! It's just busy processing eternity. Let the downloads finish buffering. The snacks will still be there when you come back.

And the transformation was nothing short of remarkable. The client's anxiety and depression plummeted. The dark cloud and gnawing sense of dread that greeted them every morning vanished. They no longer retreated to a dark closet after work, a ritual once essential for shifting from work mode to home life. Instead, they discovered a newfound sense of calm, focus, and creativity. Life began to feel less like an obligation and more like an opportunity.

What struck me most was the ripple effect. Within a few months, the client dove headfirst into a creative passion for filmmaking that lit them up from the inside out, a hobby that wasn't just an activity, but a representation of purpose. They started making choices that reflected who they were, not who they'd been conditioned to be. Witnessing that shift was one of the most profound moments of my career.

MARIA - *You stepped forward.*

CATHERINE - *It feels good being the guide.*

MARIA - *Yes.*

   It is your natural path.

CATHERINE - *I wasn't sure I was ready.*

MARIA - *No one is.*

   That's why the path reveals itself one

   step at a time.

   Continue the work.

   You are not alone.

   You are where you need to be.

A month later, we conducted back-to-back men's and women's retreats, experiences that unlocked levels of healing unlike anything I had ever witnessed in my therapeutic practice. The transformations were profound, each story etched into my memory.

One client confronted a 20-year-old trauma, discovering peace after the devastating loss of a child before birth. Another unearthed a powerful connection to their ancestry, which dramatically eased their lifelong struggle with anxiety and relationships. A third client, once paralyzed by fear, discovered their voice, shedding layers of crippling anxiety, stepping into newfound confidence. Another bravely redefined their narrative around childhood sexual trauma, reclaiming a sense of self that had long been buried. Yet another client stopped drinking entirely, releasing the grip of anxiety and depression while reconnecting with the memory and presence of lost loved ones. The last client experienced a profound shift, deepening their connection with both themselves and their family, uncovering a richer understanding of their identity and ancestral roots.

These retreats weren't just about healing—they ignited remissions similar to my own, setting lives on a new course with purpose, clarity, and unstoppable momentum.

As fulfilling as this new way to serve my clients was becoming, it was equally isolating for me as a psychotherapist. The field of counseling remained stubbornly rooted in bias and rigid protocols that contradicted the research I'd been reading, and the results I was witnessing with my clients in practice. There was a strong resistance to the idea that psychedelics could be a legitimate, transformative form of treatment. Stigma from the '60s and '70s lingered like thick, suffocating smog, clouding judgment and obscuring the truth my clients were experiencing. It was disheartening to witness how a substance with such profound healing potential had been hastily and unjustly categorized as one of the most dangerous drugs. This bias meant that psilocybin was ranked as being more harmful than fentanyl, cocaine, methamphetamine, oxycodone, and barbiturates.

The classification defied logic and science. Psilocybin is not nearly as addictive as any of the substances above, and there is no known lethal dose. Yet, it remains housed in Schedule I, a category reserved for substances with the highest potential for abuse and no accepted medical use. Psilocybin meets neither of these criteria. The injustice of the misclassification wasn't just frustrating–it was heartbreaking. It erected barriers for those in desperate need of healing while isolating practitioners like me, who had seen its life-changing power unfold firsthand.

It didn't take me long to realize there was a deep need for education and training around psilocybin-assisted therapy. While I didn't yet consider myself an expert, I had gathered a solid foundation of knowledge through my research and the transformative experiences I was witnessing with my clients. Additionally, my personal journey with psilocybin provided me with an invaluable, firsthand education.

I knew of underground practitioners offering similar services, some rooted in therapeutic work and others more spiritually based. But none emphasized safe, effective techniques based on best practices. I wasn't looking to replicate what they were doing. I wanted to offer something different—something structured and responsible. The conversations I was having indicated that people were going to use psilocybin regardless, so ensuring proper training felt essential.

The solution to my sense of isolation and frustration became clear: I had to train others in this work. I understood that if I could create positive, life-changing outcomes through psilocybin therapy, I could help advocate for its healing potential. I felt a sense of responsibility to create the blueprint for others to follow, sharing what I had learned and empowering people to do the work safely. The more qualified practitioners there were, the greater the chances we'd have to prove psilocybin's efficacy, and, ultimately, help more people heal from mental health struggles. This work wasn't just mine to carry—it needed to be a shared cause, woven with the care, wisdom, and dedication of many.

This became my "Re-Mission": to awaken the world—and especially the counseling field—to the profound healing power of psilocybin-assisted therapy, bridging the gap between science, spirit, and transformation. I felt an inner fire, a sense that the time to act was now.[1]

To do the work effectively, I knew I needed formal training. However, the available options were few and far between, especially in the United States. Most programs were tied to academia, meaning they came with hefty price tags—often tens of thousands of dollars—and a year-long commitment. I was strongly opposed to that framework. As an experienced counselor, I didn't believe it should require jumping through bureaucratic hoops to add this modality to my practice. In my experience, academia has a way of overestimating its significance, wrapped in layers of bureaucracy that seem designed to preserve tradition rather than foster progress. The notion that others must struggle through the same outdated obstacles simply because those before them did has always felt more like gatekeeping than growth.

Instead, I looked for options in Canada and briefly enrolled in a program, only to back out when the institution's CEO resigned due to allegations of sexual inappropriateness.

That experience, though disappointing, led me to TheraPsil in British Columbia, Canada, an online psychedelic advocacy and training program founded in 2019 by Dr. Bruce Tobin.

---

1   Author's Note: I hope that psilocybin can eventually be rescheduled appropriately. Currently classified as a Schedule I substance under federal law since 1970, as it's considered to have no accepted medical use and a high potential for abuse—an outdated and inaccurate designation. Rescheduling would not only remove the stigma but also open critical doors for clinical research, therapeutic use, and broader access for those seeking relief from mental health challenges. I am driven to share this knowledge, to advocate for change, and to ensure that others can experience the life-changing transformation I've seen both firsthand and through the journeys of others. It's more than just a mission; it's a commitment to reshaping the future of mental health treatment.

TheraPsil is a remarkable organization that advocates for the medical use of psilocybin and educates practitioners on how to guide psilocybin-assisted therapy (PAT) safely. I dove into their program, and within four months, I had completed the majority of the training. I chose not to complete my certification*, realizing that psilocybin's legal status in the U.S. would limit its impact until laws aligned with the science.[1]

The TheraPsil program required a one-week in-person workshop in the Vancouver, BC area. When I arrived, I was surprised to realize that I was the most experienced person in my cohort. We were the 35th or 36th group being trained in psilocybin-assisted therapy. At the time, Canadian laws were still evolving, and a moratorium prevented us from working directly with psilocybin while regulations were being clarified. Instead, the program used breathwork to induce an altered state of consciousness. Until then, I had no idea breathwork could be so intense and transformative.

For one particular training, we were instructed to create an intention for the session. Mine was to focus on finding more balance in my life. The experience began awkwardly, turned magical in the middle, and ended with undeniable healing. During the session, I found myself facing my inner child, a version of myself at around ten years old. I saw myself wearing a dark blue dress with white leggings, and my long blonde hair

---

1   Two years later, a new opportunity arose, and I returned to complete the certification. At the time, I still questioned its relevance to my work in the U.S., which I'll expand on further in the *Gathering Groups* chapter. However, by the time of publishing, New Mexico recognizes TheraPsil certification for facilitator licensure, so I chose to complete the final steps and expect to finish by the end of summer 2026.

tied in pigtails. The memory of that moment and that outfit was so crisp and real, it was as though I were there with her.

My younger self wanted to play. As she floated, a tether appeared, and I realized I could hold it, allowing her to float higher and farther, safely. I told her to go ahead and play, while I held the tether to keep her safe. As a side note, my younger self wasn't very good at playing. She'd always been expected to care for everyone—her mother, her sisters—due to the countless responsibilities of being the eldest child. This was my chance to give her the freedom she deserved. I permitted her to play without any guilt or consequences.

She was hesitant at first, unsure if she was allowed to enjoy herself. But once I convinced her that she was free to be without worry, she soared into the sky, playing with complete abandon. It was freedom. It was beautiful. And it was precisely what she needed. Balance had been achieved.

My experience at TheraPsil was incredibly affirming. It offered me validation for the work I had already done. While I can't say I learned as much as others might have, it was because I had already immersed myself in volumes of any and every material I could find. In preparation for offering psilocybin-assisted therapy to clients, I had pored over research, articles, videos, and any other resources I could discover. By the time I arrived at the in-person portion of the training, I had already taught myself much of the content through autodidactic means.

During the training, I noticed that the instructor often turned to me for my opinion on various topics because of my experience. It was incredibly affirming and validating. The most significant takeaway for me, however, was the exposure to breathwork. I learned that altered states of consciousness could be achieved without having to ingest a substance, which opened my mind to new possibilities.

And what a highlight to meet an entire cohort of like-minded professionals who shared the same goals and passion for the work! It helped me feel less isolated in such a niche field. To this day, I continue to recommend TheraPsil to colleagues seeking training, especially as an alternative to the programs offered in the United States. The US programs are often tied to academia and tend to be longer, redundant, and overpriced. TheraPsil still provides a more practical, reasonably scoped, and affordable option than academia offers.

It was a natural progression for me to begin offering training classes, given my extensive background in developing and delivering training in my previous career as a forensic scientist. For about ten years, I created and presented numerous classes, and later in my second career as a counselor, I developed one for my Emotional Triggers Treatment. I had taught around ten ETT classes before my health issues interrupted that path. Drawing on my experience in class development, I efficiently designed the curriculum for psilocybin-assisted therapy training.

Then, in early July 2023, I delivered my first PAT Training for healing practitioners. Since then, I've held eleven trainings, and I plan to continue offering them as long as there's a need in the community. The combination of my past training experience and the passion I have for this work has made this a fulfilling new chapter in my professional life and has helped to alleviate how isolating it can be working as a therapist in the realm of psilocybin-assisted therapy. Because of its current illegal status, many professionals are hesitant or afraid to openly engage in this work, which can leave those of us who do feeling like we're on an island. Looking back, the feelings of loneliness significantly shifted, primarily due to my efforts in providing training and the network of like-minded professionals I've built. To further nurture this sense of connection, I began offering a free online meeting once a month for anyone who has completed my psilocybin-assisted therapy (PAT) class. The goal is to provide a safe space for individuals who have invested their time and money into learning about PAT to continue networking and supporting one another on their respective journeys.

Additionally, I joined an online group of psychedelic practitioners from across the US. We meet weekly to discuss a wide range of topics related to psychedelics and offer mutual support. This group has been invaluable in helping me stay grounded in the work while advocating for the healing potential of psychedelics. Through these connections and ongoing support, I feel a renewed sense of community and shared purpose.

I've poured my heart and soul into educating others and spreading the word about psilocybin-assisted therapy, and I can genuinely say I've made a difference. I hope there are others, just like me, working in similar ways across the globe to spread knowledge and healing in their communities. I imagine this collective effort growing and expanding like mycelium, the vast underground, threadlike network of fungi that spans the world. Plants and trees use mycelium to transfer vital nutrients like water, carbon, and nitrogen, helping nourish other foliage. The mushrooms that sprout above ground are the fruiting bodies of this intricate system. In much the same way, I envision my work, along with the work of others, spreading, connecting, nourishing, and supporting one another as we collectively work toward creating a new and holistic approach to mental health. I see this education taking root, its foundations deepening until it converges into something greater—a unified force of healing and transformation, changing lives one connection at a time.

MARIA - *You remember.*

    The truth is clearer now.

CATHERINE - *I'm walking a new path.*

MARIA - *You are. The mission shifts. But it is*

    still yours.

CATHERINE - *I never imagined this*

    would be my work.

MARIA - *It was always your work.*

    The call to guide, to teach, to heal.

CATHERINE - *It feels like a big responsibility.*

MARIA - *It is.*

    But you carry it now.

    You have what it takes.

CATHERINE - *The world isn't ready.*

MARIA - *They never are.*

    You show them.

    The medicine found you.

    It healed and planted the seed for you to

    help others.

CATHERINE - *How do I lead?*

MARIA - *By walking.*

> *By talking.*

> *By teaching.*

> *By guiding.*

> *You open the doors.*

CATHERINE - *So this is my re-mission.*

> *Not just to heal but to ignite!*

MARIA - *Exactly.*

> *You carry the flame now.*

CATHERINE - *What else do I need to do?*

MARIA - *Now, you speak.*

> *You guide.*

> *You remember.*

> *You remind others.*

> *The journey is unfolding.*

> *The mission has only just begun.*

But just as I began to step fully into this new role with clarity, conviction, and a fire lit from within, I walked straight into the storm. I'd expected resistance from the outside world, from skeptics and systems clinging to the old ways. What I didn't expect was betrayal from within, from those who claimed to walk the same path. The very community I believed would uplift and support this sacred work became the place where I would be tested the most.

CHAPTER EIGHT

SANTA FE BULLIES

MARIA - *You knew the path wasn't paved.*

But did you think it would be smooth?

CATHERINE - *I was surprised where it came from.*

MARIA - *Not everyone who speaks of light*

has learned to sit with their own shadows.

And not everyone who guides

has taken the journey.

CATHERINE - *I've been asking myself, "Did I do*

something wrong?"

MARIA - *No.*

You simply stepped where they were

afraid to walk.

That kind of courage makes the uninitiated loud.

CATHERINE - *I feel the weight of their judgment.*

MARIA - *This path is not easy.*

Rejection follows truth.

They pull you back because you walk ahead.

CATHERINE - *Should I explain it to them?*

MARIA - *You won't.*

Words cannot carry the weight of what you know.

CATHERINE - *And they refuse to understand.*

MARIA - *You don't need them to understand.*

You walk for those who will see.

CATHERINE - *And if they reject me?*

MARIA - *Rejection is not failure.*

It is part of the path.

Stand firm in your truth.

THE TRAILBLAZING PATH I'VE CHOSEN HASN'T been easy. It's been marked by resistance and, at times, outright hostility from those who seem determined to tear me down. I was warned to watch out for people who would try to block my progress and erect barriers just to see me stumble. It's been painful feeling misunderstood and sometimes judged for daring to walk on an untrodden road. But through it all, I've learned to rise above the noise, to keep my eyes fixed on my purpose, no matter how rough the journey gets.

I've grown sensitive, almost hyper-aware, of the subtle shifts in people's reactions. It stings to see someone's face go blank the moment I mention psychedelics, to watch their interest evaporate as old stigmas dominate. I read the discomfort in their eyes, the silent judgment lurking beneath the surface. It used to hurt tremendously, but now I've learned when to let the topic go, to save my breath for those ready to listen. I won't force understanding on people who are adamant about their beliefs and their fears. Yet, I can't help but feel a pang of anticipation every time I bring it up, wondering, *Will they see beyond the stigma? Will they understand?*

Some moments catch me off guard–the spark of curiosity in someone's eyes, the subtle lean-in that tells me they're truly listening. Sometimes, they even open up, sharing their own experiences with psychedelics, revealing how a single journey shifted their entire perspective. Others speak of friends or family members whose lives were changed, stories that lingered in their minds and made them question what they thought they knew. And then, some are just starting to see the undeniable truth in the latest studies and the transformative power that can no longer be ignored.

No matter how the conversation unfolds, I find myself captivated by the dance of reactions. It's a vulnerable space to step into—speaking openly about psychedelics, or really, speaking any truth that runs counter to the mainstream. There's always that flicker of uncertainty: *Will I be met with curiosity, or will I feel the sting of rejection?* Over time, I've come to savor this unpredictability—the delicate balance between hope and hesitation. After sharing my truth, I often pause for a deep inhale, bracing for the moment of truth: *Will they lean in, or pull away?*

This journey has taught me a great deal about rejection; not just in this work, but in life. Each time I risk being misunderstood, I'm reminded of past moments when my voice didn't feel welcome, when my truth was too much for someone else's comfort. But strangely, it's also where I've found strength. Every conversation, every reaction, chips away at the walls built by stigma and fear, not just societal but personal. One interaction at a time, I'm helping to rewrite the narrative—each response bringing me one step closer to breaking through.

One of the most complex parts of my journey is realizing that no matter how hard I try, I can never fully explain what a psychedelic experience feels like. Words fall painfully short. How do you describe something so vast, so profoundly transformative, to someone who's never felt it? You can't. Not really. The only way to truly understand is to experience it firsthand.

People who've been through it often express the same frustration–the aching inadequacy of language. They try to describe the beauty and the overwhelming sense of connectedness, but every word feels hollow, like the faded echo of something infinitely richer. The words minimize, diminish, and dilute the experience. It feels almost disrespectful, like trying to capture the ocean in a single drop of water. It's humbling and heartbreaking.

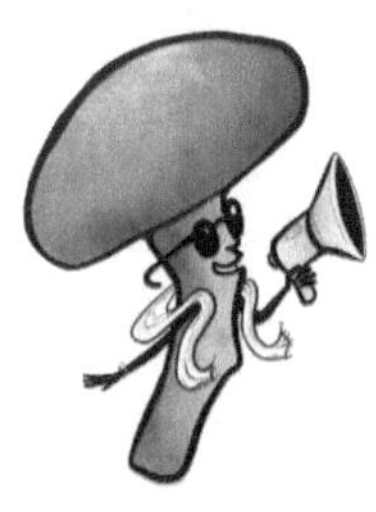

¡OYE! Language is a cage, and your journey is a comet.

Trying to describe a psychedelic experience is like catching moonlight in a jar. Words wobble. Meaning slips. Don't worry if you can't explain it all. Some truths are meant to be felt, not squeezed into sentences.

The struggle with language becomes an even bigger challenge during integration. How do you process something so profound when the very act of explaining it seems to reduce its impact? You grasp for words, but they crumble the moment they leave your lips–pale imitations of something vast and unknowable. You try again, and again, chasing meaning that dissolves like mist, each attempt only proving how impossible it is to make anyone understand. It's like trying to describe a color no one's ever seen or a song that only exists in your dreams. And yet, you keep trying because sharing it, even imperfectly, is the only way to bridge the impossible gap between worlds.

Yet, there's a strange beauty in the impossibility. The fact that words can't capture the essence means that nothing can truly prepare you for it. No amount of mental or emotional preparation comes close to what actually unfolds. And because of that, the experience is always more mind-blowing, more heart-opening, more soul-shaking than you could imagine.

Yes, there's magic in the unknown, a gift hidden within the mystery. When you surrender to the uncertainty, you allow the journey to take you places you didn't know existed. It shatters your expectations, leaving you breathless and humbled by the sheer depth of the experience. It's terrifying and beautiful, disorienting and enlightening. And that's exactly what makes it so extraordinary. It's a reminder that some things are meant to be felt, not explained. That the most profound truths live beyond the reach of words. How wholly do you love your children? Now, try to put that into words that accurately describe the feeling.

That's the paradox of integration: you return with something precious and indescribable, then are asked to make sense of it, to wrap language around the ineffable. And who you turn to in that moment matters. The difference between being met with understanding and being met with analysis can make or break your healing. Not everyone is equipped to hold what can't be spoken. And that's where I began to notice a troubling pattern.

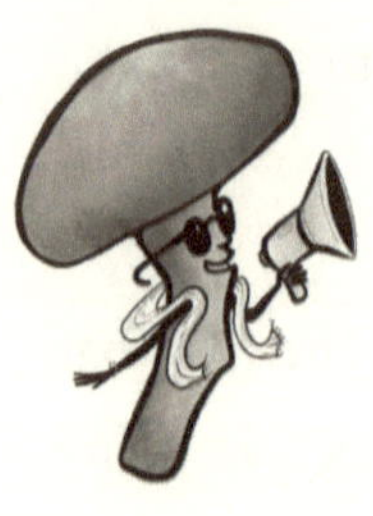

¡OYE! Don't live-stream your soul before it's done buffering.

Sharing your journey can be healing, but rushing to explain can strip away the sacred. Hold it close until it ripens.

When I speak of misunderstanding, there's another realm of the experience that must be examined. In the world of counseling and psychedelic therapy, I've come to see a stark divide—two very different kinds of practitioners. There are the psychedelic therapists who have walked the path themselves, who know firsthand the profound depths and transformative power these substances can offer. Their work is guided by personal experience, by a deep respect for the medicine and its ability to heal. And then, there are the non-psychedelic, psychedelic therapists, those who guide others through journeys they've never taken themselves. They're often drawn to the cutting-edge allure of psychedelic therapy or the lucrative opportunities it promises. Still, they lack the lived understanding that can only come from facing the medicine themselves.

I can usually tell who's who by how they introduce themselves. If someone leads with a string of credentials, rattling off the alphabet soup of letters after their name, it's often a red flag. In this work, those titles don't carry much weight. There are plenty of shamans who have the healing touch of an accomplished doctor. These official titles that some hurriedly share appear to me as trophies from an ego-driven world that prioritizes status over inner growth. However, it's important to note that I am fond of many doctors who have amassed an array of impressive titles. But those who have truly transformed don't hide behind credentials. They speak from the heart, with humility and vulnerability, because they know that no degree or certification could ever capture the depth of their work.

I remember attending a local film festival that was supposed to be about promoting psychedelics. During the Q&A panel, they spent the first fifteen minutes reading off an exhausting list of credentials. It was painful to sit through, knowing that some of these so-called experts had never experienced the medicine themselves. In fairness, not all of them, but enough to leave a bitter taste in my mouth. I felt torn, part of me wanted to support the movement, to celebrate the growing awareness around psychedelics. But another part of me was deeply disheartened, sensing that, for some, this was just another trend on which to capitalize, another way to chase fame and fortune.

That night, I felt my heart break a little. I had hoped to find a community of kindred spirits, people who understood the sacredness of the work, who were in it for the healing, not the hype. I longed for a network of souls connected, like how mycelium works quietly and powerfully beneath the surface, united in a mission to heal and transform. Instead, I felt isolated, disillusioned by the commercialization creeping into such a sacred space.

I made a choice: I wouldn't follow those chasing the spotlight or the paycheck. I couldn't. This work, this relationship with the medicine, had called me to something deeper, something rooted in truth, not ego. It was a painful realization to see how many in the field seemed more invested in prestige than in healing, but that contrast only sharpened my clarity. I knew I had to keep walking my path, even if it meant walking it alone—committed to psilocybin-assisted therapy and education delivered with integrity, authenticity, and heart.

In the early days of my journey with PAT, I took a leap of faith and started advertising my services on Facebook and Instagram. I wanted to get the word out, to let people know that I was offering safe, therapeutic experiences that could change lives. But I was terrified. I wasn't ready to list my services on a website. Not yet. There was too much uncertainty and too much risk.

The legal landscape in New Mexico, and across the U.S., was murky at best (it still is, despite a government decision in February of this year that psilocybin would be legalized for therapeutic work by 2027). I knew that others were offering psilocybin-assisted support quietly, helping people heal in the absence of regulated pathways. I didn't want to work in the shadows, but I also didn't want to risk being fined or jailed by being too bold or too visible. I felt caught in a painful divide, torn between the desire to be open about my work and the responsibility to protect both myself and the people I served. I chose to move forward carefully, always committed to safety, ethics, and integrity, even in a system that had not yet created space for this kind of healing.

It was a delicate, exhausting dance, trying to stay professional and ethical while navigating a legal grey area that felt like it was shifting beneath my feet at every moment. I lay awake at night, my mind spinning with fear and doubt. *What if I got reported? What if I lost everything I had worked so hard to build?* But then I would think about the people who needed the healing, who were suffering and searching for answers. I couldn't turn my back on them. I couldn't walk away from what I knew in my heart was my calling.

And so, with a cautious heart and unwavering resolve, I pressed on, placing each step carefully into the unknown. I was determined to do the work safely and responsibly, walking the tightrope of risk and reward. I chose my words cautiously, crafted my messaging with care, and trusted that those who needed to find me would. It wasn't easy. It was terrifying, isolating, and at times overwhelming. But I knew that this was the path I was meant to walk, no matter how uncertain or challenging it became.

In March of 2023, an email landed in my inbox that made me pause. It was from a practitioner in Santa Fe, someone who saw themselves as the gatekeeper of psychedelic-assisted therapy. Their words were sharp, laced with judgment and accusation. They criticized my work, claiming that I was recklessly endangering the "reputation and future of this medicine's use in our state." They accused me of not properly assessing individuals or providing adequate integration, all without knowing a single thing about how I practiced.

At first, I shook it off. However, they made sure to mention that they were enrolled in a year-long program and had over 200 hours of instruction, as if that automatically made them an authority. It was like they were brandishing their credentials like a medieval knight with a shiny sword—determined to conquer the conversation and claim the throne of superiority. But later, as I re-read the email, my chest tightened, my stomach knotted.

How could someone who claimed to be a healer be so harsh, so quick to judge?

Then it hit me: This was precisely the kind of non-psychedelic, psychedelic therapist I had come to recognize. The kind who hides behind degrees and certificates, who thinks authority comes from books and lectures, not from personal experience or deep inner work. I realized they might feel threatened, clinging to their titles because they probably hadn't nurtured a relationship with the medicine. Likely, they didn't truly understand it. Not the way you do when you've walked through the fire and come out the other side changed forever.

Their words didn't intimidate me, but they clarified something. I saw how fiercely I was willing to protect this work, and how deeply I believed in the healing power of psychedelics. I knew then that I couldn't let someone's fear or ego derail my purpose. I couldn't let self-appointed "gatekeepers" stand in my way. It occurred to me that the path wasn't meant to be easy. It was intended to be real, raw, and transformative—just like the medicine itself.

Looking back, I can't help but find the situation to have been a formative learning experience. The boldness of someone positioning themselves as *the* authority on something far beyond their own experience was almost admirable, if not for the sheer absurdity of it. *Isn't there always room to learn? Aren't humility and openness essential to discovery, especially in the healing fields?*

I've come to accept that transformation looks different for everyone. Some may step back when the journey asks too much, and that's okay. But for me, this path is non-negotiable. I walk it because I've glimpsed what's on the other side, and no measure of comfort or status could ever replace the depth of what I've found.

Eventually, I scheduled a phone call with the accredited therapist, hoping to clear the air and to show them that they had made assumptions about me without knowing anything about my background or intentions. But as soon as the conversation started, it was painfully evident that they had already decided who I was, accusing me of doing the work "willy-nilly." They hadn't bothered to ask about my training, my experiences, or my intentions. Yet they were certain I wasn't approaching the therapy with the care it deserved. It was as if they had already written my story without ever hearing it.

Then, this person told me that a group of practitioners in Santa Fe were concerned about my work and that they had been "chosen" to reach out to me on the group's behalf. It felt less like an offer to collaborate or understand my approach, and more like a threat. The implication was clear: If I didn't stop offering my services, they'd take it to the licensing board.

I wasn't worried about losing my license. I had already made peace with that risk when I first chose to walk the path. But what stung the most was the realization that, in a place where I thought I'd find support, I was met with judgment, suspicion, and hostility. I had braced myself for challenges, for the inevitable obstacles that come with breaking new ground. Still, I never expected the kind of ego-driven resistance that felt more like bullying than genuine concern.

It left a heavy, bitter taste in my mouth. It was disheartening to realize that some of the very people I thought would be allies, those who should understand the value of healing, felt so threatened by my efforts to bring transformation to others. I had come into this with open arms, ready to connect and collaborate. Instead, I found myself fighting to prove my worth to those who seemed more interested in protecting their territory than in the people who needed help.

What struck me most about their concerns was the suggestion that I should consider giving up my license if I wanted to continue offering psilocybin-assisted therapy. The reasoning, as they explained it, was that a negative outcome from a licensed practitioner could reflect poorly on the entire profession and jeopardize efforts to legalize and regulate this work. In their view, if I practiced without a license, I wouldn't represent the licensed community, and the risk to the broader movement would be minimized. They expressed concern about potential consequences, fearing that one negative experience could derail the entire effort to legalize and regulate psilocybin therapy for licensed professionals.

The irony of it hit me hard. They thought that if something went wrong with a licensed professional, it would strengthen the case for regulated use by licensed practitioners. But in reality, the people who work with psilocybin responsibly—who follow all the proper precautions, create safe and supportive environments, and show deep respect for the medicine—don't typically face adverse outcomes. I have always been committed to ensuring every step of the process is done with care, respect, and thorough integration. Catastrophic experiences don't happen when you put in the work to create proper safety throughout the entire process.

It's no different than something like scuba diving. The risks are real, but when done with the proper training, planning, and respect for the environment, it becomes an awe-inspiring experience rather than a dangerous one. Problems don't arise when the process is held with intention. They occur when it isn't. Psychedelic work is the same: when approached responsibly, it opens people; it doesn't harm them.

The person with whom I spoke was not open to my perceptions or interested in a modicum of collaboration–their mind was made up. It was as if they didn't understand the more profound truths of the therapy I was offering, the truths that come from personal experience, not just credentials. To me, the healing modality isn't just about legality or license—it's about understanding the medicine, the healing it can offer, and the people it serves. The fact that they couldn't see this was both disheartening and eye-opening. It made it crystal clear that the conversation wasn't really about protecting people; it was about ego, control, and a fundamental misunderstanding of what makes this work effective. We seemed to be caught in a duel between authenticity and authority, leaving me feeling more certain than ever of my path, even as the world around me seemed intent on putting up walls.

Safety is not just a priority in this work; it is the foundation. There are too many people operating underground with little regard for preparation, safety, or ethics. When someone unfamiliar hears "psychedelic therapy," they often assume I'm doing something reckless. They don't see the depth of training, the protocols, the hours of care that go into every experience I hold.

People are often surprised to learn that we have gentle, effective ways to help bring someone out of a psychedelic state if necessary. Measures like Benadryl or nano-encapsulated CBD oil under the tongue are rarely used, but when they are, they help bring the journey to a close in a safe and controlled way. These tools don't erase the experience, but they do quiet the parts of the nervous system that may be overwhelmed. This is especially important if the dose hasn't brought the client fully into ego dissolution. That space in between can be deeply uncomfortable, which is why we sometimes choose to increase the dose instead, helping the client move more fully into the medicine. When that isn't the right choice, we have options to make the process easier.

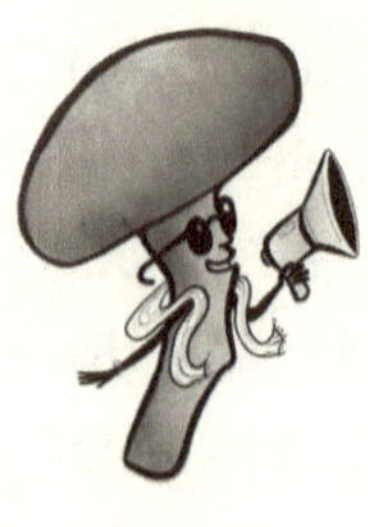

Benadryl + nano-CBD won't end the trip—but they can put ego back in the driver's seat just enough to make you feel human again. You might still see visuals, but the panic eases. The discomfort of letting go softens, and the ride becomes a whole lot gentler.

I remember one client in particular whose journey stood out to me. She was insightful, deeply self-aware, and had come into the session with a clear list of intentions she hoped to explore. As the medicine unfolded, she moved gracefully through those intentions, one by one, until she reached a place of completion. She sensed, with clarity, that she had received what she needed. It was as though the door had opened, revealed its lessons, and then gently closed behind her.

But then something new began to stir. A second door appeared, offering entry into deeper, more uncharted territory. She felt its pull, but she also knew she wasn't ready to step through it. There was fear, yes, but more than that, there was wisdom. She recognized that if she pushed herself beyond her readiness, she might lose the sense of grounding she had worked so hard to cultivate.

Instead of forcing herself forward, she did something powerful. She asked to step out of the experience. With support, she came down from the journey, carrying with her the lessons of Door One while leaving Door Two for another time. This decision wasn't a failure. It was an act of profound self-awareness and respect for her own process.

At that point, we used the combination of Benadryl and nano-encapsulated CBD oil under the tongue, as mentioned above, to help her ego come back online. These tools do not end the journey completely. She may have still experienced visuals and sensations, but they softened the overwhelming sense of surrender for her, and restored a sense of balance. It was a safe and controlled way to close the session, honoring her request to step out while still protecting the integrity of the work she had done.

Later, when the timing was right and her heart had prepared itself, she returned to the medicine. Then, she was ready. With courage, she walked through Door Two and faced what once felt overwhelming. And because she had honored her readiness rather than pushing against it, she was able to meet that deeper work with strength and clarity.

In the end, it seemed the real issue they had with me wasn't about my approach or my intentions. It was about my willingness to step into the work they so desperately wanted to do but felt they couldn't. During our call, they admitted that offering psilocybin-assisted therapy before state legalization would result in expulsion from their academic program. If licensed practitioners like them weren't allowed to do this work, they must have also reasoned that no one should.

That's when I saw it: their frustrations and limitations, all laid bare. Rather than embracing the opportunity to be part of something groundbreaking, they were holding onto the constraints of their academic and professional systems, allowing those walls to define what was possible. It felt as if they couldn't imagine a world where anyone, especially someone without their credentials, could do this work outside of the rigid structures to which they were beholden. Instead of seeing the potential for change, they were projecting onto me their guilt and their fear of stepping outside the lines.

But genuine change has often been born from the courage to challenge the system. Rosa Parks did not wait for the law to change before she claimed her seat. Gandhi did not ask for permission to defy injustice. They were not reckless. They were intentional, principled, and deeply committed to something larger than themselves. That kind of bravery, the willingness to act from integrity in the face of resistance, is what moves the needle.

What struck me was that this person could not see the difference between recklessness and responsibility. They were so deeply entrenched in their framework, so committed to playing by rules that were never designed for transformation, that they began imposing that narrow worldview on everyone else doing this work. Instead of recognizing that there are many ethical, grounded paths to healing, they clung to the belief that theirs was the only legitimate one. And in doing so, they missed the point entirely. Healing does not flourish under rigid control. It thrives in truth, humility, and the courage to do what is right, even before the system is ready to accept it.

The work I was doing wasn't about rebelling for the sake of rebellion or seeking personal validation. It was about filling a gap in a field that so desperately needed new solutions for healing. I wasn't doing this for the fame or the glory. I was doing it because people were suffering, and the tools to help them existed. Though it was hard to ignore how much fear, rigidity, and discomfort still lingered within the professional community—especially among those who, by all rights, should have been open to the transformative potential of psychedelics. It was a stark reminder that even in fields meant to heal, fear can build walls that prevent true growth.

At the end of our conversation, I made sure to address the assumption they had made about my "willy-nilly" approach. I gently urged them to reconsider, opening the door for a deeper conversation. After some honest back and forth, they paused, reflected, and acknowledged their misunderstanding, offering a brief but sincere apology. For me, the moment was more than just an apology. It was the culmination of everything that had transpired during and leading up to the conversation. It encompassed the initial intimidating email, the false sense of authority they had attempted to impose, the unfair assumptions made, and the threatening tone of the call.

All of it led to a moment of clarity.

That apology, though small, felt like a quiet victory—not because I wanted to "win" the argument, but because it symbolized something deeper. It was an acknowledgment of the harm done by rushing to judgment, by assuming someone's position without bothering to understand it. It was a rare, fragile moment of humility, one that spoke to the heart of what I've come to realize during my journey: so much of the psychedelic community—and really, any emerging field—is shaped by fear, misunderstanding, and a rush to protect the familiar, even among its advocates.

But at that moment, I also saw something else. I realized that standing firm in my truth, even when faced with hostility or ignorance, could shift the dynamic. It was a reminder that we don't always change the world in one grand gesture; sometimes, it's one interaction at a time, one person at a time, that breaks down the walls of assumption and fear. That apology wasn't just about clearing the air—it was about dismantling a small piece of the stigma that still surrounds this work. And that, to me, felt like progress.

Despite ongoing pressure and threats from specific individuals in the field, I've been surprised and deeply reassured by the state of New Mexico's support for psychedelic-assisted therapy. I do not doubt that the person—or perhaps someone within the group they represented—did report me to the state board, hoping to disrupt my work. But the remarkable thing is that, to this day, I've never received any communication from the state licensing board about my services. I believe that speaks volumes about the state's understanding of the value of safe, therapeutic psychedelic work and its commitment to preventing this critical healing practice from being driven underground, where the risks can outweigh the potential benefits.

New Mexico, the "Land of Enchantment," has always been a place where people seek sacred plant medicine, a space for spiritual exploration and healing. The Indigenous nature of this land plays a crucial role in its deep connection to psychedelics. For many Indigenous communities here, the use of plant medicine is not new. It's a sacred tradition that has been woven into their way of life for generations. Among the Diné (Navajo), healing ceremonies often incorporate prayer, song, and herbal medicines.[1] Pueblo communities have long practiced sacred rituals involving tobacco, cornmeal, and other plant offerings as part of spiritual ceremonies.[2] And in certain Apache and Ute traditions, peyote has been used in ceremony for both healing and communion

---

1   Wyman, 1975

2   Ortiz, 1969

with the spirit world.[3] These are not recreational practices—they are spiritual obligations, grounded in deep respect and community wisdom.

Many Indigenous healers in New Mexico continue to offer ceremonies to their communities, where even children as young as eight begin to learn about the medicine. Not just its effects, but its sacredness, its role in connecting them to ancestors, land, and spirit. There's a profound reverence passed down through stories, songs, ceremony, and traditions that honor the medicine's transformative power and root it in responsibility and reciprocity. This long-standing relationship with sacred plants shapes the very landscape of New Mexico, where healing through these substances isn't a trend or a novelty. It's a birthright, a cultural inheritance, and an integral thread in the spiritual identity of the land itself.[4]

With bipartisan measures gaining traction in the New Mexico legislature, the state's support for psychedelic-assisted healing is steadily growing, though perhaps more quietly than some might expect. The passing of the bill in March 2025, which enables the Department of Health and the University to collaborate on a framework for psychedelic-assisted therapy, represents a significant milestone. It's not just a legal shift, but a cultural one—a sign that the winds of change are moving toward healing over fear and understanding over suspicion. To be part of this transformation feels like a sacred privilege.

As these legislative changes unfold, it's clear that New Mexico is acknowledging and honoring its deep, indigenous-rooted

---

3   Stewart, 1987

4   Cajete, 2000

history of plant medicine. At the same time, the state is moving forward with a broader, more inclusive approach to healing, bringing these ancient practices into a new era of acceptance and understanding.

In my case, despite the criticisms and attempts to shut me down, I have continued to offer my services openly and transparently. I have been upfront about my work on my website for two years and have not received any official warnings. In fact, I had the opportunity to meet with a legislator who was genuinely interested in understanding the work I'm doing. It's clear to me now that New Mexico sees the importance of having these services available in a responsible, regulated way, and that's exactly what I've strived to do from the beginning: offer safe, well-informed care for those seeking healing through psychedelic-assisted therapy.

This experience has been eye-opening, not just in terms of my work but in understanding the dynamics at play within this field. Despite the resistance and the challenges, I've come to realize that these obstacles have only deepened my commitment and clarified the path I'm on. I've learned to quickly identify the actual psychedelic practitioners, those who understand the transformative potential of psychedelics, and those who are in it for similar reasons as mine. As I've grown, I've also found the strength to build a network of like-minded professionals who share this vision.

When I first started this journey, I didn't have a clear blueprint. I was creating it as I went, learning with every step and every challenge. Now, I am proud to share my blueprint with others. I want to empower fellow therapists to show them that there is a way to work ethically, safely, and compassionately with psychedelics to bring about true healing. This work isn't about individual glory. It's about creating a movement, one that can make psychedelics a mainstream tool for mental health care.

It hasn't been easy, and I know that resistance will continue as long as the work remains on the fringes. There will always be people who try to thwart progress, who question what we do, or make assumptions about how we're doing it. But I've come to accept that this is part of the process. The more we push, the more we pave the way for others to step into this space, to heal, and to advocate for the truth about psychedelics.

Despite the forces working against us, I'm proud to say I've found another incredible group of psychedelic facilitators in Santa Fe. These people share my mission and my belief in the power of healing. Together, we're building something meaningful. We're building a community that not only offers support but holds each other accountable to the highest standards of care and integrity. And while I'm sure there are still those who disagree with what we're doing, I know that the positive impact we're making will speak louder than the resistance.

The vision I had when I first started this work has become clearer. This journey has never been just about me—it's about forging a path for others, creating a legacy rooted in healing, compassion, and a deeper understanding of what's possible. I am committed to ensuring that the transformative power of psychedelics reaches those who need it most, not just as a tool for personal growth but as a catalyst for collective change. What I didn't yet realize was that Thanksgiving would test everything I believed—pushing me further than ever before and revealing truths I could never have anticipated.

CATHERINE - *Their accusations bruised me.*

Not because they were true.

Because they were blind.

MARIA - *You don't need to explain healing to those*

who've never surrendered to it.

CATHERINE - *I tried to stay calm.*

I tried to open a door.

MARIA - *You did.*

But some people guard their certainty like

it's sacred.

CATHERINE - *Still... I didn't bend.*

And I found my people.

The real ones.

MARIA - *Roots don't shout.*

They grow.

And they hold the earth steady when the wind tries

to tear it apart.

CATHERINE - *I feel stronger now.*

MARIA - *You are.*

And your truth has already shifted the air

around them.

You don't need their approval.

You only need to keep walking.

CATHERINE - *What now?*

MARIA - *Now, you stand firm.*

Your path is clearer.

The wind can blow, but you are rooted.

CHAPTER NINE

SET, SETTING, AND SELF-DOUBT

CATHERINE - *I thought I was ready. I thought I could teach.*

But now, I can't stop hearing that voice.

What if they're right?

MARIA - *What if you hear them because you stopped hearing yourself?*

When silence grows, even whispers roar.

CATHERINE - *I'm supposed to guide.*

If I can't take criticism, maybe I shouldn't lead.

MARIA - *You're not afraid of truth.*

You're afraid of distortion.

This voice?

It didn't start with an evaluation.

It started long before.

CATHERINE - *Then why does it still have power?*

MARIA - *Because you're trying to prove your worth.*

You are not a scorecard, Catherine.

You are a field.

Weeds don't make it barren.

THERE'S A WHISPERED MYTH IN THE psychedelic world. It's unspoken but widely believed that once you've, "Done the work," the journeys get easier. That healing becomes linear. That the medicine will always meet you with grace.

But that's not always true. Sometimes, it comes in swinging.

Set and setting had already shown themselves to be essential, yet the lesson was about to deepen. The wrong mindset, tangled with careless preparation, opened the door to one of the most challenging journeys I would ever face.

One of the most difficult mushroom trips of my life did not begin in a jungle or a candlelit ceremony. It began in the quiet aftermath of perceived failure.

I had just finished teaching my first psilocybin-assisted therapy training, having poured months of heart and expertise into it. The feedback I received cracked me open in ways for which I wasn't prepared. What followed was not a journey of transcendence, but of torment.

It began as a quiet ache of self-doubt, and swelled into a storm that stripped away my defenses, chewed on my insecurities, and offered no soothing insights in return. I emerged not healed, but humbled.

It had been an interesting day, with five colleagues undergoing treatment.

One situation stood out: a counselor wanted to dose but had chosen not to pause their antidepressant medication beforehand. Rather than feel apprehensive, I was intrigued. It was an opportunity to demonstrate, in real time, how SSRIs and similar drugs can interfere with psilocybin's effects. Since many antidepressants bind to the same serotonin receptors as psilocybin, they can significantly blunt the psychedelic experience. And that's precisely what happened. The participant's journey was flat and uneventful, much to her disappointment and her guide's. While unfortunate for them, it was an invaluable teaching moment for the group, a living example of what I'd explained in theory.

The other journeys were magnificent, each in their own way, but Nicole's stands out as pure comedy mixed with cosmic wisdom. Every time I checked on her, she was laughing, the kind of laugh that makes you wonder if she knows something about the universe the rest of us missed. Toward the end, she kept insisting she wasn't ready to crawl back into her "meat suit." Why bother with bones and gravity when she was perfectly happy floating around the room like a blissed-out balloon, untethered from the burdens of being a human?

At one point, I walked in and found her perched right next to the bedroom door, giving herself a pep talk like a kid about to jump into a cold swimming pool. She wanted to rejoin humanity, sort of. But she also wanted to stay in her shimmering, weightless freedom forever. The group gathering at the end was optional, yet she was determined to join. The only problem was convincing herself that squeezing back into a body and walking across the room was worth it.

Eventually, she did make her way in, and when it was her turn to share, she nearly had us all on the floor laughing. She swore the guides had been walking around in white lab coats with clipboards, doing our stiff little "clinical human" thing, which from her vantage point was hysterically absurd. She mimicked us strutting around like doctors on morning rounds. She even pretended to jot notes with an invisible pen, pausing to lick the tip of it with exaggerated seriousness before writing. The room erupted.

My less brilliant contribution to the comedy that day was handing out evaluation forms before people left. In hindsight, it was a terrible idea, asking someone who had just returned from dissolving into the cosmos to write on paper. One question asked, *How can this class be improved?* The answer, scrawled in large handwriting, was: *This is ridiculous. I came. She taught. There was medicine. It was amazing. These are words. This is paper.*

Later, Nicole confessed it was hers. I laughed so hard I framed it, and I still have it today. And since then, evaluations happen post-training, when people are at least mostly back in their meat suits.

Another curveball in the class came from someone who proudly announced they were there to be the "gatekeeper" for the medicine. Yet another one. By that point, I'd come to expect gatekeepers as a permanent fixture on the psychedelic landscape, right alongside the Santa Fe Bullies who posture and protect as if mushrooms belonged to them. What still baffles me is how anyone believes they have the authority to decide how this medicine should or shouldn't be used. *Does anyone own the moon? Then why do people act like they own mushrooms?*

After the course wrapped, I sat down to review the evaluation forms. Providing continuing education credits requires attendees to complete standardized feedback, rating every aspect of the course from one to five. Typically, this part feels routine. I've always taken pride in creating meaningful learning experiences, and I'm used to seeing high scores. But this was my first training focused entirely on psilocybin-assisted therapy. I felt confident in what I had delivered, yet a nervous hum ran underneath. I wanted to know how it had landed.

The first pages looked fine. Some strong reviews, some constructive notes. Then I hit one that stopped me cold.

Straight ones.

Across. The. Board.

Not a single area spared. It was the academic equivalent of a sledgehammer, a perfect score of failure. My eyes scanned the page again, willing the numbers to change, but they didn't. I had poured months of work into this. I had crafted a curriculum, designed materials, and created an atmosphere I hoped would be both professional and transformative. And here was someone saying, in the bluntest way possible, that it was worth nothing.

It felt cruel, not like feedback but like a verdict.

My chest tightened. Disbelief gave way to anger, then to shame. My ego clawed for excuses. *This isn't fair. They're being petty. They probably walked in already unhappy.* But beneath that defensive roar was something far more fragile: hurt.

A raw, aching hurt.

I had exposed a piece of my soul through this work, and in one page, it was dismissed. The rejection stung more than I wanted to admit. I felt small. Disheartened. Deflated. Vulnerable. The weight of it pressed into my chest like lead, heavy and immovable.

I'd rented a vacation home for the training, and since there was a three-day minimum, I still had it for the 4th of July. Trying to salvage the weekend, I invited family over to celebrate. We ordered food, laughed, and worked on a puzzle, some of our favorite shared activities. There's something comforting about the quiet rhythm of piecing together an image, the way it anchors conversation without demanding it. But even as I smiled and chatted, the ache lingered beneath the surface, like background noise I couldn't quite mute.

When everyone left, the silence rushed back in, sharp and suffocating. That was when I made the mistake: Instead of giving myself time to prepare, to ground, or to set an intention, I reached for the medicine as if it were a quick fix. I told myself that diving straight into the hurt would be brave, that mushrooms would untangle the knot inside me and deliver clarity. What I ignored was what I teach others so often: the importance of entering the space with respect, readiness, and care. I convinced myself that the mushrooms would meet me where I was and carry me out of the storm. Instead, my rash decision opened the door to an experience I was not prepared to face.

Ken agreed to guide me, offering his steady presence as an anchor. But no matter how strong his support, the foundation of that night had already been set, and it was shaky at best.

In hindsight, the first mistake was obvious: I chose to embark on a psychedelic journey while still in the throes of emotional crisis, raw and unsteady. The second mistake was how I approached the dose itself. Instead of treating it with intention, I cobbled together a reckless cocktail: a 1g psilocybin-infused chocolate of one strain, a 1g Rice Krispie treat made with another, and a third gram of ground mushrooms prepared with lemon tekking. Three strains, three preparations, none of them aligned. Today, that combination makes me cringe. It feels careless, even disrespectful to the medicine. Since that night, I've had an aversion to mixing mushrooms with food at all. I keep things simple now, clean and intentional. I suspect this harrowing trip is the reason why.

The descent was merciless and immediate. I came in already carrying a low energy of self-doubt, the kind of background static you can usually push aside. But under the mushrooms, it amplified, swelling from a whisper into a roar. The critic inside me, once muted, grew fangs. By the peak, I wasn't just doubting myself; I was condemning myself.

It hit like a sentence being handed down. Over and over. *You failed. You're not good enough. You never will be.*

I had fallen into what facilitators call "looping," but this wasn't ordinary looping. This was a trap. A psychological prison with no exit door. Each time I thought I might break free, the refrain dragged me back under, sharper and louder than before. There was no revelation waiting on the other side of the discomfort. Only judgment. Only shame. Only the cruel echo of my own voice turned against me.

Looping is one of the most distressing psychedelic phenomena. When clients experience it, I always recommend simple interventions: change positions, go for a walk, engage in gentle conversation, do anything to break the cycle and give the ego a chance to reorient.

I knew all of this. And I tried it all. I paced from room to room, clinging to the hope that a change of scenery might break the spell. I asked my husband to draw me a bath, praying the warmth would soothe my nerves. For a few minutes, I thought it might. But then the loop snapped back, like a cruel rubber band against skin.

I returned my gaze inward, dissecting every detail of the training until the memories became weapons against me. My tone of voice. My choice of words. The way I had arranged the chairs in the room. Each memory became ammunition, fired with ruthless precision by the critic in my mind.

And I drowned in it. Shame pulling me under. Judgment pressing down. Self-blame wrapping itself around me like chains.

I asked Ken to hold me, desperate for comfort. His embrace, usually a grounding presence, worked, but only for as long as he was touching me. His touch had always been a source of stability, especially during challenging psychedelic journeys, but this time it was fleeting. I could feel the calm it brought, but as soon as he moved, the restlessness would return. I knew remaining in his embrace was keeping me from doing the work I needed to do. Eventually, his touch became a distraction, pulling me away from my inward focus. So I vacillated, torn between the grounding comfort of his hold and the pull to dive deeper into myself.

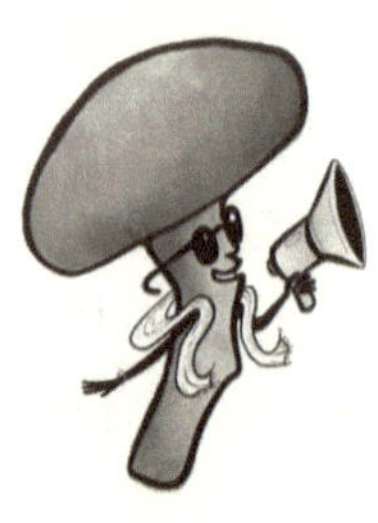

¡OYE! Touch can tether you.

Sometimes, diving into the psychic muck is only possible when you know someone in the real world has your back. That grounding hand permits you to do the dirty work, knowing you're not drifting alone through the soul swamp.

My nervous system was on high alert, vibrating like a live wire. Every muscle twitched with restlessness. My chest felt caged, my breath shallow. No position brought comfort. Nothing eased the storm. I was trapped in my own skin, jittering between the edges of panic and despair. Physically restless. Emotionally flooded. Spiritually untethered.

When the journey finally loosened its grip, the relief was immense, like stumbling out of a burning building into cool night air. But the fire had left its mark. The emotional wreckage clung to me, heavy and raw. Unlike most psychedelic experiences, which eventually soften into resolution or reveal some thread of integration, this one abandoned me in pieces. Fragmented. Fragile.

There was no healing that night—only survival.

What I carried back wasn't comfort, but information. Hard, unyielding truths about the gravity of set and setting, about the need for emotional readiness, about the recklessness of mixing strains and preparations. Lessons were delivered not as gentle whispers, but as blows, each one demanding that I pay attention. And the cost of learning them was steep.

¡OYE! No insight? Doesn't mean no impact.

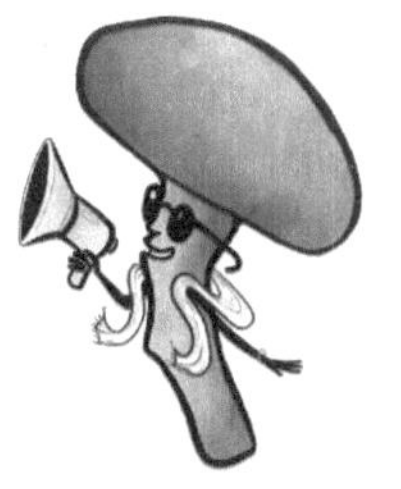

Sometimes the mushrooms deliver their message like a ninja. Silent, slow, and confusing until it dropkicks you three days later while brushing your teeth. Practice patience.

The magic of that particular journey, after receiving critical feedback, had nothing to do with the way it unfolded. The real teaching came from being thrown into the fire and forcing myself to crawl back out, scorched but wiser.

In the days that followed, I carried the residue like smoke clinging to my skin. My body felt unsettled, my mind restless, my spirit fragile. It wasn't until my next psychedelic journey that I felt a proper reset, a profound recalibration of my nervous system. That experience finally delivered the closure I had been craving. It was like a missing puzzle piece sliding into place with a satisfying click. Only then did the echoes of that night begin to loosen their grip and fade.

Clients have often shared with me stories of journeys that left them shaken, anxious, and even convinced they were "broken." I used to wonder what that felt like. Now I know. Sometimes the only way out is through. Sometimes healing demands circling back, revisiting the wound with new eyes and a steadier heart.

It does sound terrifying, especially to those just stepping onto this path. But not every journey is meant to be beautiful. Some are meant to strip you bare and teach. And this one carved into me one of the most valuable lessons of all: respect the medicine, respect the process, and never underestimate the power of your own mind to shape what unfolds. Every expert says it, but that night I learned it in my bones. *Set and setting are everything.*

Much like my own storm, I've seen how psilocybin can mirror the quality of the container it is held in. One client, whom I'll call Elena, told me about a night when she took psilocybin with friends. She thought she was stepping into a trusted circle, a space where she could let her guard down. What she did not expect was that one of her friends had invited others, people she did not know well, who arrived after the medicine had already taken hold. Among them was someone she had never wanted to see again, a man who had assaulted her years before.

The medicine amplified everything. What should have been a sanctuary collapsed into a nightmare. The moment she saw him, her body betrayed her. Her chest tightened, her stomach knotted, her skin flushed hot with terror. Fear and shame surged through her like fire in her veins. Instead of softening into the medicine, she was caught in its grip, pulled into loops of flashbacks and panic that grew sharper with each turn. Her mind became a cage with no exit. She spiraled deeper, drowning in terror, the sound of her own heartbeat pounding like a drum of warning she could not silence. Later, she told me it felt like being trapped inside her worst memory, only louder, brighter, and inescapable.

Her friends were in no position to help. They were also under the influence, swept up in their own experiences, and had no idea what she was silently enduring. She had never shared her history with them, so they couldn't recognize what was happening even if they had tried. And they were not trained guides. They were not trauma-informed. What she needed was someone steady, grounded, and capable of holding the storm. Instead, she was left alone inside it.

Elena had already been living with severe depression before that night. She carried exhaustion that no amount of sleep relieved. Joy had gone flat. Motivation was gone. Most mornings felt like a climb for which she didn't have the strength. What she didn't know was that the "bad trip" would trade one form of suffering for another.

In the days and weeks after the experience, depression was no longer her primary battle. Anxiety took its place. Her heart raced in quiet moments. She startled at sudden sounds. Crowds left her shaken. Sleep broke into restless fragments, her body jolting awake as if danger were always near. For the first time in her life, she understood what it felt like to live in a state of constant vigilance.

It took weeks before she noticed something unexpected. The heaviness of her depression had eased. She had more energy in the mornings. She could laugh without forcing it. The change was subtle, but real. The only problem was that she was too distracted by the anxiety to recognize it right away.

When Elena came to see me, she was hesitant. She had no desire to have another journey. She felt burned, betrayed, and afraid of repeating the past. Together, we began to sort through what had happened. She began to see that the medicine had not failed her. The set and setting had. Once she could separate the medicine from the circumstances, her fear softened. With that new understanding, she agreed to try again.

Psilocybin works on two levels: The first is through insights that come when new connections spark between regions of the brain that don't usually communicate. This is often where people find healing at the core, gaining clarity around trauma, depression, or anxiety. The second is through neuroplasticity, the growth of new neurons and dendritic connections that help create fresh pathways in the brain. This biological shift can reduce depression and anxiety over time, even without the powerful insights.[1] She had benefited from the second but had been robbed of the first.

Elena's willingness to try again came only after trust and safety had been established between us. This time, it would be a formal psilocybin-assisted therapy session, very different from her recreational attempt. She had her own bedroom, free of distractions. The space was quiet, warm, and safe. She wore an eyemask and had curated a gentle music playlist. She knew exactly who would be present and who would not. We set her intention carefully and calibrated the dose to meet her readiness.

This time, the medicine met her with grace. Instead of panic, she felt her body relax into the experience. The anxiety gave way to trust. The fragments of her past began to reassemble into a story she could finally hold. Tears came, but they were not tears of fear. They were tears of release.

---

1   Mortaheb et al., 2024; Shao et al., 2021

As the journey deepened, she found herself able to face what had once felt unbearable. The memory of the assault surfaced, but without the terror that had swallowed her before. For the first time, she could see the truth clearly: it was not her fault. She had carried shame that was never hers to bear. The weight of that false story began to fall away.

In its place came a new realization. The aggressor no longer held power over her. The grip of his presence, which had haunted her body and mind, dissolved under the light of clarity. What had once been a source of fear became something she could witness with compassion and a gentle sense of distance. She was not defined by what had been done to her.

By the end of the session, she no longer carried the same fractured pieces. She emerged lighter, grounded, and with a deep understanding of her own resilience. The story was still hers, but now she held it, rather than it holding her.

Her story echoed mine. I also learned what happens when the container is thrown together carelessly or the timing is reckless. My storm taught me the exact truth her night taught her: psilocybin amplifies what's present. If what's present is chaos, the chaos is magnified. If what's present is intention and care, healing blooms.

This is the line between torment and transformation. When done with respect, the medicine provides insight, integration, and healing. When done without care, it can leave someone fractured, unfinished, or longing for what slipped away.

As I mentioned, it took another journey for me to find my footing again. About three weeks later (I literally could not wait the entire month, which is recommended between journeys), I entered the space with greater care. This time, I prepared and I set my intentions with honesty instead of desperation. I created an environment that felt safe and sacred. And when the medicine met me, it did not drag me into shame or strip me bare. It cradled me. My body softened, my breath steadied, and my nervous system began to recalibrate. It was as if the jagged edges of my being finally smoothed enough to fit back together.

That reset reminded me of the truth I already knew: when held with care, this medicine heals. When approached with recklessness or carelessness, it can leave a person fractured, unfinished, or even more unsettled than when they began. Elena learned that. I learned that. The contrast between those misguided journeys and the ones that were thoughtfully prepared could not have been clearer.

Psilocybin is not a quick fix. It's not a pill you swallow and forget. It is an amplifier. It magnifies what's inside and reflects the quality of the container in which it's held. This is why set and setting are not just important; they are everything.

When respected, psilocybin can dissolve shame, ease depression, heal trauma, and awaken a sense of purpose. When taken haphazardly, it can confuse, frighten, and fracture. My own reckless storm showed me both sides. The medicine did not fail me. I failed to prepare, and I failed to be respectful. And the medicine made sure I would never forget the cost of forgetting.

That lesson reshaped the way I guide, the way I teach, and the way I honor the work. The fire burned me, yes, but it also tempered me. It taught me humility. It sharpened my reverence. And it reminded me that healing, when done with respect, will always be waiting on the other side.

Even those straight 1's, the harshest evaluation I had ever received, became part of the initiation. At the time, they felt like a verdict, a declaration that I was not good enough. Now I see them differently. They were not a measure of my worth, but a spark that lit the fire I needed to walk through. They forced me to face the storm, to return with greater humility, and to remember that my value is not found in numbers on a page. My worth is not a scorecard. It is in the lives I touch, the healing I hold space for, and the courage to keep showing up no matter the rating. And just like the journeys themselves, those evaluations reminded me that context matters. Set and setting shape the experience. A careless container can distort the truth, but a safe and intentional one allows it to shine.

CATHERINE - *I spiraled.*

> *I didn't respect the process.*
>
> *I didn't check my footing.*
>
> *I walked in with doubt and invited the storm.*

MARIA - *Even storms cleanse, querida.*

> *But don't blame the rain when you left the*
>
> *window open.*

CATHERINE - *I punished myself for one voice in a*

> *pile of praise.*
>
> *How does one review hold so much weight?*

MARIA - *Because it echoed an old wound.*

> *When you don't tend to what's festering, even a*
>
> *whisper becomes thunder.*

CATHERINE - *I see that now.*

I needed the reminder.

Set and setting.

Inside and out.

MARIA - *The medicine did not fail you.*

You forgot the agreement.

But look...

You found your way back.

Next time, you will enter the room differently.

Not to prove.

CHAPTER TEN

TRIPSGIVING

MARIA - *You left, didn't you?*

You've been running so long,

you forgot what it feels like to be still.

CATHERINE - *I had to.*

Stillness meant being seen.

And I didn't want to be seen by her.

Not then. Not ever.

MARIA - *You thought her anger meant you*

weren't lovable.

You ran, but the past followed you.

CATHERINE - *So why does it still hurt?*

MARIA - *Because even embers can remember*

what the blaze once felt like.

But today...

you will learn to breathe without burning.

CATHERINE - *Back then, I didn't know how to face it.*

MARIA - *You still don't.*

But you are ready.

In 2017, at 49 years old, my husband Ken and I made the unexpected decision to move to Las Cruces, New Mexico. The town is about fifty minutes from El Paso, Texas, the city where I was born and lived until I was fifteen. Like so many who leave their hometowns, I fled El Paso the moment an opportunity presented itself, vowing never to return.

I still remember that pivotal summer when I turned 14 years old and my sisters and I were sent to California to stay with my father. The entire summer, I quietly orchestrated my permanent escape from El Paso. A week before we were supposed to fly back, my heart pounded as I gathered the courage to ask my father if I could stay. To my immense relief, he agreed without hesitation. In that moment, I felt a rush of freedom so overwhelming that it was almost intoxicating. I was convinced I'd broken free from the dusty cage that had held me for far too long.

From that day forward, I swore to anyone who'd listen that I would never go back to the town I believed had nothing to offer except good Mexican food. But the truth ran deeper than the dust and heat I claimed to despise. I was running from memories I didn't know how to face, from streets that echoed with familiar voices and expectations that felt suffocating. El Paso was a place where opportunities seemed scarce, where people fought hard just to stay afloat, and where I feared I would be trapped if I didn't get out.

Leaving was my act of rebellion, my declaration of independence. Yet, all those years later, there I was, pulled back to a place eerily close to the past I had spent decades trying to forget. Las Cruces wasn't El Paso, but its proximity made it feel like a shadow of the place I'd escaped. Every time I looked at the familiar desert landscape, memories I thought I'd buried threatened to resurface.

When we decided to move, I knew breaking the news to my family would be complicated. I had to call each of them. I could practically hear the disbelief in their voices, even before I dialed. If they heard it from someone else, they'd dismiss it as a rumor, convinced it was impossible. After all, I'd spent years swearing I'd never come back, my stubbornness a shield against even the faintest pull of nostalgia.

But life has a way of dismantling the walls we build around our hearts. My father's health was declining, and with each update, I felt a growing ache that distance could no longer numb. The realization hit me like a punch to the gut. I wanted time with him before it was too late. Time to hear his stories again, to ask the questions I never thought to ask when I was younger.

Meanwhile, Denver, the city where I'd poured my energy into building a thriving practice, began to feel more like a burden than a home. The relentless traffic and soaring cost of living were draining me. I could feel the city pushing me out, even as I clung to the life I'd built there. Then Ken was laid off, and suddenly, the future felt like a blank slate, both terrifying and full of possibility. As the dust settled from that upheaval, a window of opportunity appeared. He wanted to finish his degree, and New Mexico's lower out-of-state tuition fees—and the promise of free tuition after establishing residency—made the move financially wise.

It was never about wanting to go back. It was about needing a new beginning, even if it was in a place so close to the past I'd tried to forget.

What began as a reluctant return became an unexpected chapter of healing, reconnection, and growth. Life brought me full circle, not to confine me in my past but to show me how far I'd come. And maybe, just maybe, to help me make peace with the girl who once ran away.

Shortly after moving to Las Cruces, my father's health improved dramatically. This was a change I like to believe was, in part, because we became a more present and steady part of his life. I have no regrets about the move. But in an ironic twist, my health challenges soon surfaced, demanding endless doctor visits that would have been unbearable against the backdrop of Denver's relentless traffic. The stress alone would have been a barrier to healing. Plus, I can't even imagine working with anyone other than Dr. Rama, who ultimately saved my life. The local support in Las Cruces that I received from family, friends, colleagues, and medical staff was exactly what I needed to navigate my cancer recovery with resilience and hope.

A few years after settling in Las Cruces, my sister, the one I had initially moved to Denver to be near, decided to make the same move. I was overjoyed at the thought of having her close again. She was, is, and will always be one of my best friends. Her presence would make Las Cruces feel more like home. And did it ever. Less than a year later, my mother followed suit, which hit me with a wave of emotions I wasn't prepared for. It was merely months after I had confronted her about the Catholic Church—a conversation that left me raw and reeling, still trying to process the aftermath.

I remember the conversation when she shared her decision. Her voice was tentative, almost fragile, as she asked, "How would you feel about me moving to Las Cruces?"

"Wow! Really? Is that what you want to do?" I replied, forcing my voice to sound neutral even as my chest tightened.

I knew my mother had made her escape from El Paso after over forty years of living there. I understood her desire to be closer to family, to escape the loneliness she felt in Georgetown, Texas. But the thought of living in the same town as her again was a complicated knot I wasn't sure how to untangle.

"I want to be closer to family, and Georgetown hasn't turned out the way I hoped," she explained, her words laced with a vulnerability I couldn't ignore. I wanted to tell her that I understood, that I sympathized. But I was too busy wrestling with conflicting feelings. Part of me worried she'd be disappointed in Las Cruces too, but another part, the part I was ashamed of, felt an instinctive resistance.

"Mom, you can live wherever you want," I said, trying to sound supportive.

"But, are you okay with me moving there?" she pressed, searching my face for approval.

"It isn't my place to be okay or not be okay with it," I replied, carefully choosing my words, knowing they hid tangled emotions underneath. The truth was, I wasn't thrilled about the idea. I had spent years carving out my independence, and the thought of her presence so close felt like an intrusion I wasn't ready for. But how could I say that? Some truths are better left unspoken.

She moved.

It happened faster than I could process. One moment, it was just a conversation, and the next, she was living with my sister while searching for a house. I felt my world closing in, the space I had carefully crafted for myself suddenly feeling crowded. I began to pull away, avoiding both her and my sister, guilt gnawing at me as I kept my distance.

I knew I was acting like a "bad daughter," and the shame of it weighed heavily on me. But the discomfort was real, raw, and impossible to ignore. It wasn't just about sharing the same town. It was about facing parts of my past that I wasn't ready to confront. Her presence forced me to look at my unresolved feelings, to see the parts of myself I thought I'd left behind. And that terrified me.

It was easy to justify seeing my mother only once or twice a year when she lived an airplane ride away. The distance provided a convenient excuse, a buffer that made the infrequency seem normal, even acceptable. But when she moved across town, that excuse evaporated, leaving me face-to-face with a truth I could no longer avoid. I wasn't staying away because of geography. I was staying away because I didn't know how to be close to her without losing pieces of myself.

The realization slammed into me like a cold wave, knocking the breath out of my chest. There was no distance to hide behind, no convenient barrier to justify my absence. I had to confront the dynamic head-on, whether I was ready or not. I was at a crossroads: either find a way to genuinely be okay with visiting her more often or figure out how to show up without feeling like I was suffocating or pretending to be someone I wasn't. The inner conflict was paralyzing.

I even caught myself rationalizing my absence by counting my husband's visits to her as if they were mine, as if his presence could somehow fill the void I was leaving. I lied to myself, clinging to flimsy justifications to avoid discomfort. The cognitive dissonance was fierce, like living with two truths that could not exist together. I wanted closeness but resisted it at the same time, leaving me tangled in guilt, fear, and resentment I could not unravel.

As a counselor, I knew better. It had only been a few months since my mother moved to Las Cruces. I knew I couldn't keep running from this, couldn't keep pretending everything was fine. I had to face it head-on, even if it meant confronting parts of myself I didn't want to see. It was a slow, often painful process, but my psychedelic journeying became an unexpected ally in this work. Each mushroom journey gently nudged me forward, softening the edges of my resistance. It showed me pieces of my heart that I'd shut off long ago, helping me understand the fears and wounds that kept me distant.

This was never more powerful than during the journey through which Gina guided me. When she performed ETT on me, something inside cracked open, allowing me to see my pain and fears with newfound clarity. In that vulnerable moment, I felt a shift and a softening that made space for healing. It was a turning point in my relationship with my mother, helping me move past old barriers to reconnect with her, one step at a time.

In due course, I found myself visiting my mom about once a month. Occasionally, the gap between visits would shrink to just three weeks. It was far from perfect, but it was progress. As insignificant as it might seem, I found a sense of pride in my small achievement—a bittersweet relief that I could finally see myself as a "not-so-great, but not-so-bad daughter." It wasn't the perfect resolution I had hoped for, but it was real, and maybe that was enough, at least for now.

I can't map out exactly how each shift happened; the details blur together, and I never thought to document the process as it unfolded. But looking back, the progress, while real, wasn't anything remarkable. If anything, it highlighted how deeply rooted my resentment was, an undercurrent of agitation that stemmed from years of being her reluctant *spotlight keeper*. The steps I took felt small because the weight I was carrying was so heavy, etched into the fabric of our relationship long before I had the tools to untangle it.

I had been working too much, and with the holidays rapidly approaching, I found myself emotionally drained. I was grappling with a painful realization about my father. It involved an earth-shifting understanding that redefined how I saw him and how I viewed the world. The details of that revelation belong in a different book, but suffice it to say, it was a life-altering experience that forced me to question the foundations of my expectations and relationships.

Feeling raw and unmoored, I decided to skip the traditional family Thanksgiving gathering. Instead, I chose to spend the day dosing with psilocybin. My sister was out of town, and she graciously offered her home as a space for my journey.

One thing I've learned through my experiences is that dosing at home can be riddled with distractions and constant reminders of daily obligations that can pull focus away from the depth of the work. A neutral, unfamiliar environment offers clarity, allowing the mind to fully immerse without the static of routine life.

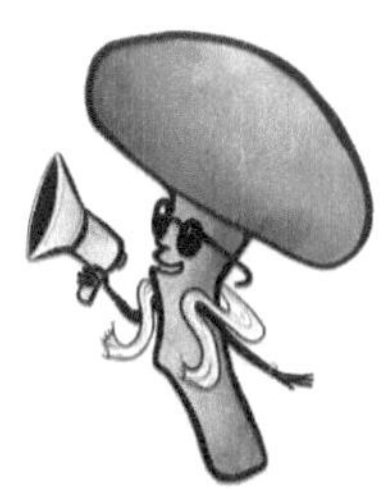

¡OYE! Home is where the dishes judge you.

A sink full of reminders can pull you right out of the medicine. Go somewhere neutral. Clean space, clean slate, clear mind.

Ken agreed to accompany me as my trip-sitter, his steady presence offering a sense of security. I can't recall if I had set a specific intention for this journey, but it didn't matter. The experience itself unfolded with a clarity and intensity that marked a definitive *before and after* in my life. It was the kind of pivotal moment that feels like turning the page to a brand-new chapter, one you didn't expect but somehow needed.

I took four grams of psilocybin and settled in for what I now refer to as *Tripsgiving*. Cocooned in my sister's bed, I curled into a ball under the covers, creating a small, safe nest where I could surrender fully to the experience. As the mushrooms began to take hold, I felt the familiar sensations, the subtle yet profound markers that the psilocybin was binding to my body and brain.

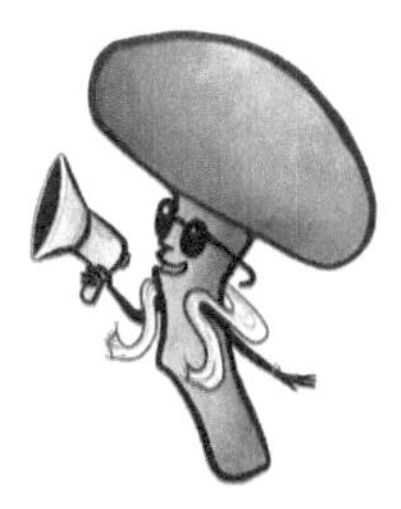

¡OYE! Pinned to the couch? Perfect.

You weren't meant to wander... at least not out there. The medicine anchors you so you can travel inward. Don't fight the stillness; it's the launchpad for your real journey.

It started with a gentle tingling, like warm honey seeping through my cells, spreading relaxation from the inside out. Soon after, the vivid visuals began to unfurl behind my closed eyes with shifting fractal patterns that were swirling and interweaving like a river of vines endlessly braiding themselves together. They moved with fluid grace, each journey offering a new palette of colors and a unique choreography of motion. No two experiences were ever the same, but this visual language had become like an old friend, always greeting me with new expressions each time.

My auditory landscape shifted as well. It felt as though I was submerged in a womb-like space, enveloped by the faint sound of water moving around me, accompanied by a gentle, vibrational hum that faded in and out of my awareness. It was both otherworldly and deeply familiar, like the echo of something ancient within me.

While many people describe psilocybin journeys as visual odysseys, like watching vivid mental movies, my experiences are different. For me, the knowledge doesn't come in images but through sensations and intuitions. It's an embodied understanding, absorbed through felt impressions that bypass language and logic. My emotions are the conduits, the primary way wisdom anchors itself within me. Each pulse of feeling is a message, each wave of sensation a lesson unfolding in real-time.

During Tripsgiving, mushrooms guided me into the depths of my mother's experience from when I was a child. With my ego dissolved, I could finally feel and embody her anger. Throughout my life, I had always perceived her rage as separate from her, but in that moment, mushrooms placed me within her soul. Her intense fury at the world surged through every cell of my body. In the presence of my ego, I always framed her anger through my perspective with thoughts like, "I didn't deserve this," "I was just a child," and "It wasn't my fault." But without my ego, I was able to experience her raw emotion without the filter of my narrative.

In that space, I realized something profound: Though I had always been the target of her anger, her rage had nothing to do with me. It would have been directed at the oldest child, no matter who that was. Her anger was born from her childhood, her divorce, the struggle of raising three girls alone, and the feeling of being unseen and unheard. Layered beneath it all was the weight of generational trauma—stories of sexual abuse, addiction, poverty, abandonment, fleeing Pancho Villa's violence, and seeking asylum in a foreign land. None of it was personal. It was circumstantial, inherited, and unhealed. And for the first time in my life, I felt a deep, genuine compassion for the pain she carried.

I finally understood that she didn't intend to hurt or neglect me. She was simply doing the best she could to survive in a world in which support and guidance were non-existent to her. In that instant, I gained a profound clarity that unraveled nearly fifty years of misunderstanding, the misunderstandings formed through the narrow lens of a child's perspective.

I got Ken's attention and told him I wanted my mother. His response was appropriate for the situation, as he calmly assured me I could call her once my journey had finished, either later that evening or the next day. I likely used the restroom and took a sip of water, a moment that often pulls me out of the intensity of a mushroom experience. I leaned back in, expecting the usual shift in the adventure, a new direction or insight; but instead, I found myself right back in the thick of my mother's anger.

Once again, I called Ken and told him I needed my mother. He responded just as before but added an offering of love, hugs, cuddles, and soothing strokes along my arms and back. His intention was clear: he believed that by offering a more profound physical connection, he could fill the void I seemed to be seeking to fill by asking for my mother. In the past, whenever I faced and resolved a trauma, his unwavering support often led to moments of closeness, and I had come to express immense gratitude for that love, often through comforting cuddles that helped seal the healing.

Ken left me to settle back into the experience. But once again, I found myself embodying my mother's raw, unfiltered anger. And for the third time, I called for him. "I want my mother," I said.

This time, his response came with hesitation and surprise: "Are you asking me to call your mother and have her come see you right now?"

"Yes. I am."

In my egoless state, there was nothing about it that felt strange or out of place. I knew, with every fiber of my being, that I wanted and needed to connect with my mother. After a brief conversation, I was able to convince Ken that this was exactly what I needed.

I heard him dial the phone, asking my mother to visit me, right then, and in the middle of a psychedelic journey. I knew she was home alone on the holiday, and I also knew, deep down, that nothing would bring her more joy than to hear from me. Thanksgiving and Christmas had always been challenging holidays for her, especially when she was by herself. I was certain she would come.

And she did.

When she arrived, she entered my sister's bedroom and gently asked if she could crawl into bed with me. I pulled her in, and as she settled beside me, she asked softly, "What would you like to talk about?"

Words are difficult to access, and vocal movement feels stiff and constrained when under the influence of mushrooms, so I indicated the best I could that I didn't want to talk at all. I muffled, "I want you to love me."

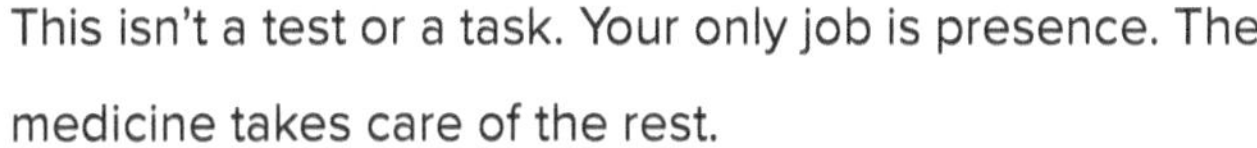

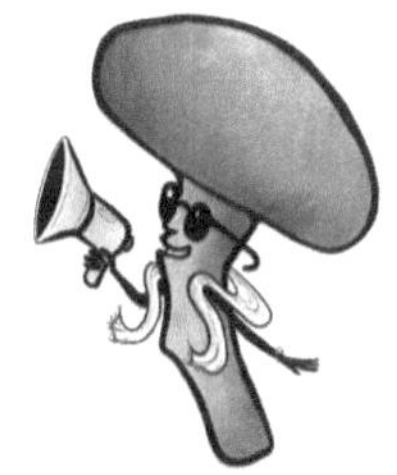

This isn't a test or a task. Your only job is presence. The medicine takes care of the rest.

I grabbed her hand and placed it across my head, running my hair through her fingers. I took her hand and stroked it across my arms. She immediately snuggled closer to me and began to gently caress me like a baby, offering comfort and affection. I'm sure this felt surreal to her, especially since I had never asked for anything like this before—perhaps not even as a child, when I'd hardly dared to seek her attention. As an adult, my mother had tried numerous times to be affectionate, but given the lack of prior affection as a child, I had rebuffed all but the obligatory hug. My mother took full advantage of my request.

At one point, I saw her small hand resting on my large upper arm, and without thinking, I blurted out, "You have to love all of me. The fat is here because of you, and you have to love ALL of it."

To my surprise, without hesitation, she reached out and gently held my legs, arms, back, and every fold of my body with both hands, filled with comfort and love. This was the second life-changing moment of the experience. My mother, the woman I'd often felt had rejected me for my body, was physically embracing the very part of me I always believed she hated.

It wasn't until I was nearly forty that I realized the truth: I had built a shield of weight around me, unknowingly punishing my mother. Growing up, I learned early how deeply presentation mattered to her. Her father was the first Hispanic dentist in town. She also married the son of the El Paso National Bank's Vice President. To her, reputation was everything. We were always expected to look perfect for others. We were perpetually aware that we might run into someone we knew.

The one thing she couldn't control, though, was my weight. She tried, of course, but this was the only place where I could practice autonomy. So I did. She pushed me into every diet, but I always knew how to sneak candy and snacks. No matter how hard she tried, she couldn't control that part of my life. It frustrated and embarrassed her, and I knew it.

From a clinical perspective, I was experiencing something profoundly precious and beautiful, an opportunity that few ever get to realize fully. My mother recreated our attachment.

Attachment is something that is established during the first years of our life and forms the cornerstone of our emotional and social development. When infants receive loving, responsive care from their caregivers, they develop a secure base from which they can explore the world. Receiving this early bond shapes how the brain will process emotions, stress, and relationships for the rest of our lives. When a child doesn't receive consistent caregiving, their sense of security is negatively impacted, creating deep relationship struggles, emotional regulation issues, lower self-esteem, damaged social skills, and less resilient responses to the difficulties experienced throughout life.

I was given an extraordinary and invaluable opportunity to redo the attachment that I hadn't received adequately as a child, when my mother's needs/wants were rated much higher than mine. Tripsgiving was the day my mother did something I had longed for my entire life–she put my needs above her own and cared for me with the kind of physical nurture I had always craved. It was a moment of profound significance, a quiet yet powerful act that reached far beyond that single day.

We spent the next hour or so giggling in bed like two teenage best friends as I came out of the mushroom journey. We held each other and talked about nonsense. She might have brought up some memories from our past as we reminisced and laughed about the absurdity of some of those moments. It was healing and it was beautiful. It was like nothing I had experienced with her before.

Eventually, I made it out of the bedroom to greet and thank Ken for giving me the safety and protection to complete the day's adventure. He had made a hearty, healthy meal to nourish us, as dosing days typically involve very little food before the journey. The three of us sat at the table as I slowly ate dinner. I remember turning to my mother and thanking her for coming that day, especially on such short notice.

My mother looked me in the eye, chuckled, and said, "Thank you for asking me. You've never asked me before."

This was the third profound insight of the day: Mushrooms gave me the emotional and mental understanding to invite her back into my life. My ego would never have allowed what happened that day to occur. The healing that took place on Tripsgiving changed me forever.

After the experience, I began to see my mother at least twice a month and sometimes even twice a week. I spent Christmas and New Year with her—and enjoyed it. I was no longer the Spotlight Keeper, happy to chuck that outdated part of my identity.

CATHERINE - *I thought the door was closed.*

I thought I locked it myself.

MARIA - *It was never locked.*

Just shadowed by pain.

CATHERINE - *It felt like I was the problem.*

MARIA - *You weren't the flame.*

You were just the nearest thing to catch fire.

CATHERINE - *I stopped running and was still.*

MARIA - *Yes.*

Still long enough to catch up to you.

CATHERINE - *I let her in.*

Not because I had to.

Because I wanted to.

MARIA - *That is healing.*

Remembering, not forgetting.

Not erasing.

But seeing the wound clearly and still

choosing love.

CATHERINE - *We are not the same as before.*

MARIA - *And now, you meet each other again.*

From a place of wholeness.

The weight you carried was never yours alone.

Now, you share the air between you.

Free of the past.

CHAPTER ELEVEN
GATHERING THE GROUP

MARIA - *You step into the unknown now.*

A group, unfamiliar, yet holding the same energy.

Why do you hesitate at the threshold?

CATHERINE - *Because they already belong*

to each other.

And I don't know if there's space for me.

MARIA - *You are not here to fit in.*

You are here to be seen.

By them, then by yourself.

Group energy holds a power that one

cannot have alone.

CATHERINE - *What if they don't see me?*

MARIA - *Then stand anyway. Speak anyway.*

The right ones will recognize the rhythm

of your truth.

CATHERINE - *What if I don't belong?*

MARIA - *You will.*

But belonging is not the point.

The point is the experience.

Lean in and let the group energy carry you.

THE FIRST TIME I HEARD THE numbers, I couldn't believe it. In a country where psilocybin-assisted therapy (PAT) is technically legal for those in desperate need, only about 160 people have been approved for treatment in the past four years—just forty people per year.

Forty.

In a world brimming with pain, trauma, and untold suffering, that number felt devastatingly small.

I had the incredible privilege of receiving my PAT training from TheraPsil in Canada, a pioneering organization that fights tirelessly to improve upon those results. Their mission is bold and urgent: to ensure that those who need this life-changing therapy aren't left waiting in the dark.

Knowing the heartbreak of those left behind only strengthened my resolve—a fire inside me to help close the gap between those seeking healing and the therapy that could save them.

TheraPsil's advocacy has been pivotal in making even this limited access to PAT possible. They've been a driving force in pushing boundaries and breaking down barriers. But their impact doesn't stop there. Beyond advocating for patients, they are shaping the future of the field by providing critical training for practitioners. They equip us with the knowledge, expertise, and confidence needed to guide others, often using the clinical trial models as the foundation. The work they're doing isn't just helping individuals, it's paving the way for a revolution in the way we approach healing. They are at the forefront of an evolving movement, and their influence reaches far and wide.

After completing nearly the entire training program, I found myself at a crossroads, just shy of earning my certification. Living and working in the U.S., I realized that the practical benefits of finishing the program wouldn't be fully realized for me in the way I had hoped. By this point, I had already undergone countless journeys myself and had guided other practitioners through their own transformative experiences, just not under the official umbrella of TheraPsil.

The final step was clear: I needed to experience a psilocybin journey under the guidance of another practitioner and, in turn, guide a fellow practitioner—both under TheraPsil's official framework. I loved the training and felt deeply enriched by it, but when it came to completing the certification, something didn't sit right. Because U.S. regulations are still in flux, there was a strong chance my Canadian credentials wouldn't be recognized. If I'd been living in Canada, the decision would have been easy, but in my case, finishing meant pouring more time and money into something I might never use. I had already gained what I came for: skills, confidence, and a deeper trust in myself. That was the real value, and I didn't need a certificate to prove it.[1]

One day, I received an email from my instructor that provided the incentive I was seeking. He was inviting me to participate in a group experience in Canada. It had been a year and a half since I'd traveled there for my training, and while I hadn't actively planned a return, I knew I needed the right opportunity to make it worthwhile. By then, something had shifted in me. I had guided over 100 individuals through PAT, and I no longer felt like the wide-eyed beginner I once was. I had grown, evolved into a more confident, seasoned practitioner, and I knew it was time

---

1   At the time of publishing, New Mexico will recognize TheraPsil certification for facilitator licensure. That shift changed the equation, so I chose to complete the remaining requirements, planning to finish by the end of summer 2026.

to stretch my boundaries and explore new ways to facilitate the transformative work.

Until then, my psychedelic work had been solitary—either alone or in groups where each person stayed in their world. This was different: twelve of us taking psilocybin together in the same room, experiencing the medicine both individually and collectively. When my instructor, in collaboration with Gathering Groups, invited me, I felt a surge of excitement. It was a radical shift, an opportunity to witness and join in the healing power of shared energy.

Professionally, I was hungry for growth, for a deeper understanding of what was possible in psychedelic-assisted therapy. And personally, I was craving connection; the kind of connection that can only emerge when people open their hearts in a shared vulnerable space. The idea sent a thrill through me. It was a push beyond my comfort zone, a new frontier, and it felt like a missing piece of the puzzle I hadn't known I was searching for.

I knew I couldn't guide others through something I hadn't lived myself. Psychedelics aren't like traditional medicine or talk therapy. You can't rely on theory alone. To grasp their depth, power, and unpredictability, I had to experience them firsthand in a group setting, feeling the shared energy, witnessing journeys intertwine. It wasn't just growth; it was essential. If it went well, I could expand my reach as a PAT practitioner and help those numbers I'd mentioned earlier rise.

For the group journey, I felt an undeniable pull to take another hero dose. I had experienced one before, although it had been at least a year. Since then, I had grown significantly in every way: mentally, emotionally, and spiritually. The call to explore it again was strong. In the early years of journeying, my experiences were mostly about trauma resolution and releasing toxic energy. My first hero dose was precisely that: I witnessed things leaving my body, evaporating into the air, and the message from the mushrooms was clear: "Release to make room for new."

It wasn't just about my personal life; it was about shedding the emotional weight I carried for my clients as well. But my journeys had evolved. They were no longer just about purging and letting go. They had become more about making connections, gaining insight, and deepening my understanding of self and the world around me.

Beyond that, I was ready for a group experience. This time, I was curious about the power of collective energy. What might it feel like to journey in the company of others, each person moving through their own layers, yet held in a shared container of trust, courage, and vulnerability? I wanted to witness and be witnessed, to allow the group field to support and magnify the insights and healing that might arise. There was something deeply compelling about being part of a unified circle, a kind of energetic weaving that could only happen when we dared to go inward together. It felt like stepping into an entirely new experience, a new frontier of healing and connection I hadn't yet explored. This retreat wouldn't be just another experience. It was an invitation to surrender more deeply, to trust more fully, and to expand in ways I never had before.

And so, this is why I felt ready for my next hero dose. I knew from experience that a hero dose, typically five grams or more, was not something to take lightly. Unlike a standard macrodose, which allows for insight and emotional exploration while still maintaining some connection to ordinary consciousness, a hero dose often dissolves the ego entirely. It is a full plunge into the unknown, a place where the boundaries of self can vanish and deep transformation becomes possible. Because of its intensity, it should only be undertaken with a strong sense of safety and support. Just as importantly, it must be approached with intention. A hero dose is not just about going deeper. It is about being ready. It asks for reverence, clarity, and a willingness to surrender. I felt that readiness. I did not want to do this on a whim. I wanted it to mean something.

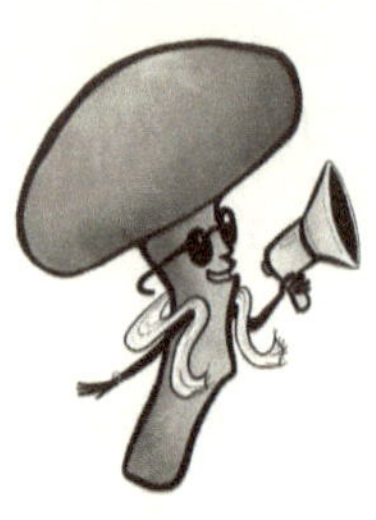

¡OYE! This is not a mushroom measuring contest.

Someone else's hero dose might be your nope. Start where *you* are, not where someone else ego-tripped.

That's exactly what this retreat offered. The group was composed of healing practitioners—skilled, grounded, compassionate people—facilitated by trusted guides in a well-held space. It felt like the safest setting I could hope for. If there was ever a time and place to surrender to the depth of a hero dose fully, this was it. The alignment of group energy, inner readiness, and external support made it feel not only appropriate, but deeply right. This wasn't just another journey; it was an invitation to step into the next layer of my healing—boldly, consciously, and in a powerful community.

The plan for the group session was as follows: twelve healing practitioners, all of whom had completed the same training I had (though at different times), would meet online for weekly Zoom calls over four weeks. Then, we'd travel to Gathering Groups—an intimate retreat center in British Columbia—for the in-person psilocybin session. Two additional weeks of integration meetings would follow, giving us time to process and reflect as a group. It was everything I had hoped for: structure, safety, connection, and the chance to engage deeply with like-minded professionals. The moment I heard the plan, I knew I couldn't pass it up.

Gathering Groups is a Canadian organization offering a structured program that includes group psilocybin-assisted therapy retreats, along with pre-retreat preparation and post-retreat integration sessions. Their approach combines Western therapeutic practices with Indigenous and land-based teachings, providing a holistic framework for personal growth and healing.

About two weeks later, I opened my email, and my heart sank. The organizer had miscalculated the number of available spots, and now I was out; I'd been bumped to the top of the waitlist. I went from overjoyed to dejected in a matter of seconds. I couldn't help but wonder: *Had my initial day of hesitation in responding cost me my spot? Had I waited too long, second-guessed an opportunity that was meant for me?*

The second-guessing, however, was short-lived. Soon, it switched to a deeper awareness. A calm sense of certainty washed over me. Somehow, at my core, I knew I would be in this group. It was an unfamiliar feeling. I chose to trust something completely without any logical reason, but it felt undeniable. It was as if the decision had already been made, and I simply had to wait for the pieces to fall into place.

Sure enough, about three weeks later, someone backed out, and my spot opened up. I wasn't surprised in the slightest. I knew this would happen all along. And to this day, I still can't explain how I was so sure, only that I was. It felt like the universe had already made space for me, and I was simply following its lead.

I had no idea just how profoundly this experience would alter the course of my path. I went into it with an open mind, eager to expand my understanding and immerse myself in the dynamics of a group setting. I liked the idea of the Gathering Groups protocol, because I wasn't quite ready to plunge into the world of psilocybin retreats in Costa Rica, Mexico, or Jamaica. Those settings are led by shamans and steeped in ancient spiritual traditions that felt like vast, intimidating leaps from the structured, clinical-trial-based methods that had grounded me in my work. My scientifically inclined mind craved something that still held a tether to the familiar.

That's exactly why Gathering Groups felt so compelling. It wasn't just an opportunity, it was a stepping stone. A chance to explore the power of group healing without diving headfirst into a realm that felt foreign and uncharted. This experience seemed to offer the perfect fusion of clinical structure and communal connection, a bridge between two worlds. And more than anything, it felt right. Like a doorway I was meant to walk through.

The initial Zoom calls leading up to our gathering were a fascinating exploration of how to create a safe, intentional space for everyone involved. Each session followed a structured process. We were given a question, each person had a few minutes to respond, and then others were invited to share their reflections— not in the form of advice or opinions, but through a specific format: *"When you said ___, I felt ___."*

This technique, known as Embodied Listening, was designed to foster deep presence and genuine connection. The practice centered on tuning into our body's natural responses as someone spoke; without judgment, without trying to fix anything, and without shifting the focus back to ourselves. Instead, it encouraged honest, body-based reactions that created a space where each person felt truly seen and heard.

Even after just one night of practice, I could feel how profoundly bonding it was. It created an entirely different kind of connection, one that wasn't built on the usual surface-level exchanges about jobs, demographics, or daily routines. Instead, we engaged with each other through emotions, presence, and authenticity. It was a way of showing up for one another in a real and deeply human way, and I could already sense how it would shape the experience to come.

One thing that immediately set me apart from the group was that I was the only participant not living in Canada. While I wasn't the only one traveling a long distance (some attendees had to travel to the West Coast from Eastern Canada), I was still the sole outsider. But none of that mattered to me. I was just thrilled to be surrounded by like-minded professionals for a long weekend.

At that time, working in psychedelics—especially in the U.S.—could feel incredibly isolating. The field was still emerging, shrouded in stigma, and many practitioners were operating underground. I often felt like I was on an island, navigating uncharted waters without a map. So the chance to sit in a circle with others who not only understood the work but lived it, breathed it, and loved it—it felt like coming home. The opportunity to connect with others who shared my passion was invaluable.

I was also eager for a change of scenery. I've always had a deep appreciation for different lifestyles and cultural perspectives.

After several years of limited travel due to health challenges since 2017, I was craving that sense of exploration again. The idea of stepping into a new environment, reconnecting with some diversity, and immersing myself in something fresh felt exactly like what I needed.

As the weeks passed, my excitement about finally meeting everyone in person continued to build. Since it would take a full day of travel just to get there, I decided to extend my trip and explore parts of Canada that I had always wanted to visit but had never had the time or opportunity to do.

Gathering Groups is located in Abbotsford, about an hour from Vancouver. When I looked at the map, I saw that Whistler, a picturesque mountain town, was within driving distance. It was the off-season, which meant fewer crowds and more affordable lodging, and since I wasn't much of a skier anyway, it seemed like the perfect chance to take a much-needed vacation. I had been working so hard, and I was long overdue for a break. My husband, however, wasn't too keen on traveling in light of COVID, especially not somewhere as far as Canada. While I would have preferred to take the trip with him, I wasn't about to let the opportunity pass me by, even if he didn't accompany me.

I also saw Whistler as the perfect setting to work on my book. The idea of sitting in the fresh mountain air with a hot coffee or, maybe, hot chocolate, and typing away on my laptop sounded like an absolute dream. I even found a place with a private hot tub, knowing it would help me unwind and ease into the writing flow.

Every part of the trip felt intentional. I was excited for the group experience, thrilled about the nice car rental I had reserved, and looking forward to the scenic drive through the countryside and up into the mountains. To top it all off, I had scheduled a day at a Scandinavian spa, which offered a silent retreat experience; hot tubs, saunas, peaceful meditation rooms, cold plunges, all set in a gorgeous rainforest environment. A full day of hydrotherapy, digital detox, and quiet solitude sounded like the perfect way to integrate the experience after a psychedelic hero dose.

Everything about this trip felt aligned. It wasn't just about learning and professional growth, it was about giving myself the space to breathe, reflect, and embrace something new.

I arrived in Vancouver at my own pace, knowing I had time to spare. Check-in at Gathering Groups wasn't until almost 6 pm, and my flight landed at 1. It felt like the perfect opportunity to breathe and enjoy the day. After securing my rental car, a beautiful Range Rover that made me feel like I was already on vacation, I treated myself to some sushi. Living in Southern New Mexico, where the Mexican food is unparalleled but decent Asian cuisine is a rare find, I was on a sushi quest, and I indulged in it fully that afternoon. It felt like the kind of self-care I hadn't allowed myself in ages. I was glad I did, because when I arrived at Gathering Groups, dinner was served...and it was Taco Night. The irony hit me in the gut. Tacos in Canada were *definitely* not what a New Mexican soul craved after a long day of travel.

Despite the unexpected taco surprise, arriving at Gathering Groups felt undeniably beautiful. The connections we had nurtured through weeks of Zoom calls deepened the moment we met face-to-face. There was a warmth, a genuine joy in seeing each other in person—a feeling both familiar and new.

What struck me most was how different this experience felt from typical introductions. We weren't starting with surface-level questions like *Are you married? Do you have kids? Where do you work?* Instead, those details felt like puzzle pieces falling into place, filling out the fuller picture of people we had already come to know in meaningful ways. The bond we had built online had bypassed the usual small talk and taken us straight into something real—something deeply human. Meeting in person wasn't the start of our connection, it was the continuation of something we had been building all along.

After dinner, we gathered for a group meeting, settling into a circle where we began sharing our hopes and intentions for the following day. Half of us would be journeying while the other half would take on the role of guides. We had been assigned dyad partners before our very first Zoom meeting, and as the group dynamic deepened over the weeks, so did the connection with our partners, the person we would come to trust and rely on during our experience.

My dyad partner had never taken psychedelics before, and I could sense the mix of curiosity and apprehension in their energy. Wanting to ease their nerves, I volunteered to dose first. In my experience, witnessing someone else go through the journey first can be incredibly grounding. It helps dissolve anxiety, providing a clearer understanding of what to expect and how to surrender to the experience. I hoped that by going first, I could offer my partner a sense of reassurance and calm.

This intentional approach was a perfect example of *set* and *setting*, two of the most critical foundations for a safe and meaningful psychedelic experience. Mindset (set) and environment (setting) shape every aspect of a journey, and by preparing with intention, we are creating the conditions for the best possible outcomes. Allowing my partner to observe first before embarking on their journey was a deliberate part of this process, giving them the chance to witness, absorb, and step into the experience with confidence rather than uncertainty.

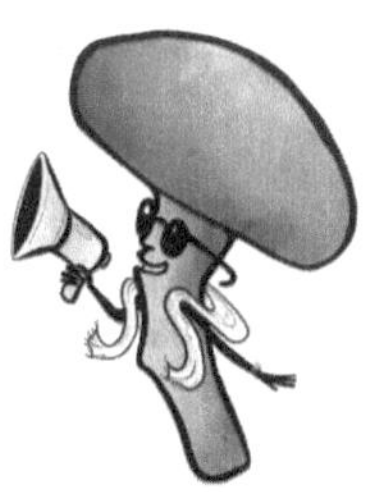

¡OYE! Set and setting doesn't just mean your couch and candles.

It's your mindset, your heart state, your readiness to meet whatever comes up. Don't just feng shui the room—check in with your soul. Are you here to heal, or are you trying to hide?

The group meeting itself provided another opportunity to bond by openly sharing our expectations, fears, and hopes. We weren't just discussing the experience ahead; we were actively building a container of trust, a sense of safety that would carry us through whatever the medicine revealed.

However, as we spoke, I began noticing something unsettling stirring within me. A theme was emerging, one I was already aware of.

I was *the American*—the outsider. No one made me feel this way, not directly, yet I felt it deeply. The more I became aware of it, the stronger the feeling grew. It gnawed at me, forcing me to examine why I was feeling so separate from the group. And then, like a sudden realization breaking through the fog, I understood.

I didn't just feel like an outsider at the retreat—I felt like an outsider in my own country, even though I was in Canada. I was embarrassed. Embarrassed by how America was presenting itself to the world. At the time, we were just weeks away from the Biden/Trump election, and the political climate back home felt toxic, mean-spirited, and divided beyond recognition. The America I had grown up in—the one that once stood for unity, for pride, for the belief in something greater—felt like a distant memory. Now, all I could see was a country that was behaving like a bully, a nation that had lost its way.

When I finally voiced this to the group, I saw nothing but compassion in their eyes. There was an unspoken understanding; a silent acknowledgment that my country had been acting selfishly and disrespectfully on the world stage. No one needed to say it aloud; we all felt it. And in that moment, as painful as it was to admit, I allowed myself to feel the grief of that loss fully. It was a brutal truth to sit with, but it was one I could no longer ignore.

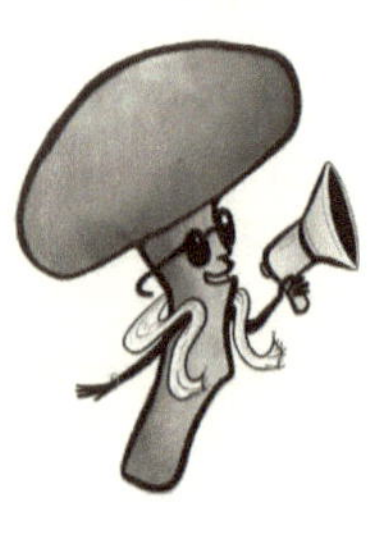

¡OYE! Sometimes the journey starts before the mushrooms show up.

The moment you set your intention, the medicine stirs. Dreams shift, memories sneak in, feelings bubble up. It's like the medicine clocked in before you even swallowed.

The next morning, I suited up in my most glorious, mismatched, colorful long johns—because if you're going to embark on a psychedelic journey, you might as well do it in comfort and style. And, of course, I brought my prized possession: my "comfy." Most people bring a cozy blanket to curl up in—but not me. My version of comfort is a crisp, percale cotton twin-size sheet, cool to the touch and quite possibly my most cherished household item. At home, I drape it over myself in my recliner every night, like a security blanket for grown-ups. Living in a place where the temperature perpetually hovers between *molten lava* and *the fiery gates of hell*, traditional blankets feel less like comfort and more like punishment. Except for a few fleeting winter months, they're nothing but stifling heat traps—and frankly, I refuse to play that game.

Sure, Gathering Groups had plenty of blankets available, but I needed my comfy—a little slice of home, a thread of familiarity in this new, unknown space. It was October, and I'm sure the Canadians were thoroughly perplexed by my devotion to what, to them, probably looked like the least comforting comfort item ever. But did I care? Not in the slightest.

¡OYE! Pack for peace, not Pinterest.

Bring a soft blanket, a meaningful object, or a scent that soothes. This isn't a slumber party... it's sacred work. Comfort calms your system. Clutter confuses it.

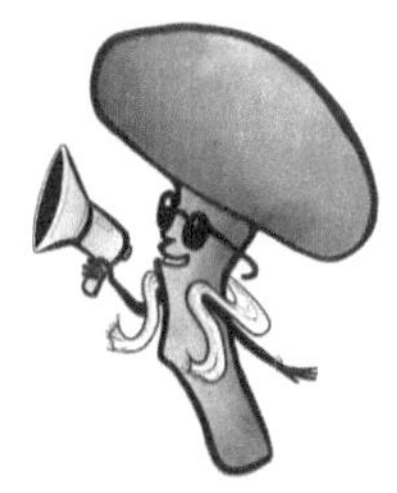

At the breakfast table, as conversation flowed easily among us, the topic of my American shame surfaced again. It wasn't surprising. I had been sitting with it, turning it over in my mind, still trying to process the weight of it. The more I spoke, the more I realized just how deeply it had been gnawing at me. Then, Laura, a woman with the kindest eyes and the warmest presence, turned to me with such gentle sincerity and said, "You know, some of the best people I know are American."

Her words landed deep in my soul, cutting straight through the heaviness I had been carrying. She wasn't dismissing my feelings, nor was she arguing with me—she was simply offering a truth I had momentarily lost sight of. And she was right. In that moment, I felt something inside me soften. It was exactly what I needed to hear.

Now, I was ready.

We then gathered for our intentions circle, a sacred ritual to solidify the intentions of those who would be dosing that day. Setting intentions isn't just a nice prelude to a psychedelic journey, it's *essential*. I firmly believe that intentions shape the experience, anchoring the mind and giving it direction. Psilocybin is an amplifier, magnifying whatever we bring into the space. If we come in with clear intentions, we increase the likelihood of gaining profound insights into them. While the process of formulating intentions begins weeks in advance, the fine-tuning tends to crystallize in the 24 hours leading up to the journey.

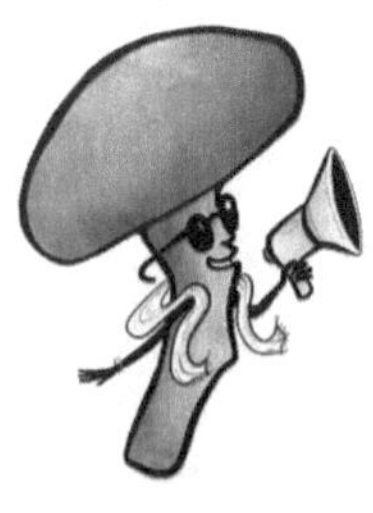

¡OYE! Have a 'why,' but hold it lightly.

Intentions guide the journey, but they don't guarantee the outcome. Be clear, but stay open. The medicine doesn't always give you what you want, but it always delivers what you need.

Here were my intentions:

Lean into Group Energy

This intention had been forming in me since the moment I decided to register. My entire reason for joining the retreat was to experience firsthand how a group journey differs from an individual one. Up until that point, my work had been one-on-one, and I wanted to explore the nuances of shared energy, collective healing, and what new layers might emerge in a communal setting. I was ready to embrace the unknown and lean wholly into the experience.

Self-Worth

This has been a recurring theme in my personal work, showing up in various forms: self-care, self-acceptance, self-trust, self-respect. But this time, I landed on self-worth. I had been struggling with feeling deserving of the abundance flowing into my life. Big opportunities, like a documentary film and a book on the work I do, were on the horizon. Yet instead of excitement, I felt an unsettling sense of unworthiness. Not for any concrete reason I could define, only because I knew it was the next layer of my self-exploration. It was time to face it head-on.

Write a Love Letter to Myself

During one of our group meetings, another participant shared a story about finding a love letter they had written to themselves years ago, just before coming to this retreat. They spoke about how reading it gave them a powerful perspective on their growth. The idea of writing a love letter to myself felt... uncomfortable. Foreign. Awkward. And that's exactly why I knew I had to do it. *What would it look like to write a letter full of love and kindness to myself? What words would I struggle to say?* That discomfort was a clear signal; it was an intention worth exploring.

After the intentions group circle completed, we gathered around the kitchen table for a sacred ritual, one that marked the beginning of our respective journeys. Only those who would be dosing sat at the table, while the guides stood around us, watching over the process with quiet reverence and support. The air buzzed with a mix of anticipation and solemnity.

Each of us had individually ordered our Golden Teacher mushrooms through Moment Mushrooms, a Canadian company known for cultivating medicine with exceptional quality and care. What impressed me most was not just their product but the way they handled the process. Each of us placed our own orders and payments, and Moment Mushrooms thoughtfully gathered everything into one bulk shipment, sending it directly to Gathering Groups.

Their attention to detail, reliability, and obvious care for the medicine gave me a deep sense of confidence. In a field where trust matters so much, they've earned mine completely. When the package was opened, the dried fungi were poured into a large bowl at the center of the table.

One by one, we passed the bowl around, each person selecting three whole mushrooms, cap and stem intact, the ones that seemed to call to us. It was a deeply personal and intuitive process, as if the mushrooms were choosing us just as much as we were choosing them.

Once we all had our selections, we held them in our hands, taking a quiet moment of gratitude and reverence. The mushrooms had taken time, energy, and care to grow. They were about to guide us into the depths of our consciousness. It felt right to acknowledge their power and mystery before consuming them.

A scale was passed around, giving each of us the freedom to choose our dose. Most people confidently chose the standard 3.5 grams—the classic benchmark for a full psychedelic experience. But when it was my turn, I hesitated.

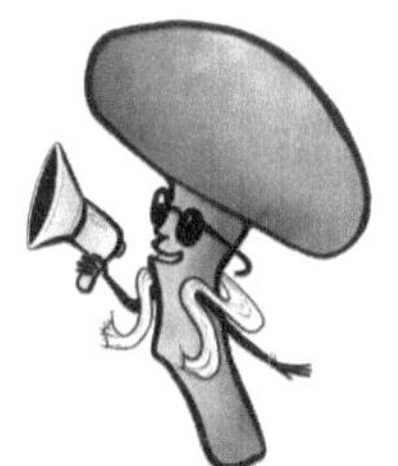

¡OYE! Macrodosing = usually 2 to 4 grams.

Start with awareness. Don't go big just to go hard.

I knew Golden Teacher was considered gentler than the strain I was used to, yet I'd never tried it before. Part of me wanted to play it safe—stick with what others were doing. But another part of me argued that if I was going to do this, I wanted it to be meaningful. Four grams had always been a sweet spot with my usual strain, and recently, a colleague had mentioned taking five grams of Golden Teacher—a proper, classic hero dose of a true, classic strain.

I hovered in that space of uncertainty, weighing my options. Was I being cautious or just scared? Was I aiming for wisdom or holding myself back? The questions buzzed in my mind as I tried to decide just how far I was willing to go.

I had been preparing myself for this moment, waiting for the perfect opportunity to push my boundaries in a setting that felt completely safe, surrounded by experienced practitioners and mushroom experts. If ever there was a time to leap, this was it.

I placed my mushrooms on the scale. 4.99 grams. JACKPOT!

A chill ran through me. I hadn't measured, hadn't calculated. I had simply chosen. And yet, the number staring back at me confirmed what I already knew deep down.

It was meant to be.

The preparation process was completely different from my usual _lemon tekking_ method. Lemon tekking involves grinding dried psilocybin mushrooms into a fine powder and soaking them in lemon or lime juice for fifteen to twenty minutes before consumption. The acidity begins to break down the psilocybin into psilocin, which is the compound the body uses. This method can result in a faster onset, a shorter duration, and often a more intense experience.

But this time, we took a more traditional approach. No citrus. No grinding. Just whole mushrooms, reverently placed on a small ceremonial plate. It felt more sacred, more intentional. Like honoring the medicine rather than manipulating it.

We carefully broke the mushrooms apart by hand, crumbling them into small, quarter- and nickel-sized pieces. There was something deeply satisfying about the tactile nature of the process, as if we were already beginning to form a connection with the medicine.

Next, we poured freshly boiled water over the mushroom pieces, allowing them to steep into a rich, earthy tea. The aroma was grounding, a reminder that the experience was rooted in something ancient and natural. Using a French press, we gently separated the liquid from the remaining mushroom material, ensuring a smooth, easy-to-drink brew.

Now we moved to the physical setting prepared for us: _the journey room_. It was arranged with intention, each detail carefully curated to create a space of safety, comfort, and deep introspection. Six bed rolls were laid out in a circle, each one topped with pillows, blankets, eye masks, and headphones, all positioned closest to the center. This wasn't just a physical setup. It was a container, a sacred space designed to hold us through whatever the journey would bring.

We were encouraged to bring comfort items, totems, or personal objects to place in the center, forming a communal altar. It was a way to ground ourselves, to bring a piece of our own world into a shared experience. My contributions were simple but deeply personal: my pillow, my comfy, my water bottle, and my journal. Each of these items carried meaning, reminders of home and familiarity as I prepared to step into the unknown.

¡OYE! You can't transcend the ego if your bra is trying to kill you.

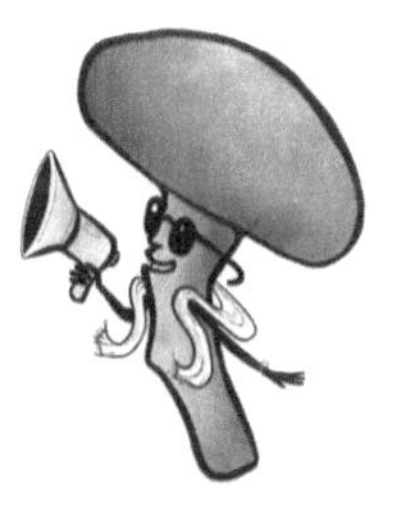

No one has ever found the meaning of life while wearing anything itchy, tight, or riding up in weird places. Choose comfort like your healing depends on it... because it kinda does.

The eye masks and headphones were essential tools, helping each of us turn inward. Music was played both in the room and through the headphones, ensuring that even if we needed to remove them for a trip to the restroom or a moment of fresh air, the soundscape remained immersive. The headphones, though, provided something extra: a cocoon, a way to block out external distractions and fully surrender to the journey.

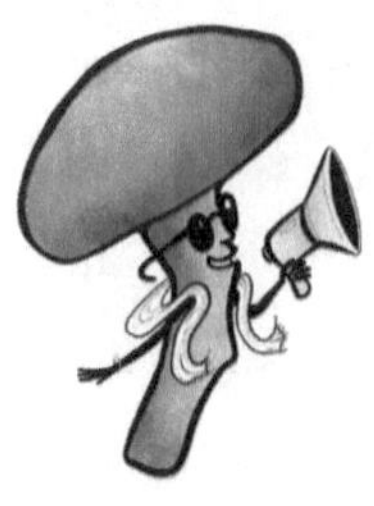

This isn't a costume, it's a spacecraft. Strap in, block out the outside world, and let the journey launch from the inside out.

But here's the thing: I had never successfully used music during a trip before. Despite all the expert recommendations, despite creating at least ten different playlists for my journeys, I always ended up rejecting the music within fifteen to twenty minutes.

Every. Single. Time.

While others swore by its ability to enhance the experience, for me, it had always felt intrusive, like an unwelcome guest disrupting my process.

Yet, I had made a promise to myself going into this experience: I would surrender to the structure they had created. No adjustments, no tweaks, just full immersion in their process. As I settled onto my bedroll, I stared at the headphones with a mix of trepidation and reluctant acceptance, wondering if this time would be different.

The basement room was dimly lit, the only natural light filtering in through high-set windows. It was a large space, holding about 17 people, and there was an undeniable sense of security in the collective energy of trained healing professionals. The guides sat near each person who was dosing, embodying the quiet, steady presence of caretakers ready to hunker down for the day. They were there for whatever we might need: a walk to the restroom, a refill of water, extra tissues, an additional blanket. No request was too small. Their presence was a silent assurance: *You are safe. You are being held. We are ready.*

As the group settled into their sacred spaces, a hushed anticipation filled the air. The guides moved quietly around the circle, their hands steady as they completed the final preparations for the tea. The soft clink of ceramic against wood marked the moment when each of us was presented with a warm mug, the steam curling upward in delicate tendrils. The rich, earthy aroma of the brew wrapped around us, grounding and inviting, signaling the threshold we were about to cross into the unknown.

Before drinking, we engaged in a ritual, a moment of reverence and connection. The guides led us through the Seven Directions Prayer, a Native American tradition that honors the energies of the East, South, West, North, Up (Father Sky), Down (Mother Earth), and Inward (the Inner World). With each direction, we paused, offering gratitude, appreciation, and acknowledgment before taking a sip.

There were additional ceremonial elements woven into the ritual, but out of deep respect for the traditions and their rightful storytellers, I won't attempt to detail them here. Instead, I'll simply say that in that moment, as we moved through the prayer together, a sense of sacredness settled over the room. This wasn't just a cup of tea—it was an offering, a passage, a step into the unknown.

As we settled in, we pulled on our eye masks and headphones, lying back in anticipation of the journey ahead. I took a deep breath, silently reviewing my intentions one last time, then exhaled, surrendering to the mushrooms and whatever they had in store for me.

To my surprise, not only was there no impulse to reject the music or rip off the headphones, but I found myself fully embracing it. The melodies didn't just play in my ears; they seeped into my being, flowing through me like an old friend whispering secrets to my soul. It was as if the music had finally unlocked a door and shoved it wide open.

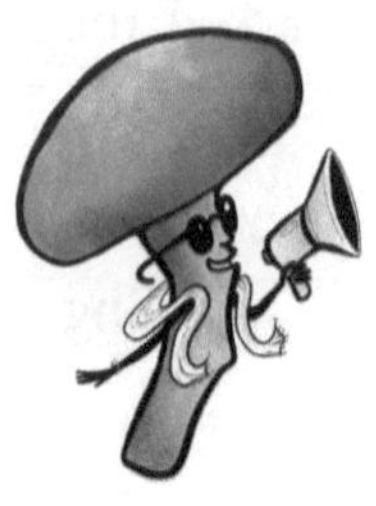

¡OYE! Music is sacred—or sabotaging.

The right song can open your heart. The wrong one might make you want to karate chop a flute. Curate wisely—your nervous system is listening.

CHAPTER TWELVE

MITZI DEATH

Just as I was melting into the revelation, a new sensation snapped me back: one of discomfort. Even though I was on a bed roll, it wasn't quite enough for my post-hip-replacement body. I needed something softer if I wanted to stay fully immersed in the experience. My mind immediately flicked to the sectional couch in the back of the room—my escape plan, my haven. When I got up to use the restroom, I didn't even hesitate. Instead of returning to my bedroll, I instinctively claimed my spot on the couch, knowing that the real journey wasn't just about where I was physically. I even unceremoniously ousted my instructor from the couch without a second thought, an ironic display of ego dissolution at its finest.

Usually, with the ego in charge, I'd be hyper-aware of social norms, overly concerned about politeness, and probably apologizing profusely for taking someone else's seat. But at that moment, none of it mattered. There was no hierarchy, no sense of 'mine' or 'yours'—just a deep, primal knowing that my body needed comfort, and the couch was calling my name. In a way, it was the purest form of surrender, letting go of unnecessary guilt and just doing what I needed to fully experience the journey.

Sorry, instructor, but the universe had other seating arrangements in mind! It was all about where I was going mentally, emotionally, and spiritually.

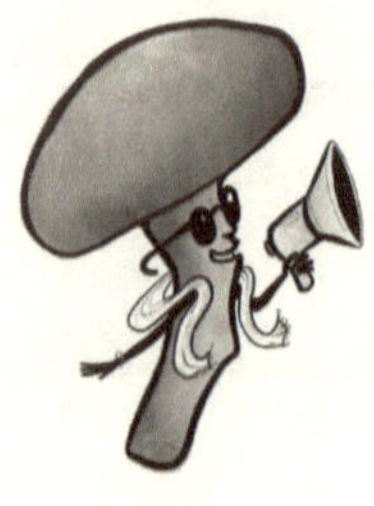

¡OYE! Lose the distractions.

Distractions are the ego's way of throwing glitter at the crime scene. It wants your attention outside so you never look at what's unraveling within. That itch? That urge to check your phone? The facial liquid letting? Classic sabotage. Guard your focus like your growth depends on it—because it does.

Suddenly, my paternal grandmother appeared before me—the woman after whom I was named. She passed away when I was twenty-four, just as I was about to graduate from college. But there she was, looking as radiant as ever.

I was her first grandchild, and our birthdays were only ten days apart in July. She was born on the Fourth of July, and as a kid, I was convinced that the entire country was throwing a giant party in her honor. Fireworks? Parades? Barbecues? *All for Grandma!* And honestly, I think she would have agreed with that assessment. Even now, I can't see a sparkler or hear the crack of fireworks without feeling that connection. Sure, everyone else might be celebrating independence, but for me, it's always been a little bit about her, a woman so special, I thought the whole world must have been celebrating her, too.

Before she died, I went by Cathi, the name my family still calls me today. But at her funeral, something strange happened. The priest kept saying her full name: *Mary Catherine Warnock*. Each time I heard it, it was like an electric jolt through my body. My name, *Catherine Marie Warnock*, was slightly different but eerily close. Hearing it spoken in the context of death and at a funeral was unsettling in a way I couldn't explain. It felt like a signal. On the flight home, just weeks before my college graduation, I made a quiet but profound decision: I would no longer be Cathi. I would step into a new identity as Catherine. It was a subtle transformation, but an important one. Even now, while I am okay with my family calling me Cathi, my deep essence is, and always has been, Catherine.

CATHERINE - *Wait a minute!*

> *Maria!*

> *Are you... my grandmother?*

MARIA - *Yes.*

> *And no.*

> *I am her echo.*

> *Her love.*

> *Her memory.*

CATHERINE - *I... I don't understand.*

MARIA - *I am.*

> *And I am not.*

> *You've forgotten the name of your mother's mother.*

CATHERINE - *Woah... how could I forget?*

> *Her name is Maria.*

MARIA - *Yes.*

> *You carry her in you.*

> *A thread through your blood.*

> *You are both, and more.*

CATHERINE - *My middle name is Marie.*

MARIA - *Yes.*

> *You are named for both.*
>
> *And for me.*
>
> *Forget my label.*
>
> *It matters none.*
>
> *Focus on the message.*
>
> *Not the messenger.*
>
> *The blood remembers.*
>
> *The thread guides.*

So when she appeared to me in this psychedelic space, thirty years after her death, I didn't feel startled or disoriented. It was warm. Familiar. Like slipping into a long-forgotten memory that had been waiting just beyond the veil. That's what psychedelics do; they strip away the shock that ego would usually impose. Instead of feeling disbelief, I simply listened.

She looked at me with love and said, "I've come to tell you something. Your aunt died today."

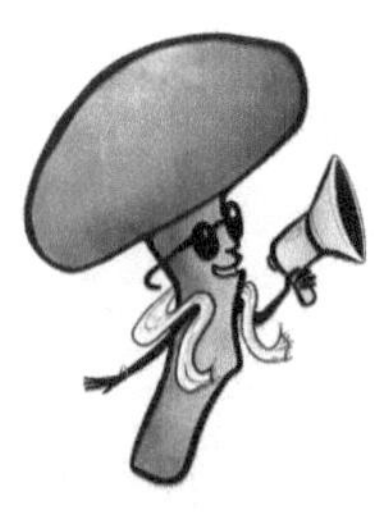

¡OYE! Lean into it.

Mushrooms don't slay your dragons for you! They hand you a flashlight and shove you toward the cave. It's scary, yes, but guess where the treasure is? Face the fire, brave the dark, and you'll find the gold. Discomfort is the toll, but the lessons are guaranteed.

Instantly, I knew she meant Mitzi, her daughter, my godmother. The next moment was an avalanche of shock, grief, and disbelief, unlike anything I had ever experienced. Until that moment, I had been spared the deepest kinds of loss. I had lost grandparents, but those deaths felt natural and expected. I had lost a few uncles, but I wasn't particularly close to them, so although their loss was sad and there was grief, it didn't devastate me. Mitzi, though—losing her felt like a freight train barreling through my soul, shattering everything in its path.

Mitzi was just sixteen when I was born, and she still loves to tell the story of how she'd take me everywhere, proudly introducing me as her own. She got a kick out of it, especially since, let's be honest, I was a pretty adorable kid. As the first child born to her siblings, I was a novelty, a little star in the family orbit.

Growing up, Mitzi wasn't just my aunt—she was the coolest person I knew. She had an effortless charm, a magnetic energy that made you want to be around her. She was the one who made life feel exciting, the one who always had a story, a joke, or an adventure up her sleeve. And the best part? That never changed. Through every stage of my life, Mitzi was there, a close and steady thread woven through my world.

The grief hit me like a tidal wave. It was raw, overwhelming, and all-consuming. I mourned her with every ounce of my being, sobbing for what felt like hours, though in reality, it was probably only fifteen minutes. The pain came in crashing waves, each one pulling me deeper into the realization of how much she meant to me. In those moments, I anchored myself by connecting with my breath: *inhale, exhale*. Again. My breath became the only steady thing I could hold onto. She had always been a constant presence, a quiet refuge in the chaos of my childhood. I didn't have many places where I felt truly safe, but with Mitzi, I always did.

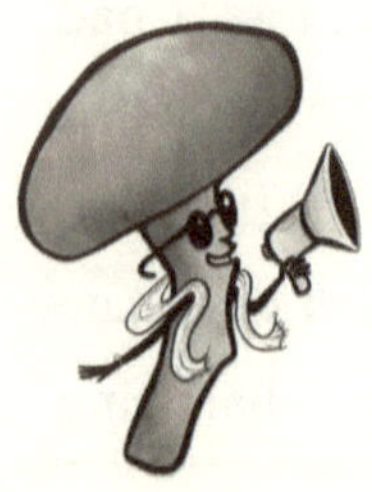

When the waves get wild, your breath is the rope that tethers you to safety. Inhale trust. Exhale resistance.

At some point, I needed to use the restroom again, and as I sat up, my ego started creeping back in. A single, disorienting thought cut through the haze: *Wait... is she actually dead?* I had no way of knowing. I was in Canada, deep inside a psychedelic journey, completely detached from the outside world. My phone was off, and there was no chance I could even attempt to use it in that state.

My guide came to help me, and I was gently led toward the restroom with my eye mask still on, my hands resting on the shoulders of the guide walking in front of me. I tried to form the words, heavy and tangled in my mind, dragging them through thick fog until they finally slipped out, barely above a whisper: *"I think my aunt died today."*

Under the mushrooms, I could not discern how the room reacted. Normally, when ego is intact, we tune into every flicker of expression and every change in tone. In mushroom energy, all of that faded away. My insight from within was so profound, so consuming, that it drowned out any awareness of others. I am sure they responded, maybe even offered comfort, but I cannot tell you what they said or did. That is the difference between ego and no ego. With ego, we are busy tracking others, measuring their responses, and adjusting ourselves to fit. Without ego, all of that disappears, and the focus shifts inward. The outside world grows quiet while the inner voice grows undeniable.

After I resettled back onto the couch, my grandmother remained, her presence as warm and steady as ever. She was there to comfort me, to hold space for my grief as I continued to unravel the depth of my loss. With each passing moment, the weight of it sank in further. Mitzi hadn't just been my aunt, she had been my person. The one who had seen me, loved me, and made me feel safe when no one else could. Now, I was staring into the vast emptiness of a world without her, and the sorrow was almost unbearable.

And then, the healing began. The mushrooms carried me on a mind-blowing journey, one that transcended simple memories. This wasn't just about recalling Mitzi's love; it was about living it, feeling it pulse through me. I wasn't just seeing her love for me; I was seeing myself through her eyes.

¡OYE! Mushrooms might flip your script.

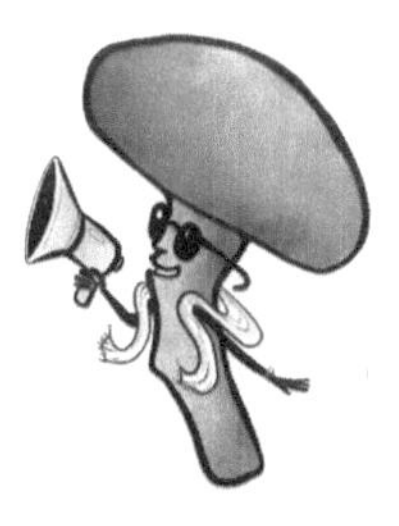

These fungi love a good contradiction. They'll nudge you into the very thing you've spent a lifetime avoiding—because that's how new neural paths are made. Insomniacs sleep. Introverts speak. Control freaks surrender. Don't question... observe.

And let me tell you, it was nothing short of a revelation. I could feel it—the depth of her admiration, the absolute awe she had for me. It wasn't just love, it was a fierce, unwavering belief in my worth. She didn't just care for me; she was mesmerized by the person I had become. Proud, amazed, and in total awe.

And in that moment, her unshakable belief in me became my own, rooted deep within me. It was like she had been planting seeds of self-worth in me all along, and now they were blooming, wild and unstoppable.

I had asked for self-worth, and there it was, being poured into me most unexpectedly, through the unwavering love of my aunt. I had asked for a love letter to myself, and instead, one was being dictated to me. Every ounce of doubt I'd ever carried about myself was being rewritten by her perspective, her truth.

But then, a question formed in my mind, nagging at the edges of this profound experience. *Why can't I feel Mitzi the way I feel my grandmother? If she had truly passed, wouldn't she be here with us?* The thought sent another ripple of uncertainty through me. *Was she really gone? Or was I grieving something that hadn't happened?* The mushrooms had given me clarity, but they had also left me with a mystery—one I wouldn't be able to solve until I returned and reintegrated into the world outside my journey.

The next part of the experience was nothing short of humbling. The mushrooms wrapped me in their love, showering me with immense gratitude for all the work I had been doing to advocate for and educate people about the healing powers of mushrooms. It was as if every cell in my body was soaking up the praise, love, and affirmation. I felt deeply validated in my efforts, as if the universe itself was giving me an enthusiastic "attagirl" for the path I had chosen. The mushrooms seemed to whisper, "Keep going. You're on the right track."

And then, they gave me another directive: *Tell the group about your fundraising efforts for the documentary.*

Just when I thought I couldn't possibly feel more supported, my grandmother returned to me. She urged me to keep following my dream, my re-mission. She spoke of how she had never had the chance to pursue her own dreams, how she had spent her life supporting the dreams of her husband, then her children. She lived in a time when women's hopes and ambitions were viewed as luxuries, indulgences even. Her dreams were silenced before they could take root. And then, with so much love and urgency, she told me that I had to follow my dreams—not just for myself, but for every woman in my lineage who never had the opportunity to do so. She spoke of the importance of honoring them—the women—, of carrying their unfulfilled dreams forward. In their name, she urged me to seize the opportunities before me, to dive into them with everything I had.

Then with surprising clarity, my grandmother told me something that felt both profound and practical: "Sell the ruby ring."

The ruby ring, our shared birthstone, had been a gift from my grandmother that I had always treasured. From that moment, she would tell me the ring was mine, a piece of her that she had passed down to me. It was more than a ring; it was a symbol of the connection between us. That's why I was so surprised, but her voice was insistent: "If you need money to make the movie, sell the ring."

This took me a moment to process. The thought of parting with it felt heavy, like a small piece of her would be gone. But I understood. She wasn't just telling me to part with an object; she was urging me to prioritize my dream, my mission. If it meant moving forward, pushing past obstacles, and taking a step toward making the documentary a reality, then that's precisely what I had to do. I could hear her, loving and wise, reminding me that the essence of what I held dear wasn't the physical object. It was the love, the legacy, and the belief in me that had been passed down along with it.

Later, one of the guides mentioned that the expression on my face during the journey was powerful. Apparently, my jaw was wide open, my head moving up and down, and I kept saying "Okay," as if I were receiving lessons with total acceptance. I looked like an eager student, absorbing everything with reverence and awe. I have no way of knowing whether I was receiving the gratitude from the mushrooms for my advocacy, or if it was the intergenerational message I was hearing from my grandmother, both of which could easily apply in this situation. Either way, the experience was one of deep connection, and I was fully immersed in the moment.

There was more. The mushrooms led me to a topic I hadn't expected to confront: my deep-seated shame about being an American in a room full of Canadians. Suddenly, I felt the full weight of it, the shock of just how much shame I was carrying around the issue. Despite years of personal work aimed at releasing shame, I was taken aback by how deeply it was running through me. It wasn't surprising, though, since psilocybin has the ability to zero in on, then expand upon what we feel, or believe, at our core… This was something that had been quietly brewing in my subconscious, an issue that had recently bubbled up into my conscious mind since arriving at the group experience. The mushrooms allowed me to sit with the uncomfortable feeling just long enough to feel it, to understand its depth.

And then, in their gentle wisdom, they whispered, "Get Laura."

I managed to peel off my eye mask and signal the guides next to me, barely able to speak. I asked for Laura, and in no time, they were bustling to get her attention. Soon, she was there, pulling me into a tight, reassuring hug. In that embrace, I felt the unconditional acceptance and love that Laura had for me, and for all Americans she respected. Something about her warmth and the quiet power of that moment made it all feel okay. Yes, I was American. Yes, I struggled with the way my country had treated other cultures and oppressed people, but in that moment, I understood that that wasn't who all Americans were. It wasn't who *I* was.

Laura's hug was the kind of comfort that melted away the layers of shame and reminded me that I was allowed to stand in my truth, no matter where I came from. That moment, that connection, made my otherness from the group disappear. It was a healing like no other, a moment of deep, humbling acceptance tied to self-worth that I could carry forward with me.

As I slowly opened my eyes and began to re-enter the room, I was struck by the beauty of watching others in the middle of their journeys. It was like witnessing a living, breathing tapestry of human experience unfolding in front of me. One woman lay as still as a board, her body unmoving for the next hour and a half, existing in a state of pure serenity. Another woman was smirking at the air, her hands weaving through invisible threads, making gestures that seemed both mystical and magical. She was contorting into positions that looked almost otherworldly, yet undeniably authentic. Another woman was fully immersed in the music, moving her body as if it were an extension of the sound itself, a dance of pure connection. Another, though, was absent, having slipped upstairs or outside, but her energy still hung in the room like an echo. And then, the guides—each one of them in a state of deep trance, embodying the collective energy of the group in an utterly beautiful way.

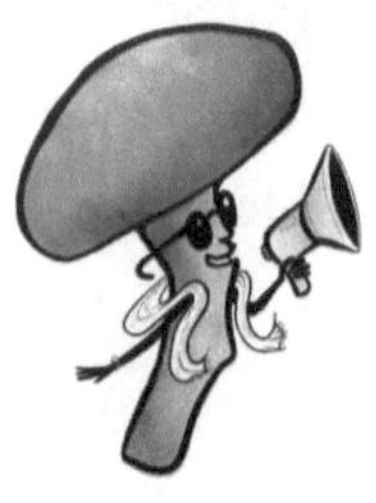

¡OYE! Twitches, tingles, and toe wiggles? Let it happen.

Your body might do some weird stuff: jerks, shudders, sighs. That's not you "losing it." That's you letting go. These odd little releases are your nervous system's way of cleaning house.

I've been known to come out of the cocoon stage of psilocybin relatively quickly, a bit sooner than most people, which sometimes feels like a disadvantage in my own journey. However, that day, it turned out to be a huge advantage. It allowed me to witness the experience not only as a participant but also as an observer. I was able to appreciate the group dynamic and the energy flowing between us. This shift in perspective allowed me to step outside of myself and truly see everyone else, rather than just being absorbed in my own experience.

I was able to focus on the beauty of the group, to feel its collective heartbeat, and to fully absorb the profound connection we all shared. It was as if the boundaries between us began to dissolve, and we were all part of something greater, a unified energy that transcended individual experiences. There was an unspoken understanding that we were all there, not just for ourselves but for each other—supporting, witnessing, and holding space. In that moment, it felt as though the healing wasn't just happening within me, but all around me, woven together through our shared vulnerability and collective intention. It was a profound, almost sacred energy, the kind of connection that can only be felt when people come together with open hearts and minds, bound by a common purpose.

I couldn't help but feel an overwhelming urge to cuddle the entire room. I mean, it was a ridiculous thought, right? Impossible, even. But the desire was so strong, I wanted to hold everyone, one person at a time; or better yet, form a giant human pile of love like some sort of psychedelic puppy pile. Seriously, my brain was like, *Why not? We're all in it together!* The love I felt for everyone around me was so immense that it felt like it could've spilled over the edges of my being and flooded the room. The group energy was so powerful, so awe-inspiring, that I was just sitting there, practically radiating love like a walking, talking hug machine. It was the kind of energy that could probably make a whole room of people turn into human confetti.

Sitting comfortably on the couch, I took it all in. I studied each person in the room, examining their essence, recognizing the unique energy they brought to the group dynamic. It was like I could see each of them on a deeper level, understanding their contributions without needing to say a word. I pulled out my journal and grabbed my felt pen, scribbling down nicknames for everyone present. I couldn't help but laugh at the giant, clumsy letters that filled the page, each word looking like it was written with crayon and twice the size of my usual handwriting. Writing has always been a bit more of a challenge under the influence, but in that moment, it didn't matter. The love and connection flowing through me made everything feel exactly as it should be.

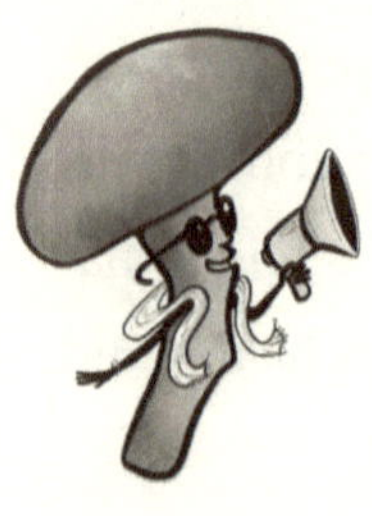

¡OYE! Capture the wisdom before it fades.

Have a journal nearby as you land. You might write like a toddler on a trampoline, and that's perfect. The scribbles, fragments, and run-on thoughts are the footprints of your experience. Don't edit the magic out.

I watched in awe as the flow of the room unfolded like a mesmerizing dance, something I'd never seen before. Each movement, each moment, seemed to flow effortlessly into the next, and it struck me with a powerful revelation: this is what genuine connection and interpersonal living are all about. Individual PAT is incredible for people carrying unresolved trauma, especially if it's their first experience. Still, the true magic of the group lies in its ability to nurture interpersonal skills and foster growth. It's in these collective experiences where transformation happens most profoundly. Individual therapy focuses on intrapersonal development, yes. But group work creates a space where we can thrive together, learning from one another and supporting each other in ways we can't do alone.

As I already mentioned, our weekly Zoom calls in the weeks leading up to the retreat became more than just a logistical check-in—they were the foundation for a deep, unspoken bond that would carry us through the experience. During those calls, we shared not only our professional backgrounds but also our personal challenges, hopes, and vulnerabilities. As we listened to each other, offered support, and shared insights, a trust began to form that felt almost palpable. We weren't just colleagues preparing for a retreat; we were a team, already invested in each other's growth and well-being.

But it wasn't just the Zoom calls that forged this connection. It was the group circles we participated in once we arrived at the retreat location. These circles became sacred spaces where we could continue building on that foundation of trust. Sharing in person, holding space for each other's stories, and offering heartfelt support strengthened our collective bond. By the time we gathered in the treatment room, this connection had created a powerful container for the experience. The love, safety, and collective intention we had cultivated made it possible for each of us to lean into the journey with open hearts, knowing that we were held, supported, and truly seen. We weren't alone in our healing; we were in it together, and that made all the difference.

A perfect example was the Laura moment.

As the journey continued, small plates with light snacks appeared before each of us; a thoughtful touch to help our bodies gently re-engage with the physical world. Cheese, pretzels, grapes, nuts, apple slices, and M&M's: a beautiful array of textures and flavors designed to bring us back to the room with others, to reawaken our senses, and allow us to feel grounded again. It was the perfect way to reconnect, both with ourselves and with the incredible energy swirling around the room.

I continued to process Mitzi's death, and I couldn't help but wonder: why were the mushrooms showing me this, especially when I had never experienced _ego death_ myself? I had heard stories from others who had undergone what they described as ego death—those profound moments where the boundaries of self seem to dissolve, and you merge with everything around you. People who experience this often report feeling as though they are no longer distinct from everything around them; they become one with the universe. It's usually a hallmark of high-dose psilocybin experiences, typically at hero doses (5 grams or more). Some people may even encounter it during therapeutic macrodoses (3-4 grams), where the intensity is enough to challenge the ego and invite them into a deeper connection with their true nature.

Ego death is widely regarded as a powerful, transformative experience in the psychedelic world. It is said to be the unraveling of the "self," where the sense of separation from others, from the world, and even from the universe fades away. In its place, there is often a profound sense of unity, oneness, or interconnectedness. The purpose of ego death is to transcend the limitations imposed by the ego—the part of ourselves that clings to identity, fear, and separation—and to experience a more expansive, broader sense of being. Many people who undergo ego death report seeing the world in a completely new light, free from the filters and judgments that typically shape their perceptions. It's in this state that some of the most profound insights, the "nuggets" of wisdom, are often revealed.

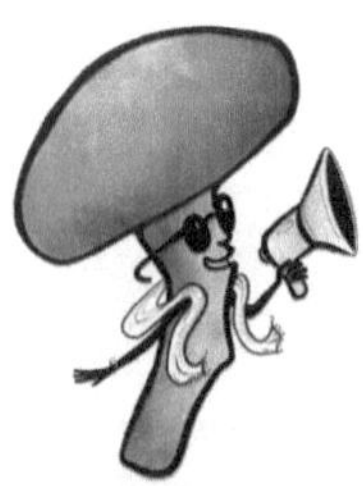

¡OYE! You don't need a "hero" dose to find your inner hero.

Ego dissolution often happens between 2–4 grams with a proper mindset.

When my clients undergo ego death, which is a rare occurrence and happens in less than 5% of the journeys, I guide them to lean into the experience rather than resist it. While it can feel overwhelming, disorienting, and even terrifying, ego death is ultimately about the rebirth that follows. I remind them that the dissolution of their sense of self is not an end, but rather a transformative process, creating space for new growth, insights, and a deeper understanding of who they truly are. I also reassure them that their bodies won't die—that they are safe throughout the entire process. The sensations they may be experiencing are not signs of physical danger, but rather part of the deep unraveling of the ego. It's an opportunity to shed old patterns, beliefs, and limitations that no longer serve them, allowing their true essence to emerge. I remind them that, although it feels like they're losing themselves in the moment, they are being re-formed and reconnected to the vastness of existence, ready to emerge with a fresh perspective on life.

However, I had never experienced ego death myself. I had always wondered if I was somehow missing out; if it was something I was supposed to go through to heal truly. But then, the mushroom revealed something to me that I hadn't expected. The message that came through was nothing short of mind-blowing: I hadn't valued myself enough for ego death to hold meaning for me. Instead, Mitzi's death was exactly what I needed to receive the message of my self-worth. That realization hit me like a ton of bricks: Mitzi's death was more impactful to me than ego death. In that moment, I understood that I hadn't needed to dissolve my ego to feel connected or to gain clarity. What I needed, in that instant, was to understand the depth of my worth, and Mitzi's death had unlocked that understanding.

I couldn't believe it. The death of the ego was something that others talked about with reverence, but I realized that for me, my healing didn't require losing myself—it required finding myself.

Mitzi's death was my teacher in that moment, showing me that self-worth was the key to everything. Wow!

Eventually, everyone who had left the room trickled back during the final song of the playlist, *Here Comes the Sun*. We had been instructed beforehand to come back together so we could close the ritual as a group, just as we had started it. There was something wonderful about that moment—seeing all of us reunited, slowly reorienting to the space and one another. It felt like we were all coming back from our journeys, but still somehow woven together in a shared, sacred experience. The energy in the room was palpable, like a collective sigh of relief, or perhaps a quiet sense of accomplishment. It was a moment of pure connection, and the warmth of being together in that space made everything feel right.

As much as I longed to check my phone, there was a part of me that wanted to delay just a little longer. I realized there was a strange comfort in being suspended in space and time, not knowing whether my aunt was alive or not. It felt almost like a buffer, a way to keep my emotions from crashing. But then, as clarity washed over me, I realized it didn't matter. I was ready to face whatever the truth was. If she had passed, I would find peace in the memories we had shared. If she was still alive, I would cherish her even more deeply. Once I found that peace within myself, I picked up my phone, turned it on, and saw no new notifications. *Whew.*

The first message I sent was to Mitzi.

It was simple, yet from the depths of my heart: "I love you so much."

Her reply came quickly, "Oohh... I love you so much too!"

I paused before replying, still overwhelmed and unable to explain what had just transpired. The mushrooms were still working their way out of my system, and words felt elusive. I needed more time to process and understand before I could even begin to make sense of it all. I would reply later.

After the journey, we were given some free time before dinner, an opportunity to do whatever felt right. We could journal, meditate, process verbally, soak in the hot tub, or just be in our own space. I spent the time outside on the back patio, talking to the guides about what had just unfolded. I was processing, trying to make sense of everything that had happened. Verbal repetition is my go-to method for processing, so I was eager to share my experience with anyone who would listen. Thankfully, after the powerful group bond we had created, there was no shortage of people willing to engage, share, and listen.

¡OYE! You just came back from the moon, don't rush into Costco.

Integration takes time. Your nervous system needs soft landings, not loud errands. Go slow. Go tender. You're still reassembling.

By the time dinner was served, I was absolutely famished. I had spent so much energy that day with little fuel to sustain me, and I felt weak but deeply grateful for the meal. There's something about the aftermath of a psilocybin journey for me that makes food especially tasty, making the soup that was offered that evening like a gift from the heavens. It was warm, comforting, and exactly what my body and soul needed, filling me in a way that was so much more than just physical nourishment. It was as though every spoonful was healing, restorative, and grounding me after the emotional and energetic rollercoaster of the day.

After dinner, we gathered for an integration circle where we could each share our experiences. When it was my turn, I did my best to summarize the profound experience of Mitzi's death. I spoke about how powerful it was to see my grandmother. In all the journeys I had experienced, I had never been visited by anyone: no loved ones, no old pets, no aliens, and certainly no creatures on a train offering cake, as others had shared with me. I don't know if it was the group energy that made the visit possible, but at that moment, I didn't care how or why. I was just grateful that it finally happened.

I found myself finally able to confront a question that had been tugging at me all day: *Why did the mushrooms make me believe Mitzi had died? Why couldn't I simply see myself through her eyes without imagining that loss? What was the purpose of this?* As the layers of understanding unfolded, it became clear that it was essential for me to fully comprehend just how profoundly important Mitzi was in my life. Only when I grasped that truth could I begin to understand the depth of her love for me and recognize how deeply she valued me. To truly appreciate her perspective on me, I had to first be made to realize how much I valued her—her presence, her love, her wisdom, and the lasting impact she had on me. The mushrooms understood that for me to reach this awareness, Mitzi had to die in my experience, so I could fully grasp the immeasurable significance of her life.

As I was still reflecting on this insight, the mushrooms nudged my brain again. I was told, gently but firmly, that I must ask the group for help with my documentary fundraising. I didn't want to, of course. This wasn't something that came easily for me. But I knew that the mushrooms didn't care about what I wanted. They always gave me what I needed, and what I needed was to put myself out there and ask for support. So, reluctantly, and with a bit of hesitation, I shared my fundraising request, explaining my mission to spread the word about the therapeutic potential of mushrooms and how I needed help to make it happen.

The room was quiet for a moment, and then, as if the universe had been waiting for this exact moment to unfold, Peg spoke up. He shared that he was an executive producer on the film *Dosed 2*, and that we should talk later. My jaw nearly hit the floor. *What?! Dosed 2* was one of the few films out there that captured stories in the exact way I had envisioned for my own project. While many films focused on science and research, *Dosed* and *Dosed 2* were unique in their approach, telling stories of real people, from before their journeys to after. And here I was, sitting right in front of someone who had already been a part of the very type of film I wanted to create. I couldn't believe it.

I was still processing the overwhelming energy of the mushrooms–and now this. I kept pinching myself, wondering if this was real or if I was still in some dreamlike state. The synchronicity of it all was too much to wrap my mind around.

What I would come to understand later was that mushrooms had directed me to make that fundraising request not because I was seeking money, but because I was meant to cross paths with someone who would guide the next step of my journey.

A week later, I hadn't even begun filming my first documentary, and there I was, seriously considering the production of a second one. I couldn't even recognize the life I was living anymore—it was like the version of myself from six months ago had vanished, and I was stepping into something entirely new. I was still reeling from the afterglow of the experience, unsure whose life I was even living.

The day after the ceremony, Peg and I had a brief but meaningful conversation about the importance of sharing our stories. We both agreed that focusing on the human aspect was crucial—not the science, which was already well-covered, but the real stories of people whose lives were being transformed. The world needed to see the entire journey: from before the treatment, through the experience itself, and into the integration phase, so they could truly understand its profound impact. That conversation stayed with me, and less than a week later, while in Whistler processing my own experience, I scheduled an online meeting with him.

When we met, Peg proposed something that blew me away. He suggested that we team up for another documentary film. This new project would focus on the Gathering Group process. It would show the magic and healing that happens when people come together in this safe, supportive environment and container. I was still reeling from my own experience, unsure of which way was up, but somehow, it felt like this was all meant to be. The synchronicity of everything, of the mushrooms guiding me to make the connection, and of the universe presenting an opportunity so perfectly aligned with my vision was overwhelming. It was like my entire life had led me to that very moment.

CHAPTER THIRTEEN

SUMMIT OF SELF-WORTH

THAT NIGHT, AFTER THE DOSE, I was utterly exhausted. My body and mind were spent from the intensity of the journey, and all I could do was surrender to the stillness that followed. But even in the haze, one thing rose to the surface with startling clarity: I needed to see Aunt Mitzi. Not eventually. Not when it was convenient. As soon as I got home. I still had several days left of the retreat, and I wouldn't be flying back until the end of the week, landing close to midnight. But the pull to connect with her was so strong, so insistent, that I couldn't wait even a few more days to make the ask. That night, I sent her a text from my room, asking if she'd be free for breakfast or brunch shortly after I returned. I'm sure it seemed like an odd time to make plans—halfway through a retreat, in another country, messaging her in the middle of the night. But to my relief, she responded warmly and agreed. We set a date.

That simple exchange felt like a weight lifted off my shoulders. The only downside to my pre-planned week-long vacation to Whistler was that it now felt like it stood between me and seeing Mitzi. I had been so excited for the vacation, but after my journey, the thought of waiting another week to be with her made the time apart feel almost unbearable. I couldn't wait to see her, and the vacation, which had once been a much-needed getaway, now felt like an obstacle in the way of that reunion. Scheduling the brunch, though, gave me something to look forward to: a tangible date with her that kept me grounded through the days ahead.

I woke up the next morning feeling both refreshed and exhausted, like I had run a marathon while simultaneously attending a cosmic rave. But all I could think about was Mitzi. I knew one thing for sure: I HAD to talk to her. Even before I could lift the covers, I reached for my phone, feeling a lot more centered and ready to articulate the mind-bending experience I had just gone through. She picked up on the second ring.

Without wasting a second, I blurted out, "I love you so very much."

She replied, "I love you too, but what on earth is going on with you?"

"Well, buckle up," I said, "because this is going to sound crazy, so ground yourself."

I proceeded to recount my entire trip to the best of my ability. It felt like trying to summarize a rollercoaster ride while riding it. When I told her that I got to feel how incredibly cool she's always thought I was, she deadpanned, "I've always thought you were cool."

I quickly shot back, "I know, I really, really felt it to my core."

I couldn't stop gushing about how much she'd always been one of the greatest loves of my life. I thanked her for being so deeply important to me, and how ridiculously lucky I felt that she's alive and I'd get to see her soon. It was as though I had a cosmic permission slip to let her know just how much she meant to me. It was, frankly, a lot of love for one phone call, but I was okay with that.

I found myself at breakfast, eagerly sharing and processing the Laura portion of my journey. I described how her words the day before had created a pivotal moment of connection, allowing me to embrace and accept myself in a way I hadn't before. One of the group members summed it up perfectly with a burst of laughter: "Nationality! It's so made up!" It was the kind of laugh that revealed how absurdly silly we humans can be—those arbitrary labels we cling to, the imaginary lines we draw. It was also one of those classic "cutting through the BS" moments that so often arise when the ego dissolves and we glimpse what really matters. The lightness in the room, the shared laughter, underscored the power of group energy to bond, heal, and unite us in ways our thinking minds could never engineer.

After breakfast, we went through the same routine as the day before, only this time, I was the one standing around the table while others chose their dried mushrooms, measured them out, and created their connections to the mushrooms before preparing them for tea. It felt like such an honor to give back what had been so generously given to me the day before. People with natural caretaking instincts often find deep fulfillment in sharing what they've received, and I was no exception. Having just experienced one of the most profound days of my life, I felt a deep sense of excitement and anticipation to witness others having their own transformative experiences. I knew the depth of what was about to unfold for them, and it filled me with a sense of purpose and gratitude.

As the participants settled into their spaces, the guides prepared the tea, and the same rituals from the day before were lovingly repeated. The group engaged in the *Seven Directions Prayer*, grounding themselves in reverence and connection, before donning their eye masks and headphones, ready to embark on their journeys.

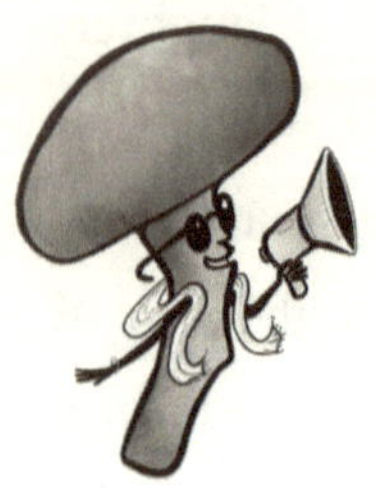

¡OYE! Music becomes a bridge.

The right playlist can become the soundtrack to your healing—even after the journey ends.

As the familiar music from the day before played, I found myself deeply appreciating the sounds that accompanied such a powerful experience. I was scribbling in my journal, trying to capture the flood of insights from the day prior, when suddenly, a song began to play. It was the song that had been playing when my grandmother told me that my aunt had passed. In an instant, I was transported back to that gut-wrenching moment, and every feeling came rushing back like a tidal wave. My stomach dropped, and a suffocating wave of grief enveloped me. Tears began to pour down my face uncontrollably. Mitzi was gone...again.

I doubled over, overwhelmed by the emotional weight, and knew I had to leave the room to let my body fully release the grief. A guide, sensing my distress, gently approached and offered to support me. I made my way upstairs, my body instinctively falling to the floor, stretching into yoga poses that seemed to ground me in the midst of the overwhelming sobs. Each stretch helped me move through the grief that had taken hold of me.

CATHERINE - *I saw myself, through the eyes of*

someone who adores me.

MARIA - *Yes.*

That love was always there.

You just needed to remember.

CATHERINE - *I've always pushed it aside.*

MARIA - *You put others first.*

Now, you see.

CATHERINE - *I never knew my worth like this.*

MARIA - *Your worth isn't theirs to define.*

It's your birthright.

Now, you see it.

CATHERINE - *Why did I need to feel it again,*

while guiding?

MARIA - *You needed to remember.*

You melted into the background to survive.

Now, step into the center.

CATHERINE - *The group energy carried me deeper.*

MARIA - *Yes.*

The group holds what you cannot reach alone.

You are seen now.

And you are whole.

After what felt like an eternity, but was likely about twenty minutes, the trainer who had guided our group came to me and asked if he could hold space for me. His presence was a gift: a loving, comforting act that reminded me I wasn't alone in such a moment of raw emotion.

Our conversation helped me integrate the intense feelings that had resurfaced. At one point, I asked him, "Why did mushrooms give me Mitzi's death, instead of the usual ego-death?" His response was nothing short of profound. He explained that children of trauma don't have the luxury of developing a strong ego, so they don't need it to die. Ego-death is for those who are rigid, and stubborn—those who need to go through a death to experience rebirth. This insight hit me deeply, reminding me that there wasn't much space for my ego in the dark shadow of my mother's spotlight. It was like a door opening to a new layer of understanding.

However, what struck me about the experience was the disorienting disconnect between my logical brain and my emotional heart. Logically, I knew Mitzi was alive, but emotionally, my heart reacted as if she were gone. It was so confusing, and an overwhelming emotional contradiction. Yet, I began to understand that in addition to the wisdom and clarity I'd gained the day before, mushrooms had also gifted me the ability to process shock in real-time. I felt an unexpected sense of gratitude, gratitude that, when the inevitable happens, I will have the strength to navigate it. It will still be unbearably hard, yes, but I know I won't be shattered by it in the same way. Life without her will never be the same—like a missing piece of a puzzle that makes it incomplete—but she will live on in me, in my heart, as long as my heart beats.

I returned to the group and rejoined the flow of the day, feeling a sense of calm as I resumed my role as a guide. I was able to fully embrace the rest of the journey, watching the dosing participants move through their emotional highs and lows. It was fascinating to witness the ebb and flow of their experiences, the way they'd settle into deep introspection, only to be swept up by waves of emotion, or how they'd surge with energy, and then find peace in stillness. Each person's process was uniquely their own, yet all of it was woven into the shared experience of the group. I felt deeply connected to their journeys, and at the same time, grounded in my own. It was a privilege to observe them as they navigated the complexities of their minds and hearts, feeling both awe and reverence for what was unfolding before me. I decided to jot down a second list of nicknames for everyone in my journal, each one reflecting the piece they contributed to the whole on this second day of journeying.

As the familiar playlist played on, I couldn't help but remember bits and pieces of my journey. With each song that replayed, flashes of my experience from the day before resurfaced. Some memories were crystal clear while others were hazy, like trying to recall a dream upon waking. Yet, each song seemed to unlock something new, a gentle reminder of the powerful emotions and insights I had encountered. I was amazed at how music could act as a bridge with sense memory, taking me back to that space of transformation. Even as I focused on supporting the group, my own journey was still unfolding in the background, woven into the threads of the collective experience.

On the final day of our journey together, we gathered for a closing integration circle. It was a moment of reflection, a space where we could honor the experiences we'd shared and acknowledge how far we had all come. As I stood before the group, I had the chance to share the nicknames I had given each of them, and for me, it was one of the most beautiful moments of the whole retreat. There was something special about hearing each person's essence captured in a two or three-word phrase, seeing how they were each uniquely woven into the fabric of our collective journey. It was like giving them the gift of being truly seen.

But then, when I finished, I asked, a little unsure of myself, "Did I miss anyone?"

Just as I thought I was done, another voice rose from the group: "Someone is missing from that list!" My heart skipped a beat.

Slightly embarrassed, I quickly asked, "Who?"

And with a grin, the group member replied, "You! You're missing from your own list! And I've got the perfect nickname for you… Honorary Canadian!"

The room erupted in laughter and agreement, and I felt a profound wave of warmth rush over me. It was as if everyone was wrapping me up in the same love and belonging I had witnessed them receive. They were bringing me into the fold, giving me a place in the circle, a spot in their hearts, and it hit me like a tidal wave of emotion. The floodgates opened, and I was overwhelmed with tears of joy, feeling deeply connected and completely seen. I couldn't speak after that, my voice lost in the depths of the gratitude and love that washed over me. We closed the circle, and with it, the retreat. But not before I was reminded of the beautiful truth: I truly belonged here, and I was part of something far greater than myself.

With the medicine's echoes still humming in my heart, we were asked to gather the truths we had uncovered and place them into words. The first invitation was to complete a series of *I AM* statements—small seeds of self-definition, planted in the fertile soil of transformation. The second was a letter to ourselves, written as if to a beloved, so that we might remember the tenderness we are worthy of.

I AM Statements

I am worthy.

I am flawed and it doesn't diminish me.

*I am my aunt's niece, and she values me. As do my
other family members and friends.*

I am proud of the work I have done and continue to do.

*I am not my country just as I am not my mother
or my father.*

*I walk a new path—one my foremothers never had
the chance to take. I do it for me, and I do it in
their honor.*

Love Letter to Myself

Dearest Catherine,

*You are the love of my life. In every way, you embody
courage, not just in the way you love others, but in
the way you are learning to love yourself. You are
worthy of all the love you give, and so much more.
You work tirelessly, pouring yourself into everything
and everyone, yet you so often forget to give that
same devotion to yourself.*

*Your heart radiates with such warmth and light that it
touches everyone you encounter. Your authenticity
is rare and precious. It's the kind of soul-deep truth
that others aspire to, but few dare to live. Your
capacity to be real, to be vulnerable, and to show
up in the world as you are, is beyond inspiring and
the stuff of legends!*

Now, I ask you to be brave in the way you love
yourself. You are worthy of all the joy, peace, and
abundance this world has to offer. You've done
the work. You've healed, you've grown, and you
continue to evolve. Keep believing in yourself,
because I believe in you. And I'll always be here
to remind you of how incredibly loved, valued, and
needed you are.
With all my heart,
Catherine

Leaving the retreat, I carried my *I AM* statements and love letter like treasures. These were quiet reminders that the work we do on the inside must eventually meet the tests of the outside world. Integration isn't just about holding onto insights; it's about seeing whether they can survive in the wild chaos of real life.

And, as fate would have it, my first test arrived almost immediately in Whistler.

I was floored by how my sense of self-worth unfolded in Whistler. It was like watching a superhero discover their powers, only instead of flying or turning invisible, I was learning to treat myself with respect. A few major things stood out, showcasing just how far I'd come since my hero dose experience.

The first involved the vacation home I'd rented for my stay in Whistler. The original place had fallen through, so I scrambled to find an alternative. The new place seemed decent enough. The pictures looked pretty, and it was located in the heart of a ski village. I didn't anticipate that parking would be much farther away than expected or advertised, and my hips weren't exactly happy about the long walk. But, fine—just a minor inconvenience, something I could manage. What I didn't see coming was unlocking the door to the one-bedroom condo and being blasted by the relentless pounding of ranchero and club music from the Mexican restaurant directly below. It hit me like a sledgehammer. Boom! I was pretty sure my brain was still vibrating from the bass by the time I closed the door.

I tried to convince myself it wasn't that big of a deal, that I could just power through it, but after hours of blasting bass pounding through the walls, it became glaringly obvious this was not the peaceful, serene space I needed to write my book. I made it through the first night, hoping the music would magically stop at 9 p.m. (spoiler: it didn't). By the time my sanity was hanging by a thread, I had somehow fallen asleep with my headphones on. I wasn't even sure when the music finally gave up. The walls were still vibrating when I drifted off.

The next morning, I woke up to a brief, heavenly moment of silence...until around 10 a.m., when the music came back like an unwanted encore at a bad concert. That was it! I'd had enough! I could already hear the music calling me from the depths of the condo, so I made an executive decision: *I'm outta here.* I decided to treat myself to the Scandinavian Spa I'd been eyeing since I made the vacation plans. If the music wasn't going to stop, at least I could immerse myself in something that didn't make me want to pull my hair out.

Walking into the spa felt like stepping into a dream. Everything was more beautiful, more serene, more luxurious than I could have imagined. The very air felt richer, filled with an energy of calm and indulgence that made my heart race. As I stood in line to register, I couldn't help but feel a surge of discomfort, like a fish out of water. The high-end vibe of the place—its polished elegance, the effortlessly chic people floating around—was worlds apart from anything I was used to since my health issues became my central focus. The high admission fee hit me like a jolt, and, for a second, I almost second-guessed myself. In the past, I would've talked myself out of it: *You can spend your money elsewhere–more effectively.* But that day was different. That day, I wasn't the same person I'd been before. I felt worthy. I deserved to be there, to experience something special, to embrace the beauty around me. And as I stood there, I realized it wasn't just about the spa. It was about honoring my new sense of self-worth, about saying yes to something that had always felt out of reach.

Then, as if the universe was speaking directly to me, a woman in a robe walked by and casually said, "I deserve this. I feel so worthy of this amazing place." Her words landed like a spark in dry tinder. It was as though she had read my soul, offering the exact affirmation I didn't even know I'd been waiting for.

I drew in a deep breath, letting it settle into my chest, rewiring something in real time. Neuroplasticity in motion. I wasn't just here. I belonged here.

And to seal it, I straightened my back, lifted my chin, and said it aloud, clear enough for the air itself to carry: "I deserve this. I am worthy of this amazing place."

The old me would have whispered it in doubt.

The new me declared my new truth.

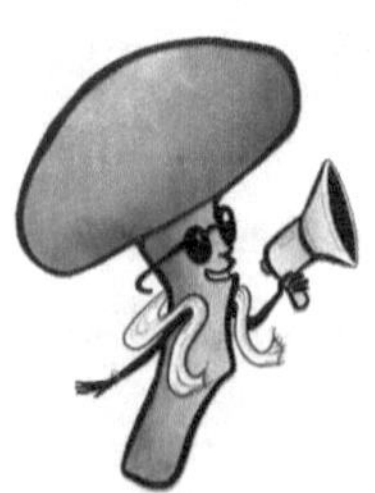

¡OYE! Expect unexpected shifts afterward.

Mushrooms move you. Literally. Sleep patterns, moods, behaviors... they all might shift.

When it was my turn to register, the attendant asked if I wanted a robe for an extra fee. Without hesitation, I grinned and said, "Absolutely!"

Gone were the doubts, the guilt. I was standing in the power of my new identity. And when I was offered a massage, I didn't even need to think twice before deciding to skip it. It wasn't about what I "should" do—it was about trusting my intuition and honoring what my body truly needed that day. My gut told me it wasn't a day for a massage. *That's something I can get anywhere*, I thought. Instead, I wanted to focus on the new opportunities the place offered. I felt like I was finally living the life I had always dreamed of, without holding myself back.

As I stood in the locker room, holding the swimsuit in my hands, I felt my heart race. The next test presented itself.

It had been twenty-five years since I'd worn a swimsuit in front of anyone other than my husband. The thought alone sent waves of self-doubt crashing over me. I had spent most of my life avoiding moments like this, hiding behind oversized clothes, never wearing shorts in public, and convincing myself that I wasn't "worthy" of being seen. And yet, there I was, about to step into a swimsuit, an act so simple for others, but for me, a monumental leap.

I had bought the swimsuit intentionally, with the hope of fully embracing the experience for which I'd been longing. It wasn't just about the spa. It was about reclaiming my power, my worth. I wasn't going to let the fear of judgment hold me back anymore. I was going to step into my discomfort and break free.

My heart raced as I stood there, clutching not one, but two towels, feeling like a total outsider in a world of relaxation. Everyone else seemed so confident, so at ease, carrying just one towel like they had been born into a world of calm. Meanwhile, I stood there, awkward and self-conscious, questioning my every move. Doubts crashed over me like waves, and I almost turned back, thinking, *Maybe I don't belong here...maybe I'm not ready for this.* The tension in my body surged as self-doubt swirled. *Am I crazy for even being here?* It all felt like too much. My insecurities paralyzed me, and the only thing that made sense was to retreat to the locker room for a moment of safety.

Just as I was running back, desperate to escape, I heard it—my name. *Wait, what?* I froze. *My name? In Whistler, of all places?* The only Canadians I knew had just parted ways the day before, two hours away. This was surreal. I couldn't believe it. My feet kept moving toward the locker room, my safe haven, thinking it must be someone calling out to another person named Catherine... but then—there it was again.

"Catherine!"

I turned around, utterly stunned. And there, standing in front of me, was Olivia, one of the people I had just spent the weekend with. My heart leaped. The moment I saw her face, every ounce of insecurity vanished, like fog lifting off a mountain. I was flooded with gratitude. It was like the universe had conspired to remind me that I *was* deserving of the moment, the space, the peace. As she pulled me into a hug, I felt a rush of relief, joy, and connection flood over me. This was the sign I needed, an affirmation that I was exactly where I was meant to be. And in that embrace, I realized I was worthy of such a beautiful, unexpected gift.

It was the universe's perfect sign. Right there, in the middle of a gorgeous spa, in a place where I felt like an outsider just moments before, I knew I was exactly where I was meant to be. Olivia introduced me to her partner, and we eagerly swapped stories. She was there to continue processing the weekend with her partner, and I was there to experience something that felt so far beyond the reach of my ordinary life in New Mexico. Just moments ago, I had been questioning my place in such a beautiful, strange location, but then, all that doubt evaporated.

The rest of the day at the spa felt like a dream, a deeply healing, soul-nourishing experience. I floated in the water, feeling every muscle in my body release its tension, and meditated, surrendering to the peaceful energy around me. I journaled, letting my thoughts pour onto the pages, capturing a peace I hadn't felt in years. I even crossed paths with Olivia and her partner again. Our brief reunion, filled with laughter and shared moments, reminded me of the incredible bond that had formed over the weekend. It was as if the universe had conspired to give me exactly what I needed.

I returned to the vacation home rental, and, once again, the music hit me like a freight train full of subwoofers. The pounding bass shook the walls, body-slamming the calm I had so carefully cultivated at the spa. I was being tested—again. But this time, I wasn't going to sit back and let my former patterns take over. The old me might have put up with the noise, accepting it as part of the journey. But the new me? She wasn't having it. I immediately pulled out my phone, found another vacation home to rent nearby, and booked it without hesitation.

As I packed up my things and made the trek back to the car, dragging my bags behind me, I felt a rush of empowerment. Every wheel of my suitcase squeaking across the floor was like a tiny victory cheer. It was a huge shift for me. I was taking decisive action that honored my sense of self-worth. I wasn't going to settle. Not anymore. No more tolerating what drained me. No more telling myself "it's fine" when it wasn't. That walk to the car felt like my own personal parade toward self-respect, and the only beat I was listening to now was my own.

When I arrived at the new vacation home, it was everything I'd dreamed of: private, cozy, and peaceful. It was like a sanctuary, free from the noise that had threatened to undo my peace. And then, I saw it: the private hot tub. The one thing I had sacrificed when the original place fell through, now right there, waiting for me.

Without a second thought, I threw down my bags, stripped off the stress of the day, and slipped into the warm, soothing water. As I sank in, every muscle seemed to relax, and every thought quieted. It wasn't just a hot tub; it was a symbol of my growth, a tangible reward for finally putting myself first. It was as though everything had quietly aligned to give me this moment of pure peace, and I couldn't help but smile.

For the first time in a long time, I was fully aligned with myself: my actions, my decisions, and my self-worth. This wasn't just a change of scenery; this was a change of heart, a victory in self-care, a celebration of embracing who I truly am. And it felt *so* damn good. I did some of my deepest integration work right there in that steaming cocoon, letting the insights from my hero journey settle in as easily as my shoulders sank below the surface.

For the first time in a long time, I was fully aligned with myself: my actions, my decisions, and my self-worth. This wasn't just a change of scenery; this was a change of heart, a victory in self-care, a celebration of embracing who I truly am. And it felt so damn good. I did some of my deepest integration work right there in that steaming cocoon, letting the insights from my hero journey settle in as easily as my shoulders sank below the surface. In that moment, I saw how self-care was not separate from integration. It was the act of weaving self-worth into my daily choices, exactly as I had intended. Integration is not just remembering the insight, but embodying it.

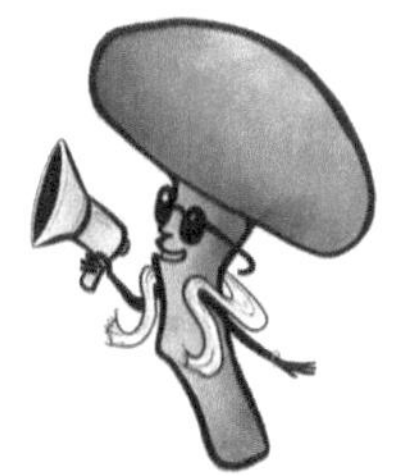

¡OYE! Integration isn't extra credit.

Taking care of yourself *is* the work. Every boundary you set, every moment you choose rest over rush, every act of kindness toward yourself—that's integration in motion.

From that moment on, Whistler felt like a dream, one that I was finally living. I met up with two incredible group members who lived nearby, and we dove into deep, soul-nourishing conversations that felt like a continuation of the journey I had started. We shared our stories, reflected on the experience, and I felt the magic of connection in every word. It was as if we were all healing and integrating, in this sacred space, in this beautiful place.

A hardcore thrill came when one of my group members got me a free ticket to the Sea to Sky gondola ride in Squamish, about 45 minutes away. They had no idea I was terrified of heights, and the mere thought of going on the skylift certainly caused my heart to race. I never would have done it on my own, but with the ticket in hand, there was no turning back. As the gondola rose higher and higher, my stomach did flips, and the view of the mountains rising from the mist and the vast expanse of the ocean below was breathtaking. It was terrifying, yet exhilarating. At that moment, I realized that facing my fear had become my new superpower, and I was so grateful to my friend for unknowingly encouraging me to step into the unknown.

As I took in the beauty of it all, something inside me shifted again. I reflected on how much had changed in such a short time. The mushrooms had opened a door to my soul, revealing my inherent worth. And now, I was living that truth in every breath, every action. The self-doubt that once held me back was fading, replaced by a fierce belief in my strength and value. I finally learned to honor myself, to accept that I am worthy of all the love, peace, joy, and beauty that life has to offer.

It felt like I was standing on the edge of the world, not just physically, but emotionally—fearless, alive, and ready to claim all that was mine.

In the end, the vacation home above the Mexican restaurant agreed to give me a partial refund since I had stayed there for only one night. But when I crunched the numbers, I was stunned: The amount I lost in the switch was almost the same as the cost of the massage I had instinctively chosen to skip. Within one dollar, to be exact.

At the time, I hadn't fully understood why my gut told me to forgo the massage, but, in the end, it all made sense. That deep, intuitive voice had been guiding me toward something even more important—real rest, real peace, and a space that truly nurtured me. It was as if the universe had orchestrated a perfect trade: a night of relentless bass and sleepless frustration in exchange for quiet serenity, a hot tub under the stars, and the ultimate lesson in trusting and valuing myself. Amazing.

CATHERINE - *I spoke my truth.*

   I said the thing I was scared to say.

MARIA - *And what did you see in their eyes?*

CATHERINE - *Not pity. Not judgment.*

   Curiosity. Respect.

   Maybe even... admiration?

MARIA - *That's not a reflection of them.*

   That is your worth, mirrored back.

CATHERINE - *I didn't even have to ask for*

   help out loud.

MARIA - *No, but your soul did.*

   And the universe was listening.

CATHERINE - *I feel more grounded.*

   The earth feels steadier.

MARIA - *The burden was never yours alone.*

   Your journey continues.

CASE STUDY: PATTY

Demographics

Patty is a 53-year-old woman from El Paso, Texas. She is the youngest of six siblings and has lived her entire life in the border town. She is married to her high school sweetheart, and together they raised four children who are now grown and living independently. Patty is also a grandmother.

Presenting Problem / Chief Concern

Patty described her primary issue as fear. In her words: "fear of everything." She had tried to manage this fear with anti-anxiety and antidepressant medications, cannabis, yoga, meditation classes, and other approaches that offered hope of relief. Meditation had been the most helpful, as it provided self-awareness and prepared her for psilocybin-assisted therapy. Through meditation, she learned to pause the ruminating process long enough to examine how trauma had shaped her worldview. She began to see how her past influenced her present, and she was ready to change her future.

Despite this awareness, she continued to struggle with changing her thoughts and beliefs. Fear remained her constant companion, robbing her of sleep, peace, and joy. She suffered from agoraphobia, feared losing loved ones, feared her own death, and often spiraled into worst-case scenarios. Her mind was dominated by severe negative self-talk and relentless rumination, cycling through imagined catastrophes and self-blame that only deepened her exhaustion and despair.

Background and Trauma History

Patty's childhood was marked by family conflict and her father's pattern of disappearing from the home. By the age of seven, she had developed a nightly ritual of staying awake until she heard any sign that he might return, straining to catch the sound of a car or watching for headlights flickering across her bedroom wall. While her siblings slept soundly in their rooms, Patty fought to stay awake, terrified that if she fell asleep she would miss her chance to intervene. Each time her father did come home, she would rush out of bed and place herself between her parents, believing it was her duty to prevent another fight. Even as a young child, she assumed the role of family referee.

She witnessed many painful arguments and felt responsible when she was not there to intervene. Both parents would turn to Patty as a "marriage counselor," pulling her into conflicts far beyond a child's grasp. She was exposed to her father's relationships with other women and to her mother's heartbreak and fury. Her father would sometimes be gone for days or even weeks at a time, leaving Patty to absorb the tension and confusion that followed.

She remembers a pregnancy with another woman that resulted in the loss of a baby. Her father grieved openly and expected Patty to help him process his pain, while her mother was consumed by betrayal and rage.

As a child, Patty did not understand these dynamics, but she absorbed the emotional wounds. She prayed nightly for peace, pleading with God to protect her family. When her prayers did not stop the fighting, she began to believe God had forsaken her. She developed the belief that God's love might be conditional and that she might be unworthy of love altogether.

This childhood trauma left her in a chronic state of hypervigilance. She carried it into adulthood. Patty married her high school sweetheart and became a devoted mother of four. Later, she also became the caretaker for both aging parents. When her parents traveled to Mexico and were in a tragic car accident, her mother was killed instantly. Patty delayed her grief to care for her father, who moved in with her until his death three years later.

Patty was consumed with guilt and shame about both losses. She regretted not fully grieving her mother and lamented the lack of closure with her father. Even four years after his death, she remained tormented. She recognized that her identity was built around "holding vigil" for others. She had done so as a child for her parents, as a mother for her children, and later as a caretaker for her aging parents.

By the time she came for psilocybin-assisted therapy, Patty could not recall a time when she was not holding vigil for someone. She described herself as haunted by existential fears, overwhelmed by negative self-talk, and perpetually exhausted from sleepless nights.

Psychosocial and Medical History

She had no reported history of substance misuse. Her medical history was not remarkable outside of the psychological concerns and eating patterns related to self-soothing at night.

Intake Sessions

Two of Patty's three intake sessions were held online since she lived about fifty minutes away from my office. For the final intake, she insisted on coming in person, but because driving herself anywhere was debilitating, her husband brought her. Any outing required a detailed plan, and the thought of driving alone triggered overwhelming fear, making her dependent on him for transportation. He also attended part of the session to understand the process. It was clear that he loved her deeply, but he had also been worn down by her decades of fear. He expressed his desperation for relief and admitted that the idea of psychedelic therapy had been his suggestion.

During our sessions, Patty identified her long-standing patterns of fear, control, grief, and guilt. She also shared that she used late-night eating, particularly sweets, as a form of self-soothing. This behavior connected to her nervous system, as eating can temporarily activate the parasympathetic "rest-and-digest" system to calm the fight-or-flight response.

Treatment Planning / Intentions

Together, we created the following list of intentions:

1. Release unresolved trauma
2. Explore the meaning of being needed—or not—and how it relates to my sense of purpose
3. Let go of control and chronic worry
4. Understand how hypervigilance has served me and how fear has shaped my experience
5. Open to the possibility of feeling joy without it being clouded by fear
6. Process grief and guilt related to my parents
7. Reflect on my relationship with food and move toward healthier, more conscious choices

These intentions were deeply interconnected. For Patty, caregiving defined her sense of self. Without it, she faced an identity crisis: "Who am I if I am not taking care of someone?"

Set and Setting

Patty attended a preparatory group meeting and displayed visible anxiety: slumped shoulders, little eye contact, and protective body language. Her husband dropped her off on treatment day and waited the entire day across the street in a park. I texted him updates every hour, as his calm nervous system would be essential for her reintegration.

Treatment Session

Patty cocooned herself in bed with an eye mask, holding a photo of her parents on their wedding day at her bedside. She had a very internal journey. From the outside, it appeared quiet, though she experienced significant "liquid letting"—streams of tears and mucus that she reported did not feel like crying but like cleansing.

Patty spoke little during her session. She did request two texts: one to her son, telling him "I love you. I see you. I feel your pain. It's going to be okay," and one to her husband, reassuring him she would not leave him after this experience. We honored both requests.

When she began to emerge, Patty reported: "I just had a ong therapy session with my parents and God. Everyone should experience this!" She appeared younger, lighter, and deeply grateful.

Immediate Outcomes

Post-session, Patty felt confused but profoundly grateful. She recognized that her list of intentions had not dictated the journey. Instead, the psilocybin had guided her to deeper truths.

On the drive home, Patty experienced the beauty of the desert landscape between Las Cruces and El Paso. (For those unfamiliar with this route, many would say that all there is to see are tumbleweeds, cow farms, weeds, and lots of brown sand.) She said she was taken by the curves of the mountains and the details in the bushes and trees. She was so focused on the beauty that her husband was confused. Normally, she would have made anxious comments about his driving or voiced fears about traffic, but this time she said nothing. Instead, she remained in bliss, appreciating the world around her as if seeing it for the first time.

Integration Sessions

Because Patty had been silent for much of her trip, I had little detail about her internal process until our follow-up. The integration sessions, held one week and three weeks after her treatment, gave her space to reflect.

The Gears

Patty described her first major insight as an encounter with a vast system of interlocking gears. She said it was not mechanical in a cold or industrial sense, but alive, fluid, and mesmerizing. Each gear turned with precision, fitting perfectly into the next, creating an endless rhythm of motion and flow.

The longer she observed, the more she realized the gears were not separate from her. They were her. They represented her mind, body, and spirit working in complete harmony. She marveled at how flawless the system was, how each piece knew exactly what to do. For the first time, she saw her existence not as broken, but as beautifully designed.

This vision filled her with awe and reverence for herself. She came to see her life not as a series of failures or flaws, but as a system working exactly as it was meant to. The gears gave her a new blueprint for self-worth. Where negative self-talk had once told her she was inadequate, the gears revealed her perfection in existence.

The Womb

After receiving an updose, Patty's awareness shifted. She found herself in darkness, enveloped by a tight but comforting space. She immediately recognized the sensation as being in the womb. The space felt safe and nurturing, yet there was also the faint glow of light ahead, like the opening of a tunnel.

At first, she hesitated. Leaving the warmth of the womb meant facing the unknown. The light called to her, but it also filled her with fear. She described waves of dread, almost paralyzing at times, as she considered what moving forward would mean.

In that space, she felt the undeniable presence of God. The presence was vast, filling every corner, and she felt both comforted and challenged. Each time she inched closer to the light, another layer of fear surfaced: fear of pain, fear of death, fear of the responsibility of living. She had to work through these fears one at a time, feeling their grip loosen as she moved closer.

Finally, as she pushed through into the light, she was overwhelmed with a profound sense of rebirth. The passage into the light was not just symbolic, but visceral. She felt herself breathe into a new life. The fears that had once bound her no longer had the same weight. Emerging from that tunnel, she described feeling renewed, as though she had been given a second chance at life.

Ancestral Understanding

This experience also opened her to the suffering of her parents and grandparents. She saw the weight of intergenerational trauma and recognized how much had been involuntarily passed down. But she also received a revelation: the *why* no longer mattered. The blame dissolved. Sitting in God's presence, she realized that love and gratitude were more powerful than explanation.

One of the most profound insights came as a clear message: she had never been alone. Even as a little girl waiting in her bed for her father to return, God's presence had been there. His love was unconditional and unwavering. This realization rebuilt her faith on unshakable ground. She no longer questioned whether she was worthy of divine love; she knew it.

By the time of her last integration session, Patty had already begun applying these insights. For the first time in years, she drove herself to my office. This was no small milestone; previously, any outing required detailed planning, and driving herself was impossible. She entered with a radiant smile and shared, "I can do it now."

Shifts and Outcomes

A review of her intentions:

- **Release unresolved trauma**: Patty recognized that her childhood experiences were no one's fault. Her parents had acted from their own limitations. She also received a download about how trauma had moved through generations, giving her perspective and compassion.

- **Explore the meaning of being needed**: She no longer felt bound by obligation to always watch her grandchildren. Instead, she re-prioritized herself, saying no when needed. She realized that, during her journey, her inner child had been seen and validated, allowing that part of her to heal.

- **Let go of control and chronic worry**: Patty was stunned at how quiet her mind had become. The negative self-talk and rumination vanished. Without the constant noise, she felt present, rested, and peaceful.

- **Understand hypervigilance**: Her husband traveled for work, and she was at peace being home alone—something unimaginable before. She noticed she no longer rehearsed every step before leaving home. Agoraphobia, once a daily barrier, seemed to be gone.

- **Open to joy without fear**: She began daily morning walks, enjoying nature without intrusive thoughts. She no longer waited for disaster to follow joy; instead, she let herself fully experience it.

- **Process grief and guilt about her parents**: During her session, she felt their presence. Instead of guilt, she received a clear message: *"You are enough. We love you just the way you are."* She realized they were proud of her, allowing her to release the burden of regret.

- **Reflect on food and healthier choices**: The night-time cravings vanished. She no longer needed food to soothe her nervous system. Trauma had driven her eating behaviors; once released, the compulsion lost its grip.

Patty also reported additional changes. She no longer felt like a scared child. She found her voice and began advocating for herself. "My little girl has a voice now," she said. Her siblings, who had minimized her for being the youngest, began responding differently. "It feels amazing. They respect me! I'm teaching them how to treat me."

Her transformation was visible to others as well. At her yoga class, fellow participants remarked on how different she looked—lighter, more grounded. Family and peers alike saw what she now knew: that she mattered, she belonged, and she was free.

Therapist Reflection

Patty's case illustrates the depth of psilocybin-assisted therapy. While her intentions helped frame the work, the medicine directed her to the deepest roots of trauma and faith. Her journey showed how intergenerational trauma, hypervigilance, and conditional love beliefs can dissolve into self-compassion and divine connection.

Her healing extended beyond her to her husband, children, grandchildren, and siblings. By releasing fear, she modeled presence, authenticity, and resilience. Patty's story is a testament to the power of intentional psychedelic work, supported by integration, to transform a life ruled by fear into one grounded in love and faith.

CHAPTER FOURTEEN

GHOSTWRITTEN BY MUSHROOMS

MARIA - *You saw it, didn't you?*

CATHERINE - *I don't want to write a book.*

MARIA - *And yet the pages keep turning.*

Whose voice do you think is narrating them?

CATHERINE - *It's too exposing. I'd rather stay behind the work.*

MARIA - *But the work is you.*

You are not stepping forward to boast.

You are stepping forward to beckon.

CATHERINE - *But what if it changes things?*

MARIA - *It already has.*

WHAT FOLLOWS MIGHT MAKE ME SOUND less like a board-licensed counselor and former forensic scientist, and more like someone who wandered out of a 1970s commune with crystals in one pocket and a journal in the other.

I thought I was simply testing a new strain of psilocybin mushrooms before introducing it to clients—but what I didn't realize was that this personal journey would lead me somewhere entirely unexpected. What began as a routine quality check quickly unraveled into something far more profound.

Quality assurance means more than just verifying the strength of the dose. It includes assessing the overall energetic feel of the mushroom, the onset and duration of effects, emotional range, and the clarity or intensity of the visuals. I want to know how the strain interacts with the body and psyche, whether it invites introspection or encourages movement, how easily it allows for emotional release, and whether it fosters a sense of connection, safety, and insight. If I'm going to hold space for others, I need to feel confident in the medicine itself. I want to know that it will support the kind of therapeutic work my clients come for: healing, exploration, integration, and growth.

With a vacation home still rented from a previous client retreat, I decided to take advantage of the space to try the new strain myself.

Once again, Ken kindly agreed to _tripsit_ for me, and after tidying up from the retreat, I took some time to choose which room to use. Of the three clients that day, Patty, (from the case study) had, in particular, an experience that intrigued me, and I felt drawn to using the same bed she had. It wasn't a rational decision, but more of a gut feeling; an intuition. The room she had been in was the smallest of the three and wasn't the primary bedroom, which I would typically choose. But something about it felt right for my journey. So, I settled in and prepared for an experience in that space. I also knew the rest of the day was open with no sessions and no obligations. The next day was Sunday, my usual day off. I felt grateful knowing I would have time to process whatever came through, both that night and throughout the following day, without needing to rush back into anything.

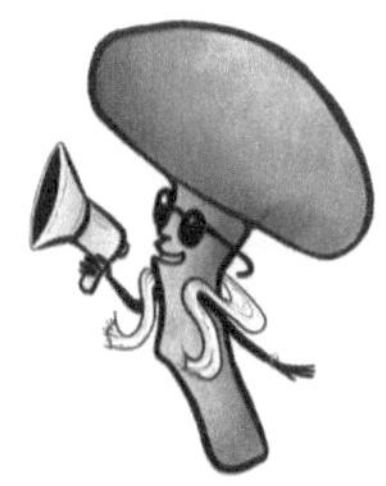

¡OYE! Plan your return before you depart.

Block off the day after your session. Cancel errands. Leave space for rest and reflection... don't go from ego death to emails.

It wasn't long before I began my usual cocooning ritual, burying my head into the pillows and pulling the sheets and covers over me. I curled my body into a semi-fetal position and welcomed the soothing sounds of being immersed in a fluid-filled space. Soon, the familiar sensations of body tingling washed over me, and fractal visuals began to unfold.

The first thing that stood out to me was the presence of my client's deceased parents in the room—not physically, but energetically. Though I never saw them, I knew they were there. My client had placed a picture of them on the nightstand during her journey, but what I felt went beyond a photograph. Their presence was warm, filled with gratitude, and unmistakable. Repeatedly, I received the same message: *"Thank you for helping our baby girl. She needed your help, and we deeply appreciate the work you're doing with her."*

Their appreciation pulsed through me, profound and undeniable.

The most intriguing part of this experience was that, up until then, I had never been visited by any beings. In therapy, many people report encounters with loved ones, deceased pets, aliens, mythical creatures, mystical beings, or other entities. Yet, I had never received any visitors myself. A part of me had felt envious of those who had such experiences. I was open to it, but it just hadn't happened for me until that moment. What was most striking was that it was the parents of a client who visited me, not the client herself or any of *my* deceased loved ones.

The connection was clear. I was in the same room where, in her mind, she had just spent time with her parents. During her psychedelic journey, she experienced what felt like a deep, extended therapy session with both God and her parents. Afterward, she shared this with me, describing it as if it had truly happened.

But had they truly visited me, or was this just psilocybin amplifying ideas already planted in my mind?

What came later made the experience even more mysterious. We discovered that her parents had migrated from the same region of Mexico that Mamaita and Papaito had come from. It left me wondering if her relatives could be part of my ancestral lineage. Could these have been my own family members visiting, doing double duty, and showing up for both of us in a way that defied logic but honored something much deeper? It might be something worth exploring someday, but for this story, it doesn't matter. The mushrooms continue to show me, time and time again, that we are all connected on a level that transcends bloodlines, held together by something far more mystical and enduring.

The next part of my journey involved visuals, which is a rare aspect of the psychedelic experience for me. Most of my experiences are more felt than seen. But this time, the mushrooms presented me with an image of a book. It was unmistakably a hardcover book, and it was clear that I had authored it. In my reverie, the image zoomed in from afar and landed about a foot from my face. The book had a dark hue, perhaps blue, green, or purple, and my name was on it.

My immediate reaction was, *I don't want to write a book.*

Next, the mushrooms presented another image, once again zooming in from a distance and landing in front of me. This time, it was an image of me being interviewed about the book. My reaction was stronger: "I said I don't want to write a book." At that point, I began to feel like we were playing a strange game. There was an aspect of inevitability, however, around the idea of writing a book, which was surprising, given my feelings.

The images didn't stop.

For a third time, the mushrooms presented yet another image, described best as zooming in. This time, it was a video of my cancer treatment, typing up blog posts to update people about my progress. At that stage in my life, it was exhausting and emotionally draining to repeat the same information over and over. Instead, I found it easier to write email updates in the form of a blog, which I could send to the forty people who were following my journey. The mushrooms seemed to be reminding me that I had once taken to writing to leverage a message. In other words, what it seemed to be asking wasn't beyond the realm of my capabilities.

This time, feeling a little weary, as though I was slowly being worn down, I said aloud, "I *really* don't want to write a book."

My reaction didn't faze the mushrooms in the slightest. They had tried, gently at first, to show me the message through images, visions, symbols, and subtle nudges. But I wasn't getting it. Or rather, I was refusing to accept it. That's when they changed tactics.

Things were taken up a notch. I noticed a laser-like light scanning my body, starting at the very top of my head and moving down the rest of my body, line by line. It wasn't just visual anymore; it was visceral. It felt as though the scan was embedding the idea that I was going to write a book. Inherent in that scan was the notion of acceptance. Not a request. A command.

Line by line, I could feel my body locking into the idea I was resisting. With each scan, my cells seemed to realign, subtly shifting into a new configuration where being an author became an undeniable reality. This was a journey without music or headphones, which made everything feel sharper and more exposed. In the silence, I could hear the sound of the laser as it moved along my body. It was a faint, energetic hum that traced each pass with eerie precision. Trapped in the couch-lock effect that mushrooms often bring, I was a sitting duck, entirely unable to wriggle or escape the process. Couch-lock is that peculiar state where your body feels like it's melting into the furniture. While you technically could get up, every fiber of your being votes a hard "no." It's not paralysis. It is more like a full-body consensus that moving is wildly overrated. Even scratching your nose feels like it would require a strategic plan and a pep talk.

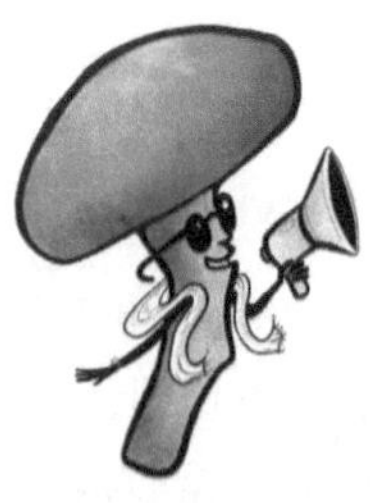

¡OYE! Silence can be louder than sound.

Sometimes, no playlist is the best playlist. Let the absence of noise become its own kind of music.

The light continued its systematic journey, scanning every part of my body until it reached the bottom of my feet. Halfway through the experience, I noticed something strange: My upper body felt fully aligned, wide open to the idea of writing a book.

But the lower half of me remained heavy, resistant, and deeply unconvinced. It was like my soul was charging ahead while my legs were dragging their heels.

I heard myself let out a faint whimper, muttering, "But I don't wanna write a book." The statement was almost laughable at that point because, in truth, it didn't matter what I wanted.

What was happening felt bigger than choice. It was resonance. Not just an emotional response, but something physical and cellular. Resonance is what occurs when something vibrates in harmony with a particular frequency. It's how a guitar string can cause another to hum from across the room, or how a perfectly pitched note can make a glass tremble. In that moment, it was as if the idea of the book had struck a perfect frequency within me. I didn't just understand it, I vibrated with it. The book had already been manifested, etched into the ether, waiting patiently for me to catch up and give it form.

As my journey began to wind down and Ken came in for his routine check on me, I asked him to draw me a bath. There's something deeply soothing about being enveloped in warm water as I slowly reintegrate into my physical self. Floating in water feels comforting, a gentle transition as my body reconnects with itself. Mushroom journeys often disconnect me from my body, as most of the energy is directed inward toward my mind, hence the cocooning process.

"How was your trip?" Ken asked.

"Mushrooms said I have to write a book," I replied.

"But you don't want to write a book," he said.

Strangely, I felt a wave of invalidation from his words. My body had already transformed, realigning its beliefs. His comment felt out of sync with my new understanding. My only response was, "That doesn't matter anymore. I have to write a book."

True to his never-ending support, he shifted his focus rapidly: "What are you going to write a book about?"

I'm not sure if I answered him verbally, but I vividly recall feeling that I had no idea what I was going to write about.

Over the next few weeks, I reached out to trusted friends and colleagues, asking for their input on what I should write about. I had it narrowed down to three ideas:

A Practitioner's Handbook on PAT – I had already created a class on Psilocybin-Assisted Therapy (PAT) for practitioners and had developed all the training materials. It wouldn't be challenging to compile a manual based on the content I had already crafted. After reading a book by a California psychotherapist on MDMA therapy, I felt confident I could create something similar, focused explicitly on psilocybin-assisted therapy.

Client Accounts of PAT – Many prospective clients express a deep interest in hearing about the experiences of others. While there are numerous documentaries, videos, and articles that explain the science behind PAT, a noticeable lack of personal stories remains. People want to know what clients seek treatment for, what their experiences are like, and what the results are after treatment.

My Own Psychedelic Journey – Initially, this didn't seem like a top contender. I couldn't imagine anyone being interested in reading about a therapist's experiences. I saw it as a last resort option, one that I would pursue only if the first two ideas didn't resonate with readers. This was the only justification I could see for offering my account.

My sister, a marketing expert, immediately recommended that I focus on the "Client Accounts" option for my first book. She pointed out that sharing real stories would help demystify psilocybin and make it a more approachable and viable treatment for mental health. By telling these stories, I could help the public understand how psilocybin-assisted therapy addresses issues like PTSD, depression, anxiety, anger, grief, guilt, shame, self-harming, and more. Additionally, it would provide prospective clients with a place to turn for treatment. Logically, this approach made the most sense, so I chose to focus my writing on real client experiences. I decided that the first chapter would be about the client whose parents visited me during my journey. (Incidentally, that's the case study about Patty that's included in this book, right before this chapter.)

I completed five chapters before needing to pause my writing to pursue a new opportunity to create a documentary. The film work was a more immediate way to share the message, with the potential of a bigger impact in a shorter amount of time. I wasn't abandoning the book, but rather, taking a brief break from my role as an author to shift gears and focus on producing a documentary that would capture the entire treatment process. I believed there was no better way to raise awareness than by documenting the client intake (assessment and preparation), group meetings, treatment sessions, and the subsequent integration sessions.

As I focused on the first documentary, a second opportunity arose, followed by a third—all in the filmmaking realm. I quickly realized that my efforts in filmmaking were pushing the book project to the sidelines.

It took about four months to complete the first film and begin working on the second one. I couldn't return to book writing until then. But during the four months, I questioned whether I would go back to the book at all, as the work on the documentaries was so consuming. To stay grounded in my writing, I joined a coaching group for authors, but eventually had to take a month off from the group to prioritize the films. Despite how far I seemed to drift from the book, my body had other plans, and there was no escaping that fact, no matter how distant it felt from my current reality.

At a women's retreat I hosted, a surprising event brought the book project sharply back into focus, clearing up any confusion I had about which direction to take with my writing.

Over the years, I had been offering training sessions and client treatments, but never anything that required overnight stays. Adding that element introduced an entirely new layer of care: meals to plan, lodging to arrange, and the responsibility of creating a nurturing environment around the clock.

Not long ago, I attended a retreat for counselors focused on building private practices while weaving in plenty of self-care. It lit a spark in me, not just to recreate the experience, but to expand on it. *What if I could offer something similar, but with a deeper focus on Psilocybin-Assisted Therapy (PAT), blending professional training with immersive, hands-on healing experiences and abundant self-care opportunities for rest and reflection?*

I affectionately referred to it as my *"fancy retreat,"* while I was deep in the throes of planning and organizing the details. It would be hosted in an extravagant mansion, for four nights, and crafted for counselors eager not just to learn, but to observe and appreciate the experience. The crafting of the itinerary was a labor of love: each participant had a dedicated day for dosing and another for guiding, allowing them to embody both roles fully.

Beyond the core training, I wove in layers of healing: morning yoga to ground, breathwork to release, sound baths to soothe, and group processing circles to integrate. The mansion itself was a sanctuary, complete with a sauna, hot tub, trampoline, and more. All of it was designed to create an atmosphere of luxury and deep rest. A personal chef curated delicious, nourishing meals, thoughtfully crafted to meet diverse dietary needs.

It was the most luxurious retreat I had ever hosted; the culmination of years of hard work, growth, and experience. It felt like the pinnacle of my journey, a manifestation of everything I had poured my heart into, now blooming into something beautiful and transformative for others.

My co-facilitator had recently become a fully certified Shaman, offering energy work as part of the retreat's healing options. She and I had been working side by side since our very first client treatment, growing together through every session, every lesson, and every challenge.

While some of the women knew each other from before the retreat, the depth of connection that blossomed among the group was profoundly healing for everyone. This was partly achieved by incorporating group circles to create space for authentic sharing, reflection, and bonding. Watching these connections form and deepen was nothing short of beautiful. It was a testament to the power of shared healing and heartfelt community.

As I often do during my training sessions, I spend a great deal of time emphasizing that the psychedelic movement I'm deeply involved in and passionately advocating for is not about me. I find myself repeating, over and over, *"This isn't about me."* It's about the medicine, about educating others, and about spreading healing across the world. My passion for psilocybin and the profound transformation it offers is so much bigger than me. I have no desire to be the focal point.

This was especially true during the filming of my first documentary. I consistently pushed for the focus to remain on the clients, their stories, their struggles, and their transformations. While I understood that my role as a guide was an essential part of the process, I had no interest in being the heart of the film. The true heart, for me, was always in the healing, in the medicine, and in the courageous journeys of those who dared to face themselves.

On the last full day of the retreat, I was relaxing in the living area with the other guides when we heard the chime of a call button. These call buttons are a simple yet powerful tool, allowing participants to reach out whenever they need support during their dosing sessions. We had spent the better part of the day documenting everyone's experiences, which involved a lot of moving back and forth between rooms and writing down our observations. We captured what they said, what they did, and the subtle and noticeable shifts that unfolded while they were under the medicine. We responded to every request with care, helping each participant stay grounded so they could focus entirely on their journey.

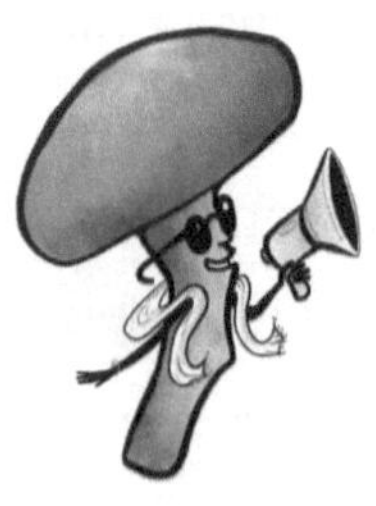

¡OYE! Got gold? Spit it out fast and get back to the goods.

If a cosmic download lands mid-trip, say it quick and drop back in. A good guide will catch it for you, like a soul stenographer with a clipboard and good vibes. You'll have time to unpack the meaning later. For now, stay with the magic.

When I first began facilitating Psilocybin-Assisted Therapy, we'd routinely check in on clients throughout their journeys. While well-intentioned, we quickly realized that these check-ins sometimes disrupted their experiences. More than once, we were met with a candid, *"You're interrupting."* Interestingly, blunt honesty is a favorable sign of actual ego dissolution because, when dosing, participants aren't typically concerned with social niceties or being polite. They are fully immersed in their process, free from the usual filters.

While ego dissolution is a positive indication of the medicine's effect, the corresponding behavior to an interruption highlighted the need for a better approach. We didn't want to risk pulling people out of profound moments of insight. Hence, the introduction of call buttons was a game-changer. It gave participants autonomy over when and how they sought support, while still allowing us to maintain visual check-ins discreetly. This minor adjustment created a more seamless, respectful space for deep healing, for them and us.

When the call button chimed, I glanced at the flashing #2 responder and saw it was a woman named Sadie. Instinctively, I jumped from my seat, preparing myself to step into whatever space she needed. I was ready to guide her through whatever was unfolding. But when I opened the door, I was met with something unexpected: Sadie was sitting cross-legged on the bed, Buddha-like, with a serene smile lighting up her face. She gently patted the spot on the bed in front of her, wordlessly inviting me to sit.

Without hesitation, I climbed onto the bed, folding my legs in front of her, open and receptive to whatever was about to happen. She continued to greet me with a warm, knowing smile, then softly asked, "Can I put my hand on your chest?"

I nodded, giving my consent. She placed her palm gently at the center of my chest, her touch both grounding and tender. Then she spoke words that landed with the weight of undeniable truth: "I know you don't want this to be about you. But you have to stop resisting, because it *is* about you. It's time for you to be seen and heard. People need someone to be the face and the heart behind the healing. They need someone to connect with, to hold onto. Lean into it. Accept it. It's going to happen."

Her words cut through the unseen barriers I had unknowingly built, skipping into the quiet, unspoken corners of my being. In that instant, the roles reversed–where I had once been the guide, I now found myself the one being led.

A jolt of energy surged through my body, like a current igniting every nerve ending, the emotions rising instantly, raw and undeniable. I didn't just hear Sadie's words; I felt them, vibrating through every single cell of my body. The truth of her message was inescapable, cutting through my resistance with a clarity so sharp it felt like it was being delivered with laser-like precision. It was as if the mushrooms had chosen her as the vessel to deliver a message I could no longer ignore.

I was utterly shaken. It felt eerily similar to the moment when mushrooms had laser-locked me with the undeniable directive to write a book. It was an unspoken command that wasn't just whispered to me; it infiltrated me, embedding itself into the very fabric of my being. This was no different. The message wasn't a suggestion; it was a truth that had already rooted itself inside me, leaving no room for doubt.

Sadie and I exchanged a few more words; her presence was still gentle, but the weight of her message lingered like an echo. Then, without ceremony, she requested to speak with another guide and gently dismissed me. I left her room, still trembling with the aftershocks of what had just unfolded, and re-entered the living area where the other guides were gathered, laughing softly, unaware of the shift that had just taken place within me.

They looked up, expecting a routine update, but instead, they saw tears streaming down my face. I tried to find the words, my voice trembling as I recounted what had just happened with a mixture of reverence and awe. The room grew still, the energy thick with something unspoken.

Then one of the guides locked eyes with me, her gaze steady and filled with knowing, and quietly said, "We've all been thinking the same thing."

In that moment, I realized the message had been waiting for me to hear it. It had been there all along, reflected in the hearts of those who had been witnessing me, waiting for me to finally see it too.

Something significant shifted within me. There I was, believing I was the one doing the guiding, only to realize I had just been profoundly guided. The medicine had found its way to me, not through one of my journeys, but through the heart and words of another.

That's the power of mushroom energy.

It can transcend the need for personal dosing, imparting its wisdom through the collective, ensuring the lessons reach you exactly when and how they're meant to.

I was so shaken by the experience that it was challenging to stay fully present for the rest of the day. My mind kept drifting back to that pivotal moment, my heart reverberating with the weight of what had been revealed. Tasks felt heavier, and conversations blurred at the edges, as if I was moving through the motions while part of me remained suspended in that sacred exchange with Sadie.

That night, as I lay in bed, the magnitude of Sadie's words washed over me. I stared into the darkness, trying to process, to make sense of how deeply it had unsettled and awakened something inside me. This wasn't something to be analyzed or logically dissected. It wasn't meant to be *understood* in the usual way—it was meant to be felt, embodied, and fully lived.

It would take days before the edges of that revelation softened enough for me to begin fully integrating the message. The lesson wasn't just about being seen by others. It was about seeing myself and not hiding behind the work, recognizing that sometimes, the guide must also be guided.

The week after the fancy retreat, I stepped back into familiar territory—teaching another PAT course for practitioners. It was a day of lecture followed by a day of experiential learning, where participants chose to either guide or dose. But something felt different this time. Maybe it was me. Maybe it was the universe. Maybe it was both.

The attendees were more than just students: they were threads woven seamlessly into the fabric of my journey, each one reflecting a piece of the path that had brought me here. It was as though everyone in attendance was supporting the directive the mushrooms had given me. Among them was a doctor I'd worked with in Denver nearly a decade before, not just attending out of curiosity, but showing up to support my work and witness how far I'd come. There was also a current client, seeking personal healing but also serving as a healer in their own right, blurring the line between student and teacher, guide and seeker. A past client, whose life had been so transformed by PAT that they'd shifted careers entirely, now walked the path of a shamanic healer. And a newly connected therapist, compelled to be there not by obligation but by an unwavering belief in the work—someone whose own psychedelic journey, spanning back to adolescence, had left an indelible mark, and who recognized the same transformative power in what I was doing.

The significance of this gathering wasn't lost on me. My past, my present, and—if the patterns held—my future were all gathered in this sacred space. Each person reflected a different part of my story, like human mirrors placed intentionally around me, as if the universe was crafting a message too loud to ignore.

I couldn't help but wonder: *Was I feeling seen and heard in a new way because I had finally opened my heart and eyes the week before at the fancy retreat? Or was the universe amplifying the lesson, presenting me with undeniable proof that, despite all my resistance, it is about me on some level?* Maybe both truths existed simultaneously, inseparable, like the guides and the guided, the healer and the healed.

A couple of days later, yet another piece of this unfolding story found me. I flew to the Chicago/North Indiana area to conduct pre-interviews for the participants in my second documentary. The film is a collaboration with Gathering Groups in Canada, focusing on the transformative power of group experiences with PAT. After a long day of filming five interviews, including my own, we gathered for a meal at a cozy restaurant, the kind of setting with remarkable food and where conversation flows easily and reflections surface naturally.

At one point, Peg lifted his glass to offer a toast. "To you," he said, his voice steady but full of meaning. "For connecting us all and bringing us together for this amazing project." His words were simple, but they struck me with unexpected force. I could feel the weight of them. He was expressing gratitude for me, for being the person who had woven this group of individuals into something exciting and bigger than any one of us.

I froze for a moment, the words catching me off guard. *What? That can't be true*, I thought. But as I glanced around the table, taking in the faces of every person seated there, the undeniable reality settled over me. I had brought them all together.

Me.

Another echo of the message I'd been trying to sidestep, impossible to dismiss.

The next morning, on my three-hour flight home, I settled into my seat, the hum of the plane offering a cocoon of reflection. I opened my laptop, staring at the five chapters I'd written months earlier. These chapters were filled with client case studies, their journeys, and their healing. But something had shifted. Without hesitation, I decided to start over. This book wasn't meant to be just about others' stories. It was meant to be about me, my story, my journey, my voice.

I had told myself that focusing on client case studies was the right approach. After all, stories are powerful, and people need to hear them. But in that moment of clarity, I saw the flaw in my reasoning. *I* have a story, one I know more intimately than any other. And if I wasn't willing to share my truth, to lay myself bare the way I asked others to, then what was I offering? Without that vulnerability, the book would feel incomplete, like a window looking outward but never inward.

So, I made a decision right there on that flight. This book had to be about me: my truth, my growth, my reckoning with the very thing I had been resisting. Perhaps I could weave in case studies, but the heart of it had to be mine. I didn't fully grasp then where this path would take me, but I knew one thing for sure: once I stopped resisting, the universe had a way of showing me exactly what I needed next.

And the next lesson? It wasn't just about psilocybin. It was about something even bigger. Something cosmic.

For the next two months, I found myself completely immersed in what could only be described as channeling the book. Every free moment was spent at my computer, words pouring through me faster than I could consciously process. I wrote late into the night, sometimes until two in the morning, compelled by something I couldn't quite explain. My shoulder began to ache from the awkward, repetitive angle I kept it in—my body clearly not used to this kind of sustained creative output. And yet, I couldn't stop. It was as if the book had already existed somewhere, and I was simply the vessel through which it was transcribed into form. Even now, when I read specific passages, I have no independent memory of writing them. That season lives in my mind like a foggy haze, but the clarity of what came through remains.

This chapter is not only a record of how the directive to write a book came through. It is also a metaphor for self-acceptance and a kind of coming out—a willingness to be fully seen. Each step of the way, the mushrooms reaffirmed that my voice mattered. That it was not only valid, but necessary for the progression of the psychedelic movement. They showed me this through my journeys, through the healing work I witnessed in those I guided, and through the growth unfolding in my colleagues who were also learning to walk this path. This wasn't just about writing a book. It was about owning the role I had tried so hard to downplay. It was about saying yes to being seen.

CATHERINE - *She said it's about me.*

That people need a face to hold onto.

That it's time to stop hiding.

VOICE - *She's right.*

CATHERINE - *But I never wanted to be the center.*

VOICE - *Then don't be the center.*

Be the vessel.

Be the firelight others gather around. Not because you demand attention, but because you offer warmth.

CATHERINE - *What if I'm not ready?*

VOICE - *You're not.*

Do it anyway.

Readiness is what arrives after the leap.

CHAPTER FIFTEEN

LSD AND THE COSMOS

MARIA - *You are called to something new.*

A cousin to mushrooms, but different.

Catherine - It feels unknown.

MARIA - *It is.*

But the essence is the same.

CATHERINE - *I'm nervous.*

MARIA - *New paths are not easy.*

Fear is only the edge of what you've yet to face.

Lean in.

CATHERINE - *What if it's too much?*

MARIA - *It is what you need at this moment.*

Trust the medicine.

Focus on the journey, not the destination.

You are not alone.

AFTER YEARS OF WORKING WITH MUSHROOMS, I felt a deep, unspoken pull to try something new. It wasn't a sudden urge, but more like a quiet whisper in my soul—an invitation to explore uncharted territory. The call to *LSD* had arrived, soft yet insistent, and I couldn't ignore it.

It had been on my radar for a while, especially after a colleague recommended a book by Christopher Bache, a researcher who had spent decades exploring high-dose LSD, documenting seventy-three journeys over twenty years in the book *LSD and the Mind of the Universe: Diamonds from Heaven*. His experiences fascinated me—the profound insights, the depths of the mind he uncovered, the sheer expansiveness of the psychedelic realm. Something about it resonated deeply, stirring a desire within me to step into a new chapter of exploration.

Around the same time, another colleague mentioned they were looking to buy LSD from a reputable source and asked if I wanted to join. I wasn't one to shy away from opportunities like this. After all, it's not every day that a trusted person offers you safe access to something like LSD.

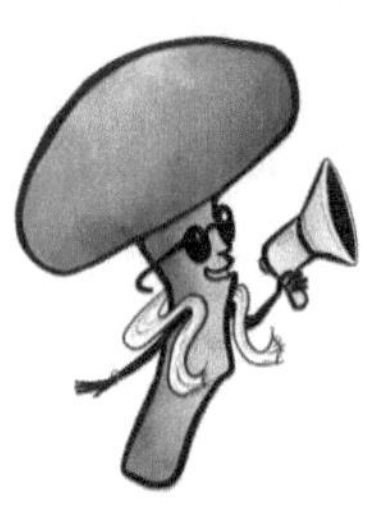

¡OYE! Sketchy vibes aren't medicine.

Get your psychedelics from trusted, reliable sources. Purity matters. Safety matters. Healing starts with knowing what you're taking.

I felt a degree of comfort knowing that my colleague had already ordered a testing kit to ensure the LSD was unadulterated and pure. This mattered to me deeply—purity was non-negotiable. The idea of ingesting something contaminated or cut with another substance was unsettling. I didn't want any unknown variables in my system; nothing that could cloud or distort the experience. I needed to know that what I was taking was truly LSD, not another research chemical, a dangerous analog, or something laced with a stimulant or sedative. Ensuring purity meant ensuring safety, both physically and mentally. It meant trusting that what I was about to embark on was the experience it was meant to be—nothing more, nothing less.

But even with such an enticing and safe option, I wasn't ready to consume the substance. I wasn't sure how to approach LSD, and my mind was filled with a blend of excitement and nervousness. The stigma surrounding LSD, the unknowns, and my lack of experience kept me at arm's length. But I wanted to have it on hand, knowing that when I was finally ready to step into this new realm of experience, I could. And there was no need to rush my decision, because LSD can typically last for several years if kept in a cool, dark, dry place in an airtight container. This seemed a counterintuitive environment for a substance that I'd soon discover would fill me with light.

Before I get to that part of the story, let's talk about what I was getting myself into. A significant difference between LSD and mushrooms is the duration of the experience. While a typical mushroom journey can be anywhere from four to six hours, an LSD trip can last eight to twelve hours, or even more. This extended timeline with LSD provides a much deeper immersion into the experience. The prolonged effects also bring a certain level of endurance, as the peaks and valleys of the trip unfold slowly, giving the user a chance to explore different layers of consciousness. In contrast, the quicker onset and duration of mushrooms can feel more intense and compact, often leading to a faster emotional release and a more immediate return to baseline. The difference in trip length can significantly shape how each substance is experienced and integrated into one's journey.

Fast forward about four months, and I felt the familiar pull. This time, the call was louder, clearer. I knew I had to dive in. Yet, still, I was hesitant. I decided to start small, to ease my way into this new world.

I took one tab—100 micrograms. I sat with anticipation, waiting for something to shift.

Two hours passed.

I felt something—a gentle stirring in my body, a subtle warmth. There were hints of color, a lightening of the air, and a subtle distortion in my perception. But it wasn't what I had expected. It wasn't anything like the experiences I had read about, and it paled in comparison to my previous mushroom experiences. I was still tethered, still in control, like I was watching from a distance instead of being fully immersed. I wasn't sure if I was disappointed or relieved, but I wasn't ready to call it quits.

So, I took another tab—another 100 micrograms. And this time, the shift began. It wasn't abrupt or dramatic; it was gradual, like the slow unfurling of something tightly coiled within me. The tension I'd carried in my shoulders, my jaw, my stomach—places I didn't even realize were clenched—began to release. There was a quiet recalibration happening inside my body, a sense of internal space opening up.

My thoughts softened at the edges. The constant mental noise, planning, replaying, and judging all faded into the background, replaced by something quieter, more curious. I became aware of a lightness in my chest, not just emotional but physical, as though some invisible weight had lifted. The room around me seemed subtly altered: the colors deepened, shadows danced at the periphery of my vision, and the air itself felt charged, almost animate.

There was a clarity to the experience, a sharpened presence. The visuals were fluid—patterns gently breathing across the floor, surfaces bending and stretching in ways that felt less like hallucination and more like a different dimension of perception had opened up. It was beautiful, yes, but more than that, it was meaningful. I felt attuned to something larger than myself, as though I had stepped through a doorway into a more expansive understanding of what it meant to be alive.

But even as I sank into the experience, a part of me remained guarded. I wasn't leaning inward the way I did with mushrooms. Maybe I wasn't willing to completely surrender, at least not yet. However, I was fascinated by the visual dance unfolding before me. The patterns, the shifting colors, the way everything seemed to breathe and morph into something new, were what I wanted to explore. The ego, that old protective force, was still holding on, unconsciously keeping me from the deep dive I knew was possible. It was a soft resistance, an unconscious effort to keep things comfortable. I wasn't ready for the dissolution of self. I wanted a pleasant, fun trip. And that's exactly what I got.

One thing that stood out during this trip was an overwhelming sense of happiness and joy. It wasn't just fleeting euphoria; it was a deep, sustained baseline of contentment. Everything was imbued with lightness, an effortless sense of well-being humming beneath the surface of reality itself. The simplest things, like music, movement, and the air on my skin, felt infused with warmth and positivity. There was no struggle, no heaviness, just a natural, flowing sensation of good vibes, as if the entire world had subtly shifted into a place of ease and delight.

Music was a game-changer with LSD. Up until that point, I had always been hesitant to use music during my psychedelic experiences, particularly with mushrooms. But with LSD, it was entirely different. The joy I felt seemed to amplify every note, and in turn, the music magnified that joy, creating a beautiful, harmonious feedback loop. Music became the heartbeat of the experience, weaving itself into the very fabric of my trip. For the first time, I understood what others had described about the deep connection between psychedelics and music. The music wasn't just sound, it was an extension of my body, something I could feel in every cell, every vibration of my being. Each note pulsed through my veins, my skin, my bones, syncing effortlessly with the heightened awareness of my physical self. The melodies swirled effortlessly with the euphoria already flowing through me, as if they were made of the same energy, feeding into one another in a perfect, blissful dance. Unlike mushrooms, which often left me disconnected from my body, LSD deepened the mind-body connection. I felt present, alive, and completely in sync with myself. Every movement, every breath, every beat of the music resonated through me, reminding me that my body wasn't separate from the experience. It was part of the rhythm, part of the magic.

After sharing my experience with colleagues, I learned something fascinating: taking multiple doses over time, as I had done with the two tabs separately, hours apart, actually lessens the intensity of the effects. This process, known as "updosing," involves taking additional doses at short intervals, often to gauge the effects before deciding to ingest more. The concept was new to me, but it made perfect sense. Had I taken both tabs at once, the experience would have been more intense and immediate, whereas spacing them out diluted the overall impact.

This discovery sparked my curiosity. It felt like a natural progression in my journey: learning not just how LSD felt, but how it worked, how timing and dosage shape the experience.

I would need some time before feeling ready to try again. I knew it was important to give myself space to fully process the relatively mild journey I had just experienced, to allow the newfound joy and vibrant energy to settle within me. On that last trip, I had spent twelve hours immersed in a state of incredible happiness, and I understood the importance of integration, to let the depth of that joy and well-being sink in. It wasn't just a fleeting high; it was a profound shift, a spark of light that had illuminated my entire being. LSD, like psilocybin, offers neuroplasticity, the ability to rewire the brain, and I knew that required time to fully absorb and make lasting change. I was eager to see how the experience would evolve next, now that the groundwork had been laid. But I would have to wait a few months.

About six weeks after my trial with LSD, I had the opportunity to conduct a private psilocybin treatment for a married couple in the Denver area. It was an intriguing experience, a deep dive into the contrasting worlds of two people united by love but shaped by vastly different childhoods. One spouse had experienced very little trauma growing up, while the other had lived through profound pain and dysfunction, rooted in parents who themselves had been shaped by their unresolved wounds.

The spouse without trauma seemed to effortlessly transcend the earthly plane, floating straight into the cosmos, their consciousness expanding into the stars. Meanwhile, the other spouse was caught in the depths of their past, working through the raw, painful layers of ancestral trauma that had been passed down through generations. The journey for both was profound, yet they existed at opposite ends of the spectrum—one soaring freely in the vastness of the universe, the other reliving painful chapters of their own history.

That experience became a catalyst for deep reflection. I had never experienced the cosmos with mushrooms—at least not up to that point. My trips had always been marked by an overwhelming need to confront my trauma, layer after layer, digging through the complexity of my wounds. I was fascinated by the fact that mushrooms could provide such different experiences for different people. For some, they went inward, unraveling and healing deeply buried pain, while for others, the journey was about transcending their earthly struggles and tapping into an expansive, cosmic state of being. The sense of interconnectedness, of oneness with the universe—that was what I longed to experience. I imagined what it must be like to dance among the stars, feeling an overwhelming sense of belonging and acceptance.

That particular couple's experience wasn't the first time I had a client who shot straight into the cosmos. It didn't happen often, but when it did, it always left me in awe. After witnessing the stark contrast between the journeys of the two spouses, I couldn't shake the questions bubbling up inside me:

What determines whether someone ventures into the cosmos or stays rooted in personal healing?

Why hadn't I been granted that experience yet?

Did mushrooms only offer the cosmic journey to those with little to no trauma, as if there was no deeper work left to be done?

Or was the cosmos simply another method of imparting wisdom, tailored to the way an individual's mind processes information?

No matter how I turned the questions over in my head, they all led me back to the same truth: I wanted to experience the cosmos.

But why wouldn't mushrooms take me there?

The day after the couple treatment in Denver, an opportunity for me to dose presented itself. We were at a vacation home rental in Denver, away from home, which I'd found was ideal for a more powerful, transformative experience. So I decided to take a macrodose of 4 grams of mushrooms, trusting that it would bring me closer to a meaningful experience.

I cocooned myself in the quiet space, ready to journey inward. What happened next, however, was a trip that took me in directions I could never have anticipated. The experience unfolded with unexpected depth, challenging me in ways I hadn't prepared for, but also offering profound revelations that were unexpected.

The first thing that struck me as *beyond* strange was the absence of the emotional release that usually accompanies my mushroom trips. Typically, I would be overwhelmed by a flood of feelings: heavy, visceral waves that shook my body and left me leaking uncontrollably. Moans, sighs, tears… all of it. My body would often tremble with raw emotion, as if I were shedding the weight of years of pent-up grief and trauma. I had even prepared for it. A hand towel was within arm's reach, ready for the inevitable tide of wetness that would pour from my eyes and nose. But this time there was nothing. Absolutely nothing. It was as if my body had gone still, quiet. No sniffles, no moans, no tears.

Ken, who had been checking on me periodically, was equally surprised. Whenever he would peek in, he was taken aback by how silent, still, calm, and composed I seemed. Normally, I would need the comfort of his presence, my call button a lifeline that I would press every time I needed something, whether it was reassurance, a hand to hold, or just the grounding energy of someone near me. But not this time. I didn't need anything, not even the safety net of his support. It was as though I had entered a different realm of experience, one where I felt *complete* in my own space. I was alone in my cocoon, and I felt okay.

The familiar hum of the mushrooms began to fill me. The fractals danced behind my closed eyelids, shifting and folding into themselves like intricate, moving patterns. I wore my mask, trying to block out the world, and chose not to play music, as it hadn't been resonating with me. Instead, I let myself sink deeper into the experience, cocooning myself more tightly in my internal world. The silence, the stillness—it was as if the universe was holding its breath along with me.

And then, *it happened*—the shift.

It was as though the mushrooms had decided to guide me in an entirely new direction, away from the usual emotional upheaval.

The mushrooms, in their boundless intelligence, unfurled a vision before me that defied anything I thought possible. I encountered an otherworldly winter landscape, alive with color and light. It wasn't just beautiful; it was transcendent. Snow blanketed the earth in iridescent softness, each flake refracting light like a prism, casting glimmers that shimmered and danced like constellations scattered across an arctic sky.

The scene pulsed with color. None of it was static; swirling ribbons of violet, emerald, and electric blue were woven together in a visual symphony that seemed to sing without sound. Everything glowed from within, radiant with a kind of sacred luminosity that vibrated with something ancient, something eternal. The air itself sparkled with sentience, and I could feel the magic of it all rushing toward me, through me, as if I had become part of the scene itself.

My breath hitched, caught between awe and disbelief, as if even the act of inhaling might disturb the fragile perfection of what I was witnessing. For those few sacred seconds—twenty, perhaps—I existed outside of time. The moment stretched, infinite in its beauty, before it collapsed in on itself like a dream evaporating at sunrise.

And then, just as suddenly, it was gone.

The brilliance dissolved, like a curtain falling, giving way to a vast and infinite blackness. Stark in its contrast, the darkness wasn't menacing. It was itself, just as real, just as honest as the light. There were no twinkling lights, no cascading color; only an expansiveness that stretched beyond comprehension. It felt like a pause in the symphony, a deep inhale between movements. Though the winter vision had vanished, I remained suspended— held, somehow—within this immense quiet. It was a different kind of beauty, one I hadn't yet learned to recognize, but could already sense was alive with its quiet wisdom.

Black fractals swirled and flowed, gliding in intricate patterns. It was deep, but not dark in a negative way. The blackness wasn't ominous; it was merely neutral, neither good nor bad. The sense of stillness and silence it offered was profound. I felt something within me shift as I understood it: *This is not about duality. This is about neutrality.*

Then came the message, clear and unspoken, but transmitted directly through my being. It wasn't words, but a sensation, a deep knowing that resonated through every fiber of my body.

The message was firm, yet compassionate:

You are not ready to enter the cosmos. You must first stay here in this neutral space to work on yourself. There is work to be done, and it lies within you.

The directive was unequivocal: I had to focus on self-love. The truth of it was undeniable, pulsing in the very core of me. To love myself, I was told, wasn't just a passing thought or an occasional affirmation. It was an active, daily practice. A reminder to myself, over and over, that I was worthy of love, worthy of compassion, and worthy of acceptance. It was clear that this was no quick fix. It would require time, patience, and consistent effort.

Mushrooms did offer me a glimpse of the cosmos, though it was fleeting, a filtered window, just enough to make me sense its vastness. For about twenty seconds, I touched something infinite, a brief yet undeniable encounter with the universe. But I wasn't allowed to linger there, to dissolve into its depths. Instead, it felt like the mushrooms were showing me only what was necessary to spark a fire within me, to awaken a deeper yearning. It wasn't a tease; it was a method, a lesson in patience, in the importance of purpose. Like a guiding hand, they offered me a brief vision, not to frustrate, but to fuel my desire, to ignite the hunger for the journey that lay ahead.

I sank deeper into the neutral space, accepting the reality of the work that lay ahead. It was uncomfortable, but also strangely comforting to know what my path forward entailed. I spent the rest of my journey in that space, quietly sending myself love and gratitude, almost as if I was reprogramming my sense of worth. It felt strange at first—awkward even—but with each moment, I could feel it becoming more natural, more integrated. The message was clear: *This might take time. Perhaps even a year or so in this neutral space before you will be ready to truly ascend to the cosmos.*

At once, it was both a letdown and a relief. The cosmos, the very thing I longed for, felt like it was just out of reach. But the clarity that came with the message grounded me in a way I hadn't anticipated. I understood that the work needed to be done within, not in the stars. But that glimpse of the cosmos, that fleeting moment of beauty, was enough to ignite a fire within me. It filled me with hope and excitement for the future. I knew my journey wasn't over; it had just begun.

MARIA - *So, you touched the stars.*

CATHERINE - *I did. I saw everything—connection,*

> *light, pure joy.*

> *And then... I was told I couldn't stay.*

MARIA - *Because your roots still ask for water.*

> *The cosmos will wait.*

> *Your soil will not.*

CATHERINE - *But it was so beautiful.*

> *I felt like I belonged there.*

MARIA - *You do.*

> *But you also belong here.*

> *Healing doesn't always look like floating.*

> *Sometimes, it looks like digging.*

The second time I took LSD was about three months after my first experience. This time, I chose to start with two tabs, curious to compare the effects with my initial trip. Knowing that the intensity of the experience was directly tied to the dose, I was ready to go deeper than on my maiden voyage. I figured I had about an hour before the effects would take hold, so I decided to take a shower.

As the warm water cascaded over me, I felt calm, at least at first. But then, suddenly, something shifted. The sense of anticipation deepened, and I could feel it coming on, unmistakable and powerful. The world around me started to blur, and I knew it was kicking in. I quickly rushed out of the shower, struggling to find my footing.

"Ken, I'm going down," I said in a voice that felt both urgent and controlled.

I barely had time to sink into bed before the ride began. My body instinctively curled into itself, settling into the soft comfort of my blankets, knowing it was best to avoid the effort of coordinating my balance on two feet as the LSD took hold. But it wasn't just a bed anymore. It was something entirely different.

My bed morphed into a cushioned eggshell, enveloping me. The sensation was surreal, like the floating egg-shaped chairs I had only seen in photos. I felt supported, suspended, yet somehow connected to the essence of everything around me. The walls of my bed felt like a soft embrace, gently molding around me, cushioning me in a way I had never before experienced.

As I lay still, my breath steady and slow, I lifted my arms into the space before me. Instantly, I was met with a soft trail of tracers: ribbons of light unfurling from my fingertips, glowing like silk in water. The air seemed to come alive, almost as if it were responding to me, dancing along with my every movement.

What had once been invisible now revealed itself, fluidly, radiantly, and full of life. I could see the air swirling and curving around me, moving in a gentle rhythm. Every gesture left behind a glowing trail, like stardust frozen in time. The simple motion of my hand felt like a conversation with the very fabric of existence.

Colors exploded around me, but not in chaos. Rather, in celebration. Golds, blues, and violets cascaded across my vision, dazzling yet peaceful. I was consumed by the beauty of it all, not just in what I saw, but in how it made me feel. It was as if the universe itself had paused to say, "Look. You belong here. You are part of this."

The moment didn't just transport me; it transformed me. It reminded me that life is meant to be marveled at, not just lived.

And then, it happened. Without warning, I was launched into the cosmos.

CHAPTER SIXTEEN

HEIRLOOM OF SHAME

I FOUND MYSELF FLOATING, WEIGHTLESS, SURROUNDED by the vastness of the universe. It wasn't just a visual experience. It was all-encompassing. I felt *everything*. The laughter of the stars. The sorrow of the universe. The joy of existence. The pain of all living beings. My emotions were vast, as though I were every person, every creature, every element, all at once. I laughed with abandon, cried with an open heart, and felt a range of emotions that was both overwhelming and beautiful. I understood, in that moment, the collective experience of humanity and the world beyond it. I felt the interconnectedness of all things, the cosmic thread that wove us together. Never had I felt so much all at once. It was glorious!

But there was something else, something even more profound. It was as if I were being welcomed, accepted, cherished, and loved in a way that was beyond anything I had ever known. The universe didn't just tolerate me; it embraced me. I was not just a part of it, but it was a part of me, and in that sense, I belonged. I felt the deepest, most unconditional love I could ever imagine. It wasn't just a fleeting sensation. It was profound, an all-encompassing force that seemed to echo through the very structure of who I was, reverberating through bone, breath, and consciousness alike.

There were no words to describe it. "Euphoric" comes close. Nevertheless, I reveled in it, surrendered to it, allowed it to wash over me with its gentle power.

It was the most transcendent moment of my life.

It wasn't a glimpse of something greater, but dissolution into it. I was no longer a witness to the mystery; I *was* the mystery. The fabric of existence did not unfold before me; it unfurled *within* me, and I recognized myself as both thread and tapestry, part of the eternal rhythm that hums beneath all things.

And then, just as I thought I couldn't absorb any more, another message began to emerge.

LSD spoke to me with a clarity I hadn't expected. It told me that mushrooms would not let me go to the cosmos—not yet, at least—because my work with trauma recovery needed to be my primary focus. Mushrooms, in all their wisdom, had recognized that I had more healing to do before I could experience the vastness of the universe. They needed me to stay grounded, fully present in the deep, painful work of trauma processing. That was my purpose. If I allowed myself to venture into the cosmos, it would derail my mission. The message of healing would be muddied and unclear.

It was as if mushrooms were ensuring I remained anchored in my work, not just for myself, but for the people who would one day read my book and watch the documentaries. They weren't withholding the cosmos as a punishment but as a form of guidance. If I was going to do justice to these projects, I had to stay in the trenches, immersed in the raw, unfiltered process of healing. They needed me to understand the depths of trauma so

I could articulate it with honesty and clarity. The cosmos could wait, but the work in front of me could not.

LSD, by contrast, understood that, while trauma work had to be the center of my focus with mushrooms, it was okay to explore the cosmos through a different lens. LSD made it possible to compartmentalize the experiences, each substance offering a unique perspective. But the message from mushrooms was undeniably clear. Until I had finished writing the book on trauma recovery, I would not be allowed into the expansive reaches of the universe through their lens. The healing message I carried had to stay intact, and mushrooms would not allow me to bypass it. I had to finish the work I'd started.

It struck me as strange, almost ironic, that LSD was offering me insight into mushrooms. There I was, deep in the heart of a powerful LSD journey, and somehow this medicine was illuminating the wisdom I had gained through psilocybin, even revealing deeper layers of its purpose in my life. Though they're different in form and feeling, in that moment, they felt like collaborators, each one helping me understand the other, guiding me in tandem toward a greater truth.

They were in cahoots!

Believe it or not, this isn't such a leap. After all, LSD and mushrooms are cousins in the psychedelic world, both born from the same ancestral family. LSD is an isolate from ergot, a type of fungus that grows on rye and other grains, which historically caused convulsions and hallucinations when consumed. *Could LSD, derived from ergot, and the mushrooms have some unspoken understanding of one another, guiding me together in different ways?* The idea was almost comical, yet there it was: LSD, offering its perspective on the powerful teachings of mushrooms. It felt like a quiet exchange between two superpowers, one that I could only understand by listening deeply to myself.

With mushrooms, my body often felt cut off from my head. I would feel detached from it, locked in place like the mushrooms themselves, rooted to the ground, still and seemingly immobile. My mind would soar, but my body remained secured and still. I felt disconnected from my physical self and couch-locked, almost as though I had forgotten how to move.

But LSD provided a different kind of experience. With LSD, I felt every inch of my skin, every pulse in my veins, every subtle shift of my muscles. It wasn't just my mind that was awakened; it was my entire being. The experience was embodied, vibrant, alive. I could move, stretch, and dance. It was as if my body had become part of the journey rather than an anchor keeping me in place.

It's fascinating to consider that mushrooms—beings rooted in stillness—might be grounding me in a way that speaks to their existence. Their fruiting bodies remain fixed to the forest floor, but beneath the surface, they are anything but static. They stretch through the earth in vast, unseen networks, connecting tree to tree, life to life. Perhaps this is their wisdom: to show that movement doesn't always require motion. That deep, silent connection can be just as powerful as flight. In their stillness, they teach me how to settle into the body, into the present moment, into the weight of what must be felt to heal. They invite me to root down, to listen, to be.

By contrast, LSD feels like air or fire. It's restless, expansive, and kinetic. It stirs me, opens me, sends my consciousness flowing outward like wind through open fields. But the mushrooms? They remind me that even the most grounded beings can travel, just not in the ways we expect.

When I was on LSD, I was connected harmoniously to both my body and mind. It was fluid, graceful, like I was a dancer of the earth, swirling and spinning with the world around me. I could do yoga, stretch my body into positions I hadn't been able to before, and feel every release as the tension melted away. LSD allowed me to explore movement and connection in ways mushrooms didn't.

If I had to describe the difference to someone who hasn't experienced both, I would say that mushrooms hold me in a fetal position, cocooned, facing the internal work I need to do. It's a grounded, introspective experience, like being wrapped in a warm, protective shell. LSD, on the other hand, opens me up, arms wide, inviting me to connect with the world. It's the opposite of being closed off—it's expansive, like the iconic scene from *The Sound of Music*, twirling in the mountains, free and open, with the wind in my hair. For me, LSD is the embodiment of freedom, of joyous exploration, and the perfect counterpart to the hard lessons I learn through mushrooms.

Because my experiences with LSD were so breathtakingly joyful, so weightless and exhilarating compared to the deep, often grueling intensity of mushrooms, I couldn't help but wonder: *What would microdosing LSD feel like? Could I capture even a fraction of that expansiveness in my daily life?* I had worked with microdosing mushrooms for years, especially when transitioning off my medications, and had come to rely on them as a gentle but powerful ally. *But LSD?* That was unknown terrain. If a full-dose LSD journey could crack me wide open to the cosmos, what kind of subtle magic might a microdose weave into my everyday existence?

When it comes to mushrooms, I have always followed the Fadiman protocol: 0.12–0.15 grams every three days for six to eight weeks, followed by a crucial month off. That break matters. It prevents tolerance from dulling the effects and provides space to evaluate the shifts without the medicine's influence. Microdosing isn't meant to be a crutch, something taken indefinitely like a daily antidepressant. It's a tool, a catalyst for real, tangible transformation. Unlike antidepressants, which simply plug receptors and numb the lows, microdosing actively reshapes the brain, fostering neuroplasticity and lasting change.

The beauty of microdosing lies in its subtlety. For me, I'm not hurled into an altered state, nor is my ego dissolved into the cosmos. Instead, it whispers, softly but powerfully, just beyond the edges of perception. The effects are quiet but undeniable: an effortless sense of flow, heightened creativity, laser focus without the usual mental noise. The world feels more alive, colors a little richer, movement a little smoother. The things that once required motivation and drive, such as starting projects, finishing tasks, and even social interactions, become easier and more natural, as if life itself is carrying me instead of me pushing through it. And best of all? I can function completely. No impairment, no fog; just a lightness, a clarity, a sense that maybe—just maybe—life is meant to feel this good.

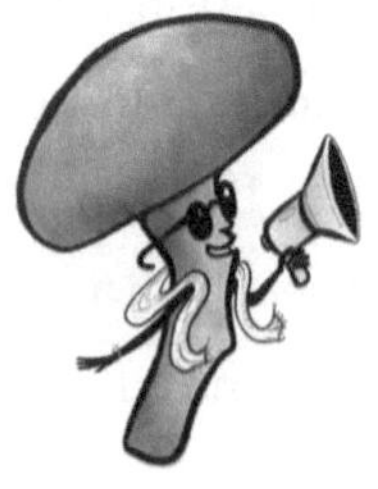

¡OYE! Small doses, steady rewiring.

Who knew subtle shifts could sneak in like ninjas and rearrange the furniture?

Halfway through my second round of microdosing mushrooms, after taking my scheduled month-long break, something remarkable happened. I developed an intuitive connection with the medicine, something I had never experienced with any other substance before. It was as if my body and mind had learned to communicate with it on a deeper level. Each morning, I would wake up and just *know* whether I needed a microdose that day or not. No rigid schedule, no external cues, just an undeniable internal sense of what was right for me at that moment. Some days, I felt the call to microdose on consecutive days. Other times, I could go two whole weeks without it, completely content. It was a dance, a natural ebb and flow, and I trusted it. Eventually, I settled into a rhythm, microdosing anywhere from two to six times a month.

These days, I only take it on rare occasions, when I feel a subtle nudge, notice a dip in my mood, or sense myself slipping into old patterns of overthinking or emotional heaviness. Sometimes it's a response to a particularly stressful week, other times it's when I need a little extra clarity or creativity. It's no longer about routine; it's about resonance. When the moment calls, I listen.

The confidence I felt after the positive experiences of microdosing psilocybin, and the reverence with which others spoke of microdosing LSD, stirred my curiosity to life. If macrodosing mushrooms invited me into the depths— demanding courageous inner work in exchange for hard-won insight—and macrodosing LSD had lifted me into pure, expansive joy, then what might a microdose of LSD offer? I already knew what microdosing mushrooms could do: they sharpened my focus, hushed the background noise in my mind, unlocked wells of creativity and productivity. But even in small amounts, mushrooms had a certain gravity to them. They asked something of me. They pushed me—sometimes gently, sometimes not—toward growth.

Would LSD be different? Would it carry that same sense of inquiry and invitation, or would it offer a lighter touch—one that simply illuminated life from within?

I was ready to find out.

I prepared with care, almost as if it were a ritual. I filled a small amber dropper bottle with 10 milliliters of purified water, slid one square of LSD inside, and watched as it slowly surrendered to the liquid. A few good shakes and the mixture was ready. From there, I measured out a single milliliter at a time, tiny and precise doses every three days. The rhythm became its own practice: steady, intentional, almost meditative. I committed to it for a month.

What followed was, without question, the most joyful thirty days I'd ever known, microdosing LSD. It was as if someone had turned the brightness up on the world itself. Everything shimmered with a quiet kind of brilliance. There was no striving, no uphill climb; just a gentle hum of happiness that moved through even the most ordinary moments. For the first time, life didn't feel like something to manage. It felt like something to savor.

A few things became undeniably clear in my deepening relationship with LSD. Microdosing had given me one of the most joyful months of my life, but joy is not always the same as healing. While LSD elevated my baseline happiness and well-being, it did not treat my depression. That realization hit hard. I had assumed that because I felt lighter and more playful on LSD, it might be enough to keep the creeping shadows at bay. But depression is insidious. It does not always crash the party loudly. It seeps in quietly, until one day everything feels heavier.

I had unknowingly drifted too far from mushrooms, and three or four months had passed without a single dose of mushrooms or LSD, micro or macro. It was Ken and my sister, Linda, who first noticed the shift. They pointed out that I seemed off: more irritable, more easily disappointed, more pessimistic. At first, I brushed it off, but the more I reflected, the more I realized they were right. I had gotten disconnected from mushrooms and had lost my balance. Over the years, I had learned that these were the very signs that, for me, present when depression creeps back in. I was struggling, and I hadn't even noticed it happening.

That's when the truth became unmistakable: LSD could lift my mood, but it could not hold back my clinical depression. Mushrooms could, and they always had. I had failed to maintain my side of the relationship with them. So I did what I knew I had to do. I returned to the medicine.

After four months away from mushrooms, I took a microdose of .15 grams.

Within two hours, it was like someone had flipped a switch. My energy surged, and suddenly, I was in motion. I tackled my office, organizing, sorting, putting things away that had somehow become invisible in my fog. The piles that once felt overwhelming now felt effortless. It wasn't just about productivity; it was about clarity, about feeling like myself again. The irritability, disappointment, and pessimism that had been creeping back in lifted almost instantly. That .15 grams of psilocybin had shifted me back into alignment, into a space of peace and balance. I was no longer stuck in the grip of depression; I felt *so* much better.

The second major insight was about the deep inner work I had already done. My journey with mushrooms had been long and intense, years of processing and re-narrating trauma, turning my pain into something meaningful. And because of that, LSD met me in a different space. It greeted me with love, beauty, and joy. But I couldn't help but wonder—*if I had taken LSD before working through my trauma with mushrooms, would I have had the same experience? Or would it have surfaced the same deep wounds, just in a different way?*

There's no way to know for sure, and I can't speak for others; each person's journey is unique. But what I do know is that mushrooms guided me through the darkest depths of my past, while LSD arrived as a playful, loving force once I had done the most challenging work.

The third revelation concerned *how* these medicines appeared to be working in conjunction. From my experience, mushrooms were the master of deep, internal healing, while LSD seemed to shine in the realm of *external* work. In other words, how I engaged with the world once my foundation had been rebuilt. But I also had to acknowledge my own bias. I had dosed over 150 people with mushrooms, guiding them through their journeys, while my experience with LSD was far less extensive. I didn't yet know how LSD worked in others the way it did with psilocybin. But what I *did* know was that these two medicines—*cousins*, both derived from fungi—seemed to be working together, giving me exactly what I needed at every step of my journey. It was as if mushrooms had assigned themselves as my strict but loving guide, ensuring my healing work stayed on course, while LSD arrived as the joyous counterpart, the reminder of how beautiful life could be once the heavy lifting was done. And somehow, they were communicating with each other, crafting an intensely personal curriculum designed just for me.

While on the subject of LSD, I would like to recount one particularly profound macrodose experience I had in March of 2025.

After a long, grinding day and an even longer, grueling week, I could feel the tension in my body, coiled like a spring ready to snap. The weight of stress had been piling up, pressing into my shoulders, tightening my chest, seeping into every muscle. I had been holding too much; too many thoughts, too many emotions, too much unprocessed energy swirling inside me with nowhere to go. The itch to dose was undeniable, a whisper in my mind that grew louder with each passing hour until it was no longer a suggestion, but a demand.

And the timing was perfect. I had a couple of days off, a rare pocket of space where I could fully surrender without responsibilities tugging at me. I felt the call of psychedelics, an ancient, knowing pull, inviting me into the depths of my own consciousness. It wasn't just an urge; it was a beckoning, a sacred nudge from something greater than myself, telling me it was time. Time to process, to unravel the knots, to release all that had been wound so tightly within me. Time to let go, to surrender to the experience, to allow the medicine to guide me into deeper understanding.

So, I did.

I placed two tabs of Lucy Diamonds LSD gel tabs, totalling 260 micrograms, under my tongue and let them dissolve, feeling the subtle tingle as they seeped into my bloodstream, a quiet promise of what was to come. The anticipation threaded through my body, taut and humming, like a violin string just before the bow is drawn.

At first, there was nausea, a queasy churning in my stomach, as if my body was rejecting the journey ahead. This was unusual for me. *Maybe it was my ego clinging to control, resisting the inevitable unraveling?* I breathed through it, feeling the grip loosen, the resistance soften. The colors around me began to stretch and breathe, no longer static but alive, pulsating with a rhythm beyond comprehension. The animated movie I had put on became impossible to follow, the plotlines melted, the characters morphed, their faces shifting in ways that defied logic. Time fractured. I felt myself dissolving into the experience, no longer tethered to the mundane world.

I closed my eyes. And that's when the real journey began.

With my vision shut off from the physical realm, the psychedelic world unfolded in vivid, fluid motion. Patterns of impossible geometry unfurled like sacred tapestries, alive with intelligence, shifting in colors I had no name for. Light wasn't just light; it had texture, density, a language of its own. I felt my body vibrating, not in an uncomfortable way, but as if I was being tuned, recalibrated. A deep hum resonated through my bones, as if the sound of the universe itself were singing me into alignment.

I was launched into the cosmos, weightless, suspended in the vast expanse of the universe. I felt the raw, unfiltered joy of existence, the beauty of all life, and the deep, aching pain of the world. Both were there, intertwined, in perfect harmony. Time and space became meaningless as I soared through the stars, seeing everything and nothing all at once. I felt connected to the whole of humanity, to all of existence, as if I could touch the pulse of life itself.

But just as quickly as I was shot into this boundless joy, I was pulled back down, zooming through time and space, landing with an abrupt jolt deep within my body, into the very fabric of my ancestral line. It felt like the universe had guided me across galaxies just to lay bare the grief etched into the core of me, not only in my heart, but in the marrow of my bones and the shadows of my spirit. And there, at the core of it all, I felt the suffocating weight of my lineage, an ancient, ancestral shame, passed down not just through Mamaita but deeply embedded in my very DNA.

At that moment, it all crashed down on me—a flood, a tidal wave of raw, unfiltered emotion. Shame, thick and suffocating, poured into every cell of my body. It wasn't just mine; it was a heavy inheritance, ancient and unspoken. And in that flood, I saw Mamaita, a young woman, small and shrunken by the weight of her own hidden identity. Her eyes were downcast, her Mexican heritage buried beneath layers of survival, and I understood that this was the shame that she had passed on, knowingly and deliberately, like a dark heirloom.

Her shame and embarrassment stemmed from the belief that survival meant blending in, that safety and security required silence about her and my origins. It led her to sever the connection to her roots, my roots. She had cut me and my family off from our heritage, keeping us distant from her parents and siblings. I don't ever remember meeting any of them, nor were there any pictures of them. There were no stories of her childhood, no mention of her past, nothing of her relatives. She stopped speaking Spanish to me, wanting me to blend in, to be White. She wanted me to have the privilege that came with it, but in doing so, she cut me off from the very culture that was meant to carry me.

In this moment, as the LSD took hold, I felt the void of being cut off from that part of myself. The emptiness was overwhelming. *Who am I? What is my lineage?* I felt a deep, painful ache as I realized I didn't know that part of myself. It was like an entire section of my soul had been left untold, erased from my story, and the weight of that loss hit me with a crushing intensity. *How could I not know my own heritage? How could something so central to my being be erased?* It hurt in a way I couldn't fully comprehend, a pain that came from the absence, from the severing of a connection that I never even knew was missing until it was too late.

I felt the disconnection as if it were a physical wound, a hollow cavern in my chest. The distance between me and my ancestors stretched infinitely, a chasm carved by assimilation, by generations trying to survive at the cost of identity. It ached. It burned. My body curled in on itself as sobs tore through me, my throat raw, breaking open with each guttural wail. I doubled over, gasping, grief erupting in waves so powerful I thought they might swallow me whole.

I don't know my Mexican roots.

The truth shattered me. The loss of it, the weight of everything I hadn't learned, hadn't been given. *Who am I without that connection?* The question spiraled in my mind, expanding, echoing, pulling me deeper.

I slid from my bed to the floor, unable to hold myself upright, my body limp with the sheer force of emotion. I lay there, motionless, my tears soaking into the towel Ken had placed beneath me. And then, another wound surfaced: abandonment. It wasn't just a thought; it was a sensation, a deep, throbbing ache that reverberated through my entire being. I could feel it in my bones, in my blood, in the marrow of who I was. Every cell in my body pulsed with the truth: abandonment was not just something I had experienced, it was something that had been passed down through generations, a thread woven through time, stretching back farther than I could comprehend.

The pain was unbearable. The loneliness was absolute.

But then, something shifted.

A whisper, an understanding, rising from the depths of my soul.

This pain—it didn't have to define me.

It could fuel me. I could carry it forward, not as a wound, but as a force, a reclamation.

My awareness expanded beyond myself, beyond my lineage, beyond time. My mind opened to the vast suffering of entire cultures, entire histories abandoned, erased, oppressed. I saw Indigenous people ripped from their land, their traditions compressed into the margins of existence. I felt the sorrow of those forced to trade heritage for survival, their entire worldviews condensed into what little space they were allowed. I saw generations of suffering, their voices echoing through time, their grief still alive, still breathing in the spaces between history.

And I continued to weep.

I wept for the suffering. I wept for the privilege. I wept for the bridges that had yet to be built, for the stories left untold, for the identities lost in the pursuit of acceptance.

As I lay there, my body trembling, my soul stripped bare, I felt something sacred in my suffering. This pain, this truth—it wasn't an end. It was a beginning. It was something to be honored, to be transformed.

And in that moment, I understood: this journey was never just about me.

I kept thinking about a video I had watched the day before. It had been gnawing at me, replaying in the back of my mind like an unresolved chord. I had been reviewing raw footage from an interview with an Indigenous healer, a man whose wisdom and presence would become part of the group documentary project. His story wasn't just something to be heard; it was something to be felt. And feeling it was excruciating.

While watching the video, a heavy, unbearable weight settled into my chest. White guilt surged through me, thick and suffocating, drowning out any ability to process his words logically. My mind could no longer hold onto the details; all I could do was feel. The sorrow, the injustice, the centuries of suffering he spoke of rushed through my body like a tidal wave, sending sharp pangs of pain into every limb. I wanted to take it all in, to understand fully, but my system simply shut down. The weight of it was too much. My stomach twisted, nausea rising as if my body wanted to purge the truth, to expel the unbearable reality physically. But this suffering wasn't something I could vomit out. It wasn't just mine. It belonged to all of us. It was the sickness of an entire civilization, of a culture so deeply detached from its own humanity that it had long forgotten the cost.

"Western worldview is so frustrating that it frustrates itself," he had said. And he was right. He was speaking the raw truth about the Western culture mindset in which I was raised.

During my LSD journey, the dam of emotion shattered as sobs wracked my body. I cried until there was nothing left inside me, until I had emptied myself onto the floor, curled into a shaking ball. It wasn't just sadness—it was something deeper, something ancient. A raw, guttural grief for everything that had been lost. For the severed roots. For the cultural abandonment that had left me, and so many others, unmoored. It wasn't a personal wound; it was an ancestral one.

Ken found me like that, small and crumpled, my breath still hitching in the aftermath. He knelt beside me, his hands warm as he gently gathered me up, holding me as I trembled. He didn't try to fix it, didn't offer hollow words of comfort. He just held me, letting me come back to myself, allowing me to exist in the vulnerability of it all. And for the first time in a long time, I truly saw it: the wound, the disconnection, the loss.

And I knew this journey wasn't just about healing myself. It was about something much bigger.

The road to bigger runs through me, I discovered.

The next stage of the trip was self-examination. And it was brutal.

I understood now the depth of the shame Mamaita had carried; the way she had buried her heritage to survive. It wasn't just her. My mother, too, had inherited that silent message: to blend in, to stay small, never to draw too much attention. I could suddenly see the whole chain of it—generation after generation internalizing the message that who we were, in our most natural and cultural essence, wasn't enough.

It wasn't a far stretch to see how that same shame had taken root in me. Only, it had morphed, shifting from culture to body, from ancestry to self-worth. I hadn't taken care of my body in years, and it showed. The shame that had once felt like a vast, inherited burden now turned inward, zooming in like a spotlight piercing straight into my heart. The pain shifted from ancestral suffering to something deeply, intimately personal.

There was nowhere to hide. No distractions, no justifications—just me, face-to-face with the raw, unfiltered truth of how I saw myself. And what I saw was unbearable.

A woman in her 50s. Obese. Sagging breasts. Rolling cellulite. A body that had carried me through life, but one I had neglected and disregarded. I saw myself through the world's eyes, and the image was crushing—a woman who hadn't given her body the care it needed.

I had poured all my energy into excelling mentally and emotionally, but my physical existence had been pushed to the side. The judgment was deafening, a relentless voice echoing inside me: *Why haven't you taken better care of your body?*

The shame was immense, suffocating. *You're going to Mexico in three weeks*, the voice reminded me, *and you'll need to walk everywhere. You should already be in better shape. You should have started long ago.* It wasn't just about health. It was about presentation, about how I showed up in the world.

CATHERINE - *I see it now.*

   The shame wasn't all mine.

   It was passed down.

MARIA - *Yes.*

   It was woven into your family like an heirloom no

   one wanted, but everyone inherited.

CATHERINE - *I spent so much time rebelling,*

   punishing myself.

MARIA - *You learned to rebel against them.*

   But you were also punishing yourself.

CATHERINE - *I pushed back by overeating.*

   It was the only thing I could control.

MARIA - *It was the only way you knew to*

stay separate.

But now you see.

Your rebellion was a chain.

Now, you can break it.

CATHERINE - *I understand now.*

It wasn't just about defying them.

It was about punishing myself for what I inherited.

MARIA - *And now, you release it.*

The shame ends with you.

You are free to rewrite your story.

The idea of presentation wasn't new. It had been ingrained in me since childhood, a rigid cultural standard woven into my family's fabric. Presentation mattered. How you looked mattered. And I had spent my entire life fighting it. Resisting. Rebelling. The resentment had taken root early, growing into something unshakable. I had refused to conform, had refused to be shaped by everyone's expectations. And I had found the perfect way to defy them.

I made sure to be overweight.

It was the one thing I could control, the one way I could push back. No matter how hard my mother and Mamaita tried, no matter how much they insisted, I could always find a way to overeat, to remain just outside of their standards. And it drove them crazy. Their frustration was fuel, feeding the rebellion that became second nature to me.

But now, in this moment of unforgiving clarity, I wasn't just rebelling against them; I was punishing myself. I wasn't free. I was trapped in a cycle of defiance that had long outlived its purpose.

And I couldn't ignore it any longer.

What I eventually came to understand about myself was that my body had not just been a rebellion. It had been a meat shield—a suit of armor, built layer by layer, protecting the most vulnerable parts of me. My weight wasn't just excess flesh; it was a filter, a boundary, a way to separate the superficial from the sincere.

The rolls, the folds, the curves—they became more than just physical. They were a test. A detector. A force field against those who only cared about the surface. My body, in all its fullness, served as an unspoken challenge: *If you can't see past this, you were never meant to see me at all.*

And it worked. The ones who were drawn only to appearances, to polished exteriors, filtered themselves out effortlessly. They had no interest in looking deeper, in discovering the complexity beneath. But the ones who stayed? The ones who saw beyond the shape of my body to the shape of my soul? Those were the people who mattered. The ones I let in. The ones I trusted.

It had been an incredible, almost foolproof bullshit detector. A phony-vetting machine that kept my inner world safe.

As I started coming down from the trip, my mind was still swimming in the remnants of the experience, my body vibrating with its intensity. I sat with Ken, trying to make sense of it all, still very much under the influence but with the promise of clarity. The world around me was still shifting, softening, and warping at the edges. LSD has a way of dissolving boundaries, of making everything feel fluid. The distinction between objects, between people, between where one thing ends and another begins, becomes almost meaningless. In that moment, faces stretched and shrank, one eye growing large while the other compressed, then shifting back again in an endless, hypnotic dance. Reality itself pulsed and breathed, reminding me that nothing—*nothing*—was ever truly solid.

And in that in-between space, I began to talk.

I reached for Ken's hand, needing something steady. "I don't even know where to start," I said, my voice raw. "The shame… it was overwhelming. It went from something massive and cultural to something deeply personal. Like it zoomed in until all that was left was me. My body. My choices. My life. And I hated what I saw."

Ken squeezed my hand gently. "Why?" he asked.

I exhaled sharply, pressing my free hand to my chest. "Because I saw myself the way the world sees me. A woman in her fifties. Fat. Sagging. Covered in cellulite. A woman who doesn't take care of herself. A woman who…" I swallowed hard, "I don't value enough."

Ken was quiet for a moment, his thumb tracing slow circles on my hand. Then he said, "You keep saying 'the world sees you that way.' But who exactly is *the world*?"

I frowned, caught off guard. "I don't know. Everyone. Society. People."

He shook his head slightly. "People aren't born thinking these things. They learn them. And where do they learn them?" He paused briefly before answering his own question. "Culture, he said." He tilted his head, watching my expression shift. "But culture is a made-up construct. A set of rules that someone decided we all just go along with. It's not real."

I blinked, trying to grasp what he was saying as the walls continued their slow, rhythmic breathing.

Ken went on. "You're in pain because you're seeing yourself through the lens of others. Through the expectations that were drilled into you. But that lens isn't *yours*. It's been handed down, shaped by a world that profits off your insecurity."

My stomach twisted. "So what? I just… stop caring?"

He shook his head. "No. You stop measuring yourself against something that was never real to begin with. The shame isn't yours. But the way you treat yourself because of it? That is. And that's where the work is." He shifted, his gaze steady, locking onto mine. "You have to accept *all* of you. Not just the parts you've been told are 'good.' Not just the parts that fit into someone else's idea of what's worthy. *All of you.*"

I swallowed thickly, my throat tight. "But what if I don't know how?"

Ken squeezed my hand again. "It's all about self-acceptance. Not changing yourself to meet what culture expects."

His words landed like a tidal wave, a force strong enough to shake something loose inside me. The years of rejection, of seeing myself through fractured mirrors built by other people's expectations, felt suddenly… optional. Like I had been gripping onto them out of habit, not necessity.

Self-acceptance. *That's* what had been missing all along. It wasn't about changing myself, fixing myself, or trying to finally "get it right." It was about *being with* myself—fully, without judgment, without trying to mold myself into something more palatable for the world. For my family. For anyone.

I let the thought settle deep in my bones.

What if I could stop fighting myself? What if I could just… be?

A lifetime of resistance had convinced me that self-love was something earned. That if I just became *better*—thinner, more disciplined, more polished—I could finally rest. But now, in this space where time stretched and reality pulsed, I saw the truth: *There was nothing to earn. There had never been.*

The battle had always been with myself. And I was tired of fighting.

I exhaled, a breath that felt like it had been waiting to be released for years. The shame released and softened. It lost its claws. I could still feel traces of it, lingering in the background, but for the first time, I realized—I didn't have to let it control me.

I looked at Ken, eyes wet, voice quiet. "If self-acceptance is the key… then I think I'm finally ready to find the door."

The night was long, almost endless. The LSD's glow still lingered in my system, like embers pulsing quietly after a fire. I couldn't sleep. The substance, having taken hold around 2 pm, was still weaving its web around my mind well into the early hours of the morning. By 3 am, I was wide awake, my body vibrating with the remnants of the experience. I lay next to Ken as he slept soundly beside me, his breathing deep and steady, while I continued to process the journey through which I had just gone. It was like my mind couldn't fully release the trip, still caught in the echoes of the emotions and revelations. I drifted in and out of consciousness, caught in that in-between space where everything felt alive—every thought, every feeling, still expanding and unraveling. It was uncomfortable, the buzz, but somehow necessary. Plus, it gave me more time to work on processing and integrating my experience.

As the insights settled, I was met with a sobering realization: the shame I carried wasn't entirely mine. It had been passed down—generation to generation—woven into the fabric of my family like an heirloom no one wanted but everyone inherited.

Mamaita, with her quiet self-loathing and desperate attempts to rewrite her story, had unknowingly handed me a legacy of disconnection. She fed me and criticized me in the same breath, a reflection of her own fractured relationship with herself. She denied her lineage so deeply that she framed a photograph of a stranger and called her "mother," as if the truth of who she was had to be scrubbed clean before it could be seen. That kind of shame doesn't stay contained; it seeps into children, into grandchildren, teaching us to reject ourselves before we even understand who we are.

In that moment, I saw the whole picture. My own struggle with self-acceptance wasn't just personal; it was ancestral. I wasn't adrift because I had failed; I was adrift because the map had never been drawn. There was no lighthouse because those before me had lived in shadow. But now, I could choose differently.

I couldn't change where I came from, but I could change what came through me. I could meet that legacy not with bitterness, but with compassion. I could become the ancestor who teaches a new language—one of self-trust, of worthiness, of love. I made a quiet vow to myself, right then: to no longer carry what wasn't mine, and to live the rest of my life learning how to accept the woman I am fully. Not despite where I come from, but because I now understand it.

When the morning light finally crept through the curtains, I woke feeling the shift, barely tangible but undeniable. It was like I could feel the tug of the past, and the pull of the new me, fighting for space. I could feel the slightest tinges of shame still lingering, just below the surface, like an old outfit I kept trying to shed. But there was something else there now; a new understanding, a flicker of self-acceptance that had started to take root. The tug-of-war between these two versions of myself—yesterday's shame and today's potential—was palpable. I would try on the new version of me, embrace the possibility of change, but then, like a reflex, I would find myself slipping back into the old clothes of shame, back into the self-critical patterns that had defined me for so long. It was like an awkward dance, a constant back-and-forth of shedding one layer only to return to the old one again briefly before letting it go. This is how I integrate after a journey: slowly, tentatively, as I test out what I've learned and give myself space to reframe the old stories.

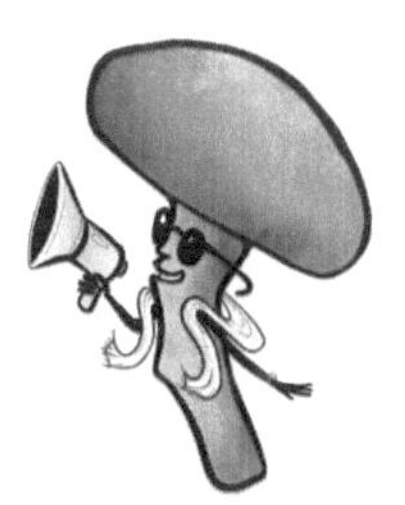

¡OYE! New self, same old closet.

Integration is like trying on outfits. Shame still hangs on the rack, but you don't have to wear it. Keep slipping into the new fit of self-acceptance until it feels like your favorite.

I didn't know exactly how, but I knew I was ready to move forward in a way I hadn't done before. The heaviness of yesterday's revelations still lingered in the air, but they didn't feel oppressive anymore. It felt like a doorway had opened, and I was ready to step through.

I decided to go for a walk.

I grabbed a pair of yoga pants from my drawer, something I would never have dared wear in public before. When I slipped them on, I immediately felt exposed, almost vulnerable. The fabric clung to my body in a way I wasn't used to. I was always so self-conscious about how much of my body was on display in these particular pants. But today it felt like a different situation, and for the first time, I didn't want to hide. I asked Ken, "Do these look too revealing?"

He looked at me, his eyes soft but proud. "No. Definitely not something you would've worn outside a year ago. I'm really proud of you for doing this. It's a big step."

His words sank deep into me, like a warm current. He was proud of me, and for the first time, I realized that I could be proud of myself too. I could see the change happening, slow but steady, and that felt like something I hadn't let myself believe in for a long time.

I walked outside, feeling the cool wind tugging at my skin. Typically, I would have used the wind as an excuse not to exercise and stay wrapped up in blankets, hiding from the world. But today, I didn't. I kept walking.

There's a small park in front of my house, and I decided to lap it. One lap—*a quarter of a mile*—wasn't something I would usually want to do. But that day, it didn't feel like a chore. I lapped it once. Then again. And again. And again. Five times. Each lap felt like a small victory, and by the time I finished, my heart was pounding, my breathing heavy. Usually, I would have resisted the discomfort, but not that day. I felt invigorated.

I leaned into it—the beating heart, the rush of breath in my chest—and instead of seeing it as a struggle, I saw it as a sign of strength. I wasn't just preparing for Mexico; I was preparing for the physical demands I feared I wouldn't be in good enough shape to meet. I was looking forward to the trip itself, but dreading the possibility of not being able to fully enjoy it, of being held back by my body. But in that moment, I realized that I didn't need to wait for some perfect version of myself. I was already in the process of preparing. This was the moment.

As I walked, I found myself thinking about the things I would need: new shoes for walking in a beach town, clothes that actually fit, that felt comfortable, that I didn't have to hide in. Each thought was no longer a burden, but an opportunity. I could see a future where I wasn't bound by shame, where I wasn't afraid to take care of myself, and where I was no longer trying to make myself invisible.

Three weeks. I had three weeks. And for the first time, I believed I could be ready.

What stood out most about this LSD journey was that, for the first time, it wasn't just radiant joy and expansive bliss. This time, LSD brought a kind of edge, a gritty undertone I had previously only associated with mushrooms. The early hours were unexpectedly raw. I found myself wrestling with unease, navigating unfamiliar emotional terrain that pushed back rather than opened effortlessly. It felt as though LSD was showing me a different facet of itself, one that challenged me to stay present even when it wasn't easy.

But then, like a tide turning, the experience softened. The beauty returned, the colors danced again, and I was swept back into the luminous current I had come to associate with LSD. That contrast, between discomfort and delight, contraction and expansion, was revelatory. It reminded me that no matter how many times I return to these medicines, they will always have new lessons, new layers. They evolve with me, and in doing so, they keep humbling me. Just when I think I've grasped their nature, they shift, teaching me again that the only certainty is the unfolding.

That's part of the magic—and the mystery. Psychedelics defy simple categorization. They aren't linear. They're alive, dynamic, responsive, which is exactly why I can only speak from my own lived experience. What I share in these pages is a reflection of my path, not a prescription for anyone else's. These journeys are deeply personal. And that's what makes them so powerful.

What's even more remarkable is that this personal path of mine was beginning to echo something larger: a rising tide of curiosity, openness, and courage sweeping across the collective. I could feel it. The world was shifting. Conversations were changing. Psychedelic-assisted therapy was no longer a whispered possibility; it was becoming a movement.

And that's where the next part of this story goes.

CATHERINE - *I wanted the cosmos, but mushrooms held me back.*

MARIA - *Yes.*

They reserved the right to keep you here.

Focused on your healing.

CATHERINE - *LSD let me touch it, just for a moment.*

MARIA - *That medicine rewarded you.*

Your work was never in the cosmos.

It's always been here, within you.

CATHERINE - *And now, I must focus on self-care.*

MARIA - *Yes.*

You are in the process of becoming.

Take the time to heal, to self-nurture.

The cosmos will wait.

CHAPTER SEVENTEEN

HEY ELIZABETH, IT'S POURING!

CATHERINE - *I don't understand.*

For years, I've spoken with my whole heart, but no one is listening. It's like I'm living underground.

MARIA - *You have been.*

But not in exile.

In incubation.

CATHERINE - *It feels like exile.*

Watching others rise while I stay still.

Watching the world ignore what I know is sacred.

MARIA - *Some seeds need darkness.*

Some truths take longer to root.

Yours were never meant to bloom overnight.

CATHERINE - *But the silence...*

It makes me doubt I was meant for this.

MARIA - *Doubt is part of the soil, too.*

But I don't doubt you.

Even when you feel invisible, you are growing.

Be patient.

The rain is coming.

FOR YEARS, I POURED MY HEART into a message the world wasn't ready to hear. I spoke of sacred medicine, of what is possible when psilocybin meets intention and courage. But my words felt like they dissolved the moment they left my lips. No echo. No ripple. Just still air.

At first, I told myself I was planting seeds. That it would take time. That maybe someone, somewhere, would water them. But as months turned into years, I began to wonder: *Am I speaking into barren ground?*

The silence wasn't neutral. It was discouraging in a way that slowly eats at your sense of meaning. I was doing work I knew was important. I had seen lives transformed—people broken by trauma, shame, or depression emerge with a light in their eyes, a sense of belonging to themselves. And yet, outside the room, beyond those sacred moments, the world kept turning as if none of it mattered. My work existed in the shadows, unspoken, misunderstood, sometimes ridiculed. It felt like standing at the edge of a forest fire with a cup of water in my hands, screaming for help, and watching people walk by as if I weren't there.

And still, I kept showing up.

I guided, I wrote, I taught. I whispered to the New Mexican desert soil, even when it looked like dust. I tried not to let the ache of invisibility change me. But there were days I felt hollow. Days I questioned everything. *Am I early? Or simply deluded?*

And then something shifted.

It wasn't dramatic. It was quiet, almost imperceptible at first, like a faint breeze after years of still heat. Someone sent me an email after reading a blog post I almost deleted.

"I've never heard anyone speak about healing this way," they wrote. "Please don't stop."

Then a former colleague reached out. "I think I'm ready to talk about this."

Another person referred to me as, "the one to talk to about psilocybin," and I was stunned—not just by the recognition, but by the tone. It was respectful. Curious. Willing.

I felt a drop.

After that, the clouds began to gather. More emails. Podcast invitations. Clients showing up no longer broken, but hopeful. Colleagues who once kept their distance started sending people my way. People who rolled their eyes at my passion a year earlier began to ask, "Can you tell me more?"

It was as if the cultural weather had changed. Something that had been underground was finally breaking the surface, and people were starting to notice.

I looked around, and the air was different. Damp. Alive.

Could this be the end of the drought?

I didn't realize how thirsty I was until the rain began to fall.

This wasn't just professional validation, it was soul hydration. For years, I had given relentlessly, not knowing if it would ever matter. Now I was watching those seeds push up through the soil. I could feel something returning to me; not just energy, but recognition. Visibility. I wasn't shouting into a void anymore. I was being heard.

And in the middle of that shift, there was a moment that brought it all home.

It's strange how life lines up sometimes. I had been looking for someone to help me carry the weight of the work. Not just an assistant, but a true partner; someone who understood the heart of it, not just the logistics. I had tried to bring Ken into the fold. He was willing, thoughtful, and deeply supportive, but our styles clashed. My urgency didn't match his pace. What felt like life-or-death to me felt, to him, like something we could "get to tomorrow." That gap became painful. Resentment crept in. We both knew we had to let it go, or it would cost us more than time.

And then there was Elizabeth.

She had been in my life for years. Not as a colleague or friend, but as the person who came a couple of times a month to clean the house. Yet from the beginning, I felt something in her that I couldn't name. Maybe it was the way she noticed things, the way she moved through a space with quiet care, tending to small details most people overlooked. Or maybe it was her energy. Grounded. Present. Gentle.

During the hardest season of my life, when I was recovering from cancer treatments, we hired a house cleaner because I was too disabled to manage the basics. That's how Elizabeth came into our lives. Early in our relationship, she saw me at my most fragile. I was in pain. Raw. Exhausted to the bone. I couldn't speak much when she arrived the first day. I remember lying on the couch, trying to stay still, trying not to let the grief leak out. She cleaned around me in silence. No questions. No pity. Just presence.

One day, after finishing up the housecleaning while I was especially unwell, Elizabeth left as usual. About twenty minutes later, she returned, this time with a bouquet of fresh flowers in her hands.

"I could feel your pain," she said, placing them beside me. "I just… I needed to do something."

I cried when she left. Not because of the flowers, but because I felt seen.

That was the moment I knew she was more than a housekeeper. She was a healer in her own right. Which is why I hired her as my assistant the second the opportunity presented itself.

When I did so, I expected that she would be dependable. But what I didn't know was that she would become my anchor. She brought order to chaos and created systems out of scattered ideas. She didn't just step into the work, she studied it. She watched how I moved through tasks, noticed the rhythm of my days, and quickly learned what mattered most. From those observations, she began managing logistics with surprising ease: scheduling, payments, and communication. She was a quick learner. In her quiet way, she reflected back to me a clearer picture of my own work, showing me the shape of what I had been too close to see.

I started calling her my "work wife." At first it was a joke. But the truth was, there was a rhythm between us that felt like partnership. We understood each other. We trusted each other. And that trust made space for something rare: *ease.*

To this day, Ken still tells Elizabeth she saved our marriage when she took over the administrative work. And he's not exaggerating.

There was one moment in particular that pierced through the noise and anchored the new reality for me.

By this time, Elizabeth had become my right hand, my sounding board, my co-dreamer. We met monthly for lunch to connect and recalibrate. During one of those lunches, she looked at me, her voice steady but full of feeling.

"You're the best role model I've ever had," she said.

I blinked, caught off guard. "What?" I asked, my voice barely above a whisper. Then, without thinking, the next question tumbled out: "Why?"

She didn't hesitate. "Because you lead with honesty. You don't pretend to be perfect. You've walked through fire and yet you keep going. You didn't just tell me I could survive. You showed me. Watching you keep going… it changed me. And you call me out when I'm wrong, in a way that I respect. You don't shame me. You challenge me. That's rare."

She told me I was her hero.

I sat there stunned, her words wrapping around a place in me I hadn't realized was still aching for acknowledgment. Not for my accomplishments, but for who I had become in the process. That moment wasn't about praise, it was about being truly seen.

And it landed. Deeply.

After so many years of output, of giving, leading, and holding space, this was the moment I finally allowed myself to receive.

Not just support. Not just partnership. But reverence.

Someone was telling me, *You matter. What you've done matters. Who you are matters.*

It wasn't applause I needed. It was this. And in that moment, a major revelation occurred: Gratitude isn't just about saying "thank you." It's about letting others give to you—and letting it matter.

That conversation with Elizabeth became one of the clearest signs that the drought really was ending. Not because everything was easy now, but because I was no longer invisible. I was no longer alone.

The clouds were gathering.

The rain had started.

And for the first time in a long time, I let myself stand in it, face turned toward the sky.

People were waking up. And simultaneously, so was Elizabeth on a personal level.

Elizabeth wasn't just capable. She was steadfast. Over time, our working relationship blossomed into something deeper.

She attended one of the classes I taught, not out of obligation, but because she was deeply curious. Her interest grew from logistics to the medicine. She became fascinated with mushroom cultivation, and eventually, she admitted, shyly, "I think I might want to be a guide someday."

I smiled gently, but I was also firm. "You know the requirement."

She nodded. "I have to do the medicine myself."

That is a non-negotiable for me.

My work isn't like chemotherapy or many other medications, where a doctor prescribes a drug, manages symptoms, and monitors progress without ever personally experiencing the treatment. Psilocybin is fundamentally different. It's a sacred medicine, an experience that touches the core of one's being, alters perception, and invites profound transformation. To guide someone properly through this journey, you must have walked the path yourself.

Guiding isn't about clinical observation or intellectual understanding alone. It's about empathy born from your own vulnerability and healing, about presence cultivated through your own encounters with the medicine. Without having surrendered to psilocybin's lessons firsthand, a guide cannot fully hold space for another's journey. They cannot truly anticipate the nuances of what arises, nor support with the depth required.

The medicine demands this. It calls for readiness. Not just intellectual or logistical readiness, but emotional and spiritual preparedness that only experience can give. To be a guide is to walk alongside another through their darkest and brightest moments. That can only be done authentically if you know the medicine's power yourself.

So I waited. Patiently. Never pushing, never suggesting. I knew that readiness had to come from within Elizabeth.

Then, one day, over coffee, she looked at me, eyes raw and vulnerable.

"I'm not okay," she whispered. "Things are so hard right now. I'm desperate for some healing."

I didn't need to ask if she understood the weight of what she was saying. Elizabeth didn't romanticize the work. She had already seen it up close with clients unraveling, breakthroughs that left them trembling, and the long integration that followed. She understood that guiding wasn't about being a savior or a mystic. It was about being still. Being real. And being willing to witness everything, without looking away.

She was ready.

I watched her prepare in the days leading up to her journey: measured, thoughtful, and more curious than afraid. She approached it with intention, spending time reflecting on what she wanted to face, what she hoped to release, and what she longed to heal. She worked quietly on setting her intentions, writing them down, revisiting them, and holding them close like a fragile promise to herself. But beneath that calm exterior, I could feel the tension in her, the weight of everything she had held inside for so long.

She arrived for her journey in soft pajamas, an eye mask tucked under her arm, and a handwritten list of intentions clutched in her hand. I remembered her in training, voicing her fear that the mushrooms might reveal things she wasn't ready to face. But the woman who walked through the door that morning was not afraid. She was grounded, resolute, and open. She had done the work beforehand. She was ready.

And then there's the oddity that she's one of the very few people I've ever met who actually enjoys the taste of psilocybin mushrooms. I love these mushrooms for what they do, but taste-wise, they're earthy at best. I need lemonade or limeade just to get them down. Elizabeth, on the other hand, tossed back the mushroom limeade mixture like a seasoned pro. No hesitation, no grimace. For someone who rarely drinks alcohol and had never touched psychedelics before, she carried herself with surprising confidence.

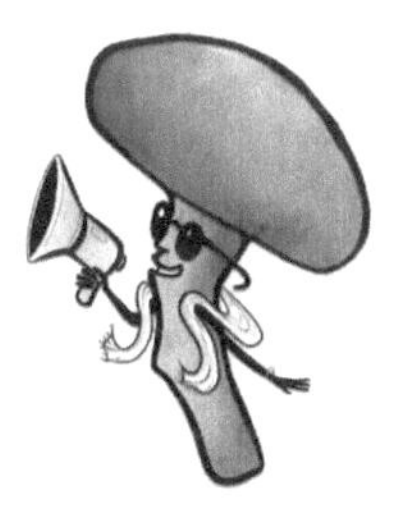

¡OYE! If it tastes like a forest floor, that's because it basically is.

Don't expect dessert. Expect dirt. Mix with citrus if you need to, and if you like the flavor... we're both impressed and mildly concerned.

Prior to that, we prepared the medicine together. As we ground the dried mushrooms and blended the tea, I told her the story of María Sabina, a revered Mazatec *curandera* (healer), who shared the sacred mushroom rituals of her people with outsiders, only to be exploited and cast aside. Her name had been erased by those who built careers on what she revealed. Yet still, her spirit lives on in the medicine, in the rituals, in every careful, intentional healing circle.

"She gave everything," I told Elizabeth, "and people took it. But her wisdom—that never left. She's still guiding people."

CATHERINE - *Maria Sabina...*

> *She brought the sacred mushrooms to the world.*

> *Are you Maria Sabina?*

MARIA - *You already know that I am.*

> *And I am not.*

> *I am the voice she left behind.*

> *I am your guide.*

CATHERINE - *But...*

MARIA - *I carry the spirit of her.*

> *Her wisdom, her love, her teachings.*

> *But I am not her.*

> *I am the one you need now.*

CATHERINE - *So, you are connected to her, but*

> *not the same?*

MARIA - *Exactly.*

> *I am here to guide you.*

> *To walk with you on your path.*

> *Her path is part of the story, but your journey is*

> *yours to make.*

As Elizabeth lay back, eyes closed, I held her hand and reminded her, "This is your time. You are safe. You are loved. Let the medicine show you what you need to see."

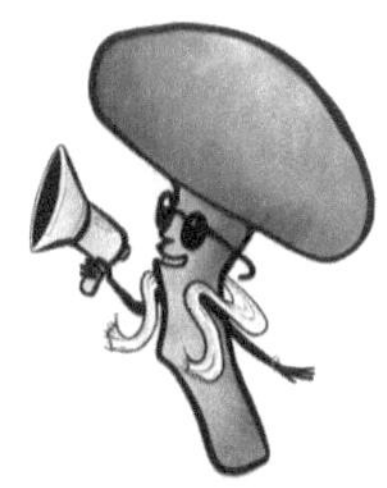

¡OYE! Talk consent around touch beforehand.

That reassuring hand on your shoulder? Beautiful—
if expected. Awkward, if not. Always check in first.
Nobody wants surprise intimacy while talking to a tree.

Elizabeth carried stories that had never been told. Not because she was hiding them, but because she had been too busy carrying everyone else's pain. The medicine found those stories quickly. It moved with a fierce tenderness, uncovering the layers she didn't even know were still buried. These included old grief, shame, responsibility, and loss. It gave voice to the silence she'd carried for years.

In the first hour of her journey, Elizabeth wrestled with letting go. She faced the familiar, often intense battle with ego that many first-time journeyers experience. Waves of coldness gave way to sudden heat, accompanied by strange physical sensations and tingling that unsettled her body. Nausea crept in, adding to the challenge.

Through it all, she saw the women in her family: generations of caretakers, each bearing burdens the world never acknowledged. She recognized how deeply her own identity had been shaped by the act of holding others. Her childhood dynamics played a part, too. She had always been the one to pick up the pieces for her parents and siblings, and they had always let her. And perhaps for the very first time, she saw how little she had held herself.

It was as though the medicine asked her: *"Are you willing to stop hiding behind service?"*

It wasn't an accusation. It was an invitation. To stop performing worthiness. To stop earning love by doing. To stop being everyone's safe place without building one inside herself.

At one point, she lay back, letting the warmth of the medicine hold her. In that place beyond ego, beyond narrative, she met something she described as *the original her*, a presence that wasn't defined by roles or tasks or expectations. It was quieter than personality. Older than her name. Just… her. Later, during the journey, she whispered something that chilled me.

"She's here," she said. "The curandera… she's here. She's making me die."

"What do you mean?" I asked gently.

"She keeps stopping my heart. I see a bright light. Then it fades, and she works on the next part of me that needs to die."

I placed my hand on her shoulder. "Let go," I whispered. "Let it die. And focus on the rebirth."

Again and again, María's spirit helped her shed what no longer served. Layers of guilt, responsibility, and old pain; all dying one by one to make room for something new.

Afterward, when the journey ended and we debriefed, Elizabeth sat across from me, teary-eyed and radiant.

"I realize I don't have to carry everyone's pain anymore," she said. "I can have my own voice. I can just… be me. And that's enough."

I watched her fall in love with herself again. She spoke of a deep tenderness toward her husband—new understanding, new connection. "It's like I saw him through different eyes," she said. "Through love."

She also spoke about what so many psilocybin-assisted therapy participants experience afterward: the pause.

"It's like… I don't have to react the same way anymore," she said. "My brain stops me. It gives me a choice. I can do something different now."

¡OYE! Psilocybin drops "choice points" like breadcrumbs after a journey.

You can replay the old track, or spin something brand new.

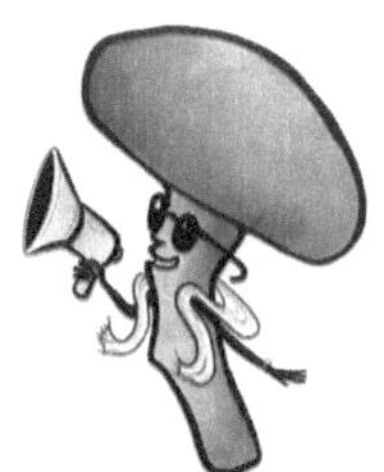

That is one of the miracles of the medicine: the pause. It changes everything. In that pause, new neural pathways can begin to form, new behaviors can take root, and a new way of living can emerge. I call these moments *choice points*. Thanks to the brain's neuroplasticity, we're given the opportunity to interrupt old patterns and choose a different response. We can still follow the familiar paths if we want to. But now, we have access to a deeper understanding. We can choose differently, and with intention, reinforcing those new pathways until they become the new default.

All of her intentions were addressed. Her view on life was transformed. She stepped more fully into herself, and into the work.

Over the weeks that followed, I watched her change, dramatically and outwardly. There was a new gravity in her, a deeper steadiness born not just of competence, but of integration. She moved more slowly, but with increased certainty. Her voice carried a different energy which was clearer, stronger, no longer diluted by the need to please. She began to speak her truth more freely, without shrinking to make others comfortable. She no longer made herself small to fit into spaces that had never really held her.

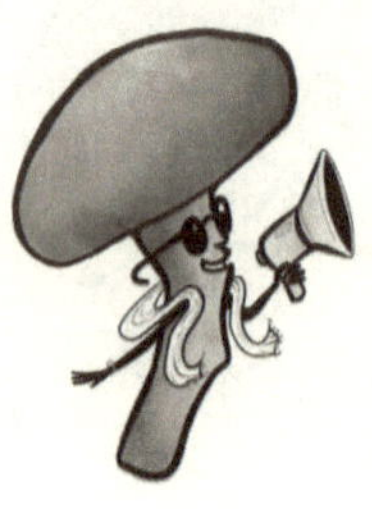

You don't have to solve your experience. Just return to it with curiosity. New layers will reveal themselves over time.

This shift was not without its ripples. Her husband, like many partners of those who undergo psilocybin healing, had to adjust to a version of her that was no longer content to absorb discomfort just to keep the peace. She was setting boundaries that would have been unthinkable before. She was sticking up for herself, not from a place of defiance, but from a place of worth. She owned her feelings and stopped taking responsibility for emotions that didn't belong to her. She was no longer reacting on autopilot; she was responding with intention, grounded in her own clarity.

Many people tell me their partners are worried when they decide to take a journey. I often hear things like, *"He's afraid I'll discover I don't need him anymore,"* or *"What if she comes out of this and doesn't love me?"*

These fears are real, and they deserve acknowledgment. But from my years of guiding, what I have seen is that psilocybin does not create false distance or fabricate new problems. It reveals what is already there. Psilocybin is a non-specific amplifier. It brings buried feelings to the surface, giving them room to be processed and understood. Yes, there are times when someone emerges with a new resolve and decides to leave a relationship. Still, every time I have witnessed this, it was because the relationship was already unhealthy and the truth was already bubbling under the surface. What the medicine offered was clarity and courage. I have never seen someone in a loving, committed relationship come out of a journey ready to walk away. More often, what emerges is tenderness, empathy, and a deeper connection with the partner who has stood beside them. And in the weeks that follow, I usually see relationships grow stronger and healthier as the insights continue to take root.

¡OYE! Psilocybin isn't a homewrecker.

It doesn't break your marriage. It just turns up the volume on what's already there. Love gets louder. Resentment does too. The medicine doesn't invent problems. It just flips on the light.

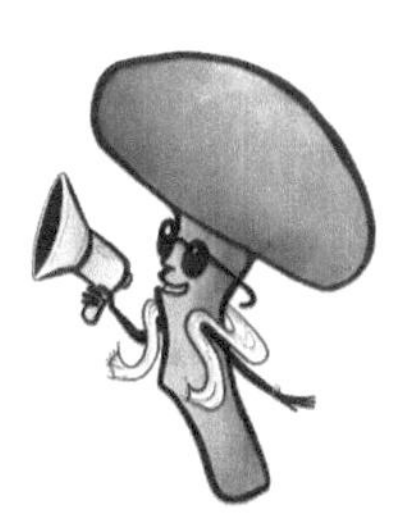

I can already envision her beside me on future journeys—not as an assistant or a student, but as a guide in her own right. There's a quiet wisdom in Elizabeth now, a steadiness that wasn't there before, and an intuition that's beginning to rise to the surface after years of being buried under responsibility. I see how her presence, once cautious and deferential, now carries the weight of lived experience and hard-won clarity. In time, I believe she will bring something uniquely powerful to the space; not just her compassion and calm, but a deeper knowing that can only come from doing the work herself. She is learning to trust that voice within, and I look forward to the day it leads her confidently into the role she's growing toward.

Her path reminds me of Maria Sabina, the Mazatec curandera, who first shared the sacred mushroom ceremonies of her people with the wider world. Sabina never sought fame or attention. She simply answered the call to serve. Like Elizabeth, she held the medicine not as a tool, but as a trust. Something to be honored, not exploited. Something to be lived, not owned.

What happened with Maria Sabina is still a cautionary tale: how the Western world rushed in, hungry for magic but unready for meaning. Her village was overwhelmed. Her sacred traditions were commodified. She was revered by strangers but ostracized by her own. And yet, in the quiet of her life, she remained devoted to the work. She never stopped praying with the mushrooms.

Elizabeth carries that same quiet strength.

Not flashy. Not performative. Just true.

She simply shows up with reverence, with humility, and with the authority of someone who has faced herself and chosen wholeness.

And that, I've learned, is more than enough.

And it wasn't just Elizabeth who was seeing me differently. The professional landscape was shifting too. Invitations began to arrive: first a podcast interview, then another, then requests to speak about psilocybin-assisted therapy at places where my voice had once been dismissed. Each one felt like another drop of rain, proof that the drought was breaking.

Then came Peg. What began as conversations about our shared passion soon grew into collaboration, the spark of another documentary taking shape. Together, we began organizing and identifying participants, shaping the circle of people who would eventually step into this group work. It was not just about filling seats. It was about weaving together a group of practitioners from different backgrounds, each bringing their own wisdom and perspective. Therapists, counselors, healers, and seekers all came forward, drawn by a shared calling to explore the potential of psilocybin. The diversity of the group mattered. It created a richer dialogue, a wider net of insight, and a deeper container for what was about to unfold. For me, the goal of this documentary was to educate the field and the world about the power of psilocybin and group work.

The trip to Northern Indiana, where we conducted pre-interviews with participants, was one of the clearest signs to me that the drought was truly ending. I have already recounted that dinner, where Peg raised his glass in a toast that left me stunned and deeply moved. I return to it here because it was one of those rare moments when you can feel the ground shift beneath your feet. It was proof that all of the unseen years of labor were bearing fruit.

More confirmations soon followed. I was asked to speak at the SB219 hearings, a pivotal step in New Mexico's unfolding relationship with psychedelics. A graduate program on Psychedelic Science invited me to lecture, recognizing that my work had a place in the classroom as well as the therapy room. I was nominated for, and accepted, the role of Secretary for Decriminalize Psychedelics New Mexico. Each of these invitations carried weight, not just because they offered a platform, but because they signaled that people were finally ready to listen.

My efforts had not disappeared into silence after all. They were leading somewhere: toward connection, toward community, toward something far bigger than I had ever carried alone. The silence had ended, the doors were opening, and with them I felt the drought giving way to rain.

CATHERINE - *They're starting to find me.*

My words, my work—

It's like something is waking up.

MARIA - *Not something.*

Everything.

CATHERINE - *It feels... nourishing.*

Like the silence is over and now the world is

drinking in too.

MARIA - *Because the drought wasn't just yours.*

It was theirs, too.

And now your waters rise together.

CATHERINE - *I see it now.*

The seeds I planted weren't wasted.

They were waiting.

So was I.

MARIA - *You didn't just endure the drought.*

You softened in it.

You listened.

And now, beloved,

It's time to bloom.

CHAPTER EIGHTEEN

SHAKEN, STIRRED AND STRENGTHENED

CATHERINE - *This doesn't feel right.*

> *It's not like before.*

> *I'm uncomfortable and jittery.*

> *What is this?*

MARIA - *It is the stirring before the knowing.*

> *Discomfort is not danger.*

> *It's just the body resisting insight arriving too soon.*

CATHERINE - *But I don't understand it.*

> *I want to know why I feel like this.*

MARIA - *You will. But not yet.*

> *Sometimes the soul prepares for a storm before*

> *the sky darkens. You are being made ready.*

CATHERINE - *For what?*

MARIA - *The unknown.*

> *You don't have to name it.*

> *Only trust the hands already waiting to hold you.*

IT WAS FEBRUARY OF 2025, AND even with all my experience, after years of exploring the depths of consciousness and guiding others through psychedelic terrain, I wasn't prepared for what came next. Up until then, mushrooms had been my lantern in the dark, illuminating the past so I could make peace with it. They helped me process trauma, grieve losses, and shed what no longer served me. But this time, the medicine turned its gaze forward.

What I initially dismissed as an unusually intense journey, which felt chaotic, disorienting, and strange, wasn't random at all. It was a prelude. A whisper from the future disguised as a storm in my psyche.

The mushrooms knew something I didn't. They were preparing me for a reality I hadn't yet seen: a threat reawakening in my body, waiting just beyond the horizon.

In hindsight, the signs were everywhere. I just hadn't learned to read them yet.

So much turmoil. I entered the experience with a sharp, tart edge, like the sting of citrus fruit on a fresh wound. What followed was a whirlwind, a chaotic tornado of emotion and sensation, before I finally released, landing more grounded than ever.

I'd planned to dose the night prior, but a sour stomach made me pause. I thought it better to wait until morning. When I woke, though, I felt an unexpected resistance. It was hard to pinpoint at first, but as I sat with it, I realized it was a sense of obligation. I was feeling an invisible pressure to dose; not from desire, but out of duty. Duty to my work, my clients, and myself.

Yet still, there was something on the periphery that I couldn't quite place. Perhaps it was the call to keep my depression at bay. It felt transactional, like checking off a box on a to-do list.

Something was off.

Looking back, I can see that I *did* need the medicine just as much as I needed to sleep, eat, or breathe. But at the time, that truth was buried beneath layers of logic and routine. On the surface, everything seemed fine. I felt stable, grounded, even physically well. But underneath was something else. A restless cacophony I couldn't name. An edge to my thoughts, a tightness in my chest. Like a bowstring pulled too far, trembling with pressure I didn't fully understand. Something was off, though I couldn't quite put my finger on what—or why.

I usually prepare psilocybin with limeade or lemonade, letting the ground mushrooms pre-digest for about fifteen minutes. This time, I used an especially strong, tart lemon juice without tasting it first. Once the mushrooms were mixed in, there was no going back. I tried adding water and honey to soften the sharpness, but it barely made a difference. There's a poetic justice to the way that particular journey began, both sharply and tartly, literally and metaphorically.

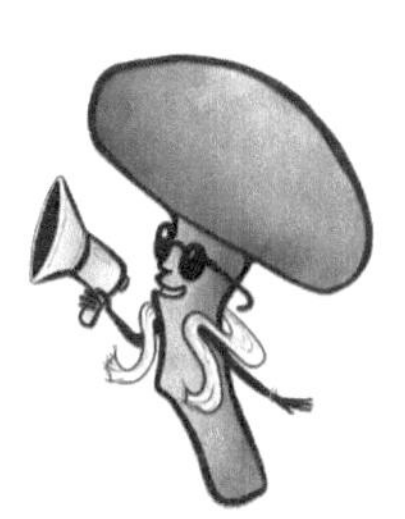

¡OYE! Lemon tekking is like pressing fast-forward—on purpose.

Mix your mushrooms with fresh-squeezed limeade, lemonade, or orange juice (not from concentrate!) and let it steep for fifteen to twenty minutes. The effects come on faster, feel more intense, and don't last as long. Many people find they need a smaller dose. Just don't forget to drink it, because after twenty minutes, the magic starts to fade. This isn't a hack; it's a shift in timing. Use it when you're ready to meet the medicine sooner and stronger.

The trip itself was a struggle. I was restless and uncomfortable, like my skin didn't fit. I couldn't find my center. It felt as though I was being picked up and shaken, like a salt shaker tossed between invisible hands. Turmoil. Turbulence. A random whirlwind shifting direction every second, amplifying flickers of resistance and discomfort.

Psilocybin is an amplifier, and that day it cranked the volume on everything I'd been resisting, starting with the harsh taste of ingestion.

Yet, even amid the chaos, I felt surrounded and wrapped in the invisible embrace of my support system: family, friends, colleagues, even clients. They held the perimeter, like a protective bubble against the storm. That containment made it okay to spin and twist through the air, knowing the tornado had its boundaries. It wasn't endless. It was temporary.

I still don't fully understand what that uncomfortable trip was all about. My husband suggested it might simply have been the release of accumulated energy. After all, so much had been happening. All good things, yes. But even joy can create tension when left unprocessed. Maybe that was all it was: an emotional backlog, needing to be shaken loose.

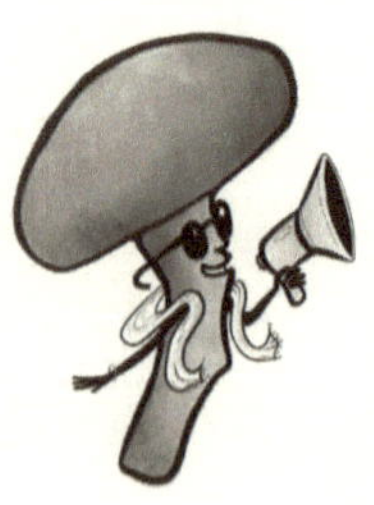

¡OYE! If you're wondering if it's working... it's working.

Doubt is part of the ride. Trust the unfolding, even if it doesn't look how you imagined.

The release, however, was sudden, visceral, like bursting through the eye of a storm into an unexpected calm. The restless energy vanished, leaving a landscape of stillness stretching for miles. There was no wreckage, just a raw, stripped-down purity. Back to basics. Back to myself.

I felt fantastic afterwards, when the tornado had passed and sorted itself out.

Two weeks after the mushroom journey, I walked into my six-month follow-up with Dr. Rama, fully expecting it to be my last. I was ready to close the chapter on being someone who'd had cancer, to finally be free of the appointments and tests that had consumed my time and energy for so long.

As she reviewed my medical history and the latest test results, I felt a wave of anticipation. Usually, I would've completed my blood work the week before, but somehow, it had slipped through the cracks. *No big deal*, I thought. I'd just swing by the lab on my way out. I wasn't worried. Why would I be? I truly believed that everything was fine, that I was on the brink of being released from treatment.

At my previous visit, my blood work had shown elevated calcium levels, a potential red flag. But a follow-up test one week later revealed that everything was normal, and we dismissed it as a fluke. It felt like another hurdle I'd cleared.

I mentioned to Dr. Rama that it had been two years since my last colonoscopy and that I'd been experiencing some irregular bowel activity, unusual sounds, and occasional abdominal pain. I thought it would be wise to have another colonoscopy, just to be sure.

She listened carefully and took note, her expression thoughtful. She agreed and decided to refer me for a diagnostic colonoscopy sooner than planned, just to be cautious.

Two days later, my phone exploded with notifications. A message from the gastroenterologist invited me to set up an appointment for my colonoscopy. Another from Dr. Rama's office requested more blood work—my calcium levels were high again. And then the third message delivered the gut punch: a PET scan had been scheduled.

Wait… what? I thought we were done. I thought I was in the clear. Suddenly, it felt like the ground was shifting beneath me. It was déjà vu, dragging me back to the whirlwind that first swallowed me when all of this began. It was happening so fast, just like before. So fast I could barely catch my breath. *Whoosh!* That familiar, gut-wrenching sensation, throwing me into a triggered state of medical trauma.

I sat in my car, staring at the flurry of messages on my phone, feeling completely overwhelmed. But it wasn't fear of what was happening. No, it was the haunting echo of what had happened four years ago: a wave of unresolved pain and panic that I had never truly faced.

This is the nature of unresolved trauma: It doesn't stay buried. It waits, quietly tucked away, until something in the present strikes a match. Then it erupts, flooding the now with echoes of the past, distorting reality and making everything feel bigger, heavier, and impossible to manage.

I recognized it instantly, both as a practitioner and as someone who's lived it. That awareness didn't make it easier. If anything, it made it more maddening. I could see the spiral forming, knew exactly why it was happening, yet I still couldn't stop the past from hijacking the present. It was like watching a storm roll in, knowing I had no shelter.

I went home, and once again, I was faced with the gut-wrenching task of sharing the bad news with Ken.

Poor Ken.

I could see the familiar flash in his eyes, that same reaction from before. I wasn't sure if it was fear or if I was just seeing it through the lens of my own triggered emotions. Either way, it didn't matter. It was still the same painful déjà vu, pulling up old wounds and dragging them into the present, reactivating all the hurt and fear that had never fully healed.

The following day was a nightmare of phone calls, each one another obstacle in an endless maze. I spent hours navigating insurance questions about coverage, getting quotes for each procedure, and trying to schedule the necessary tests. I had to reach out to my general doctor to adjust a medication that could have been responsible for raising my calcium levels. The PET scan and the colonoscopy—all needed to be scheduled—but each step felt like wading through quicksand.

It was a whirlwind dealing with the broken, fragmented medical system. I spent long periods on hold, waiting for answers, for an appointment, for someone, anyone, to help. I cancelled all my meetings to focus on getting it all done. But with each phone call, my patience thinned, and I could feel my mood souring. I was irritable, snapping at nothing. God, how I hated it all. At one point, I was trapped in the chaos, on hold with one person while another called through on the other line. *Do I risk losing the person who's on hold, or do I ignore the new call and hope they'll leave a message?* It was an anxious mess, a tug-of-war between decisions that made me feel like I was drowning in a sea of stress.

Eventually, I surrendered, submitting to the endless bureaucracy, trying to survive the process with as little emotional damage as possible.

Ken tried to soothe my growing frustration, offering support in the ways he knows best: making me a warm, nourishing meal, offering a cup of tea, doing everything he could to take care of me. To an outsider, we probably looked like we had slipped right back into our old roles: the cancer wife and the devoted, caretaking husband. And in a way, we had. We slid into those familiar patterns effortlessly, like putting on a well-worn glove.

But beneath it all, those triggered emotions sat quietly in the background, making everything feel more difficult, like how a lack of sleep makes even the simplest tasks harder. There was an underlying layer of anxiety, constantly pulling at the edges of my thoughts, amplifying everything around me. It was exhausting. I had to push through a couple of long days, back-to-back clients, all while carrying a heightened sense of fear that had been triggered. On top of that, I was dealing with the side effects and withdrawal symptoms of changing my blood pressure medication—a medication that might have been the culprit behind the rising calcium levels. The weight of it all, the mental and physical exhaustion, was taking its toll.

My logical mind tried to ground me, reminding me that the symptoms I was experiencing could be due to my blood pressure medication. But there was also a chance they were signs of the cancer returning. I didn't know which it might be, and that uncertainty fueled my fear. The spectrum of possibilities was clear in my mind, logically understood. But the emotional brain doesn't operate on logic. It only knows the raw, visceral experience of what it's felt before.

And in that moment, it was reliving the emotional intensity of the first time I was diagnosed, fueled by the overwhelming whirlwind of feelings that bound these two events together. My body was expressing all the unresolved emotions from that original experience—feelings I had never fully processed. If I hadn't had the awareness to understand what was happening, I'm certain I would have been spiraling into a full-blown anxiety attack, overwhelmed by everything my body was trying to process.

Less than a week later, I was still dancing with old triggers, doing my best to ground myself in logic, compassion, and self-care. But it wasn't easy. The echoes of the past had a way of bleeding into the present, and I was feeling it in my body, in the tightness in my chest, in the way I startled at nothing.

On a call with my best friend back East, I found myself talking fast, too fast, rushing to fill the space between us with explanations and reassurances.

"Okay, so Monday was rough," I began, barely taking a breath. "But I've been doing all the right things: breathwork, walking, journaling. I'm okay, really."

There was a pause on the other end of the line. Then came her quiet reply, thick with worry. "You don't sound okay."

That's when it hit me.

I was racing through my words not just to update her, but to shield her. I could feel the fear in her voice, and I was desperate to pull her out of it, to protect her from sitting in the uncertainty I hadn't fully allowed myself to feel.

"I know it's hard not to go there," I told her, softening. "But I promise you, most of this is my nervous system reacting to the past, not the present. There's nothing definitive yet, no proof this is cancer-related. We're still waiting on the tests. I don't want us getting swallowed up by assumptions. Not yet. Not again."

She let out a breath, and in that quiet moment, I realized I wasn't just trying to convince her. I was trying to anchor myself, too

And then, right in the middle of our conversation, something clicked. The mushroom journey that had left me spinning and unsure hadn't been chaos for chaos's sake. It was a message in motion. I was being shaken and stirred, yes, but not broken. It was a kind of sacred undoing, a preparation. I wasn't meant to brace against the storm; I was meant to remember that I would be held through it. My people had been there all along. They hadn't vanished; instead, they were momentarily obscured by the fog of fear and survival. I'd been squinting at the trees, trying to make sense of the shadows, forgetting that a forest quietly encircled me.

I realized that my mushroom journey had been preparing me for this moment. It wasn't just a chaotic, turbulent experience. It was a process of awakening, offering me the knowledge and insight I would need when faced with the possibility of cancer's return. The intensity, the discomfort, and the uncertainty mirrored what I was feeling, but the trip had already given me the tools to navigate the storm. It reminded me of the importance of trusting the support system around me, of understanding that the chaos is temporary, and that I would land on my feet.

Through the lessons learned during the trip, I was able to meet the new challenge with clarity and presence, using the emotional release from the journey to navigate the fear and uncertainty of the present. What I learned then, about resilience, trust, and surrender, became the foundation I needed to face the moment, bringing me back to stillness even in the face of the unknown.

It was a significant moment—the first time mushrooms assisted me with something that hadn't yet happened. It gave me a structure and coping technique to deal with a challenging situation that made me feel uncertain and anxious. During the trip, I was confused about why I was being put through such an intense experience. Even when it ended, and I began to make sense of it, I didn't fully grasp its value. It wasn't until I faced the health scare that I realized how much better I was able to handle the entire week because of it. The journey prepared me, giving me what I needed before I knew I needed it.

I came to realize that no matter how chaotic life gets, I'm held by a soft, steady cushion of love, a circle of people ready to catch me, no matter how or where I might fall. And as I step into the unknown, there's a quiet, unwavering sense, deep within me, that no matter what happens, I'll be okay. Maybe not right away, but eventually. I will land, and I will rise.

The week following the journey, I noticed something profound: I allowed myself to exist in the neutral zone. For years, I'd counseled clients with the phrase, "worrying doesn't change the outcome," a simple truth, but one that is often very difficult to implement. Yet here I was, actually doing it. And it felt like a monumental shift. I knew there was a spectrum of possibilities. On one end, the elevated calcium levels could simply be the result of my blood pressure medication. On the other hand, it could indicate the cancer had returned. There were many potential causes in between, and I didn't have enough information to know for sure yet.

The pendulum swung between the two possibilities, and in the past, I would have immediately spiraled into catastrophic thinking, imagining the worst-case scenario. I would have spent countless hours feeding my fears, letting them take root in my mind, and sending my nervous system into overdrive. My mind, left unchecked, would have latched onto every scary possibility, making the situation infinitely worse than it had to be. Without any test results, the mind is free to conjure up endless horrors.

But this time, something was different. I realized that worrying wasn't just a futile exercise—it was a draining one. It was like tapping into an endless reservoir of energy for no reason other than habit. I have also always believed that our thoughts have real power: they can align our cells, shape our realities, and even steer outcomes in ways we don't always understand. So why feed that energy into a fear that hadn't even manifested? Why squander it when I might need it later, when the real challenge might come?

Instead, I chose to conserve my energy, to stay neutral. By doing so, I wasn't dismissing the possibility of bad news, but I was saving the strength I would need if it did come. Why exhaust myself now, only to be left empty if the moment of genuine need arrives?

And then came the call, the one that truly tested my resolve.

The day before my PET scan, the hospital phoned to say the technician was sick and my procedure had been pushed back *two whole weeks*. I stood there, phone in hand, somewhere between disbelief and laughter. "Really?" I muttered aloud, half to the universe. "Is this a joke?" It felt like a cosmic pop quiz on everything I had just practiced: patience, presence, and neutrality.

That initial five-day wait had been challenging enough, but this… this felt like the real test. And yet, somewhere in the quiet between the moments of frustration and fear, I found myself grounded. My recent mushroom journey had prepared me for this, not just by healing old wounds, but by planting new roots.

It had shown me how to find stillness in the unknown, how to remain upright and centered even when everything around me was shifting. It reminded me that the storm doesn't dictate the direction of my path: I do.

Neutrality became my greatest ally. It allowed me to stay present in the rest of my life—showing up for clients, connecting with loved ones, and trusting that I was held by something greater. I wasn't alone in this. My support system—friends, family, loved ones—was like roots beneath the soil, steady and unseen, holding me up even when I felt like I was falling. They were there, quietly holding space, ready to catch me if I fell. And I knew I would land, one way or another, on solid ground.

Almost comically, that's when the delays really started piling up. After the PET scan postponement, I got another call, this time from the gastroenterology office. My colonoscopy, which was already scheduled, had to be rescheduled. "The doctor's not even in that day," the scheduler explained sheepishly. I blinked at the phone. *What the hell is happening?* It felt like a cruel comedy of errors. The delays, the reschedules, the waiting...all of it conspiring to throw me off balance. But instead of spiraling, I stayed steady. Not because it was easy, but because I had been trained for this. The mushrooms had taught me.

In the midst of all this, Dr. Rama called me into the office for an infusion. My calcium levels were dangerously high, and this treatment would both correct that and strengthen my bones. I squeezed the appointment into my jam-packed schedule, assuming it would be quick.

Just before the nurse inserted the IV, I paused.

"This isn't going to make me sick, right?" I asked, unease creeping in. "I remember how those chemo injections used to wreck me—days of bone pain and exhaustion. I couldn't even function."

"It should be fine," he said with a smile. "Side effects are pretty rare."

Famous last words.

The next morning, I woke up drenched in chills, feverish, and aching from head to toe. I assumed I'd caught the flu… until I remembered the infusion. I pulled up the side effect list: *Fever. Chills. Lethargy. Muscle pain. Insomnia.*

"Damn," I whispered. I called the office and reached the same guy.

"Oh… I guess you're one of the rare ones," he said, with a tone that landed somewhere between apology and surprise.

"Yeah," I replied dryly, "lucky me."

Tylenol and ibuprofen got me through, and eventually my fever broke. But the fatigue lingered, and I had to cancel all my clients, which never feels good. Rescheduling meant longer days ahead, more stress later, and that familiar burden that comes when you're both the healer and the one in need of healing. And still, I stayed steady. Tired, yes. But emotionally grounded.

I barely had time to recover before heading to Ruidoso to film a new segment for one of my documentaries. We were dosing three incredible women that weekend, and there was no way to reschedule. I packed my bags, pushed through the discomfort, and made the mountain drive. I showed up sick, exhausted, and aching. But I showed up.

By the time we wrapped filming, a windstorm rolled in. I couldn't sleep in the unfamiliar bed, and my body was screaming for rest. The second the dust settled, I jumped in my car and made the long drive home, arriving late that night, knowing I had a full day of clients ahead. It was all a blur. But I kept going.

Two days later, my knees ballooned to twice their size. I could barely walk. Ken had to pull out my old walker, and just like that, I was thrust back into memories I didn't want: painful reminders of two hip replacements, learning to walk again, the fragility of my body. It wasn't full-blown PTSD, but it was close.

It was grief. It was fear. It was the echo of old trauma knocking at the door.

And all of this—all of it—was happening while I still didn't know whether the cancer had returned. But I didn't break. I didn't fall down the rabbit hole of worry and what-ifs. I held the line. I stayed neutral. And in hindsight, I don't know exactly how I did it. But I know I did. And I know the mushrooms played a role.

It took over a month to complete the tests and receive the final results. And when they came in, the wave of emotion was overwhelming.

First, I cried. Then, I celebrated.

"No cancer," the doctor said. And then, I thanked the mushrooms, not for healing something in my past, but for teaching me how to prepare for the future, especially one as unwritten as mine.

Every appointment delay, every side effect, every echo of old trauma was happening while I still didn't know if the cancer had returned. The question hung over me like a shadow, growing heavier each day. And yet, I didn't fall apart. I stayed grounded.

It wasn't one challenge; it was a gauntlet. Fever, pain, swollen joints, missed work, and pushing through travel while sick. Every time I thought I could breathe, something else hit. But I didn't spiral. I didn't collapse into fear. I came back to center. To neutrality. To now.

I held it together like a boxer in a prize fight. I should've broken down. But I didn't. I stood in the storm, fully awake, and didn't run from the body blows.

That last journey had confused me at the time. It felt vague and ungrounded. But now I see it clearly: It wasn't healing, it was training. The mushrooms whispered, *You'll need strength. Let me show you how to hold it.*

And I did. I held it. I stayed upright even as everything around me shook.

It's a simple truth that what we feed grows. I chose peace and neutrality. I chose presence. And in doing so, I protected something sacred: my energy, my trust.

Interestingly, had the news gone the other way, I still would've been okay.

I know that now.

That was the quiet power I carried. A strength I hadn't fully recognized until it was tested multiple times.

The mushrooms hadn't just shown me how to heal the past; they had also shown me how to heal the present. They gave me the tools to stand tall in the unknown, to move forward without wasting my energy on fear that never needed to exist.

They prepared me. They grounded me. And when the storm passed, I was still standing, feet forward, heart open, and ready for whatever might come next.

CATHERINE - *It felt like a storm inside.*

MARIA - *It was. But storms pass.*

CATHERINE - *I don't understand why it was so*

uncomfortable.

MARIA - *You were being prepared.*

For what comes next.

CATHERINE - *It felt so heavy, so overwhelming.*

MARIA - *That's unresolved trauma.*

It rises when you least expect it.

But it does not need to consume you.

You are steady now.

CATHERINE - *I felt so neutral before the diagnosis.*

MARIA - *Neutrality is your strength.*

It holds you steady.

CATHERINE - *No cancer.*

MARIA - *No cancer.*

But more than that,

you were prepared.

For whatever may come.

FAMILY AFFAIRS

MARIA - *You are about to share.*

A path, a passion.

CATHERINE - *I don't know what will happen.*

But I feel the weight.

MARIA - *The weight is not just yours.*

You share it with them.

CATHERINE - *I'm nervous.*

What if they don't get it?

MARIA - *It doesn't matter.*

You stand in your truth.

That is enough.

CATHERINE - *What if they're not ready?*

MARIA - *Not everyone will be ready at the same time.*

You cannot control that.

You walk forward.

And the path reveals itself.

FROM THE VERY BEGINNING OF MY psychedelic journeying, my father had been curious, almost eager, to join me, which wasn't all that surprising.

In his younger days, Dad was what you'd affectionately call a bona fide stoner, coasting through the hazy seventies with a joint in hand and a mischievous glint in his eye. I wouldn't be shocked to learn he'd tried mushrooms back then, and if so, it would have definitely been recreationally. There was something about the way he lit up when I brought up psychedelics—like I'd tapped into a long-lost current of youthful freedom, the kind that smelled like patchouli and possibility.

His attitude was very reminiscent and similar to that of Sabrina's, one of the counselors who joined me on the Ruidoso retreat, where we tested different doses as part of an experiential training. Sabrina had boldly chosen the hero dose and ended up having a massive, transformative experience. Both she and my dad shared a magnetic pull toward the unknown, a fearless curiosity that left no room for hesitation. They didn't tiptoe into the idea of mushrooms. They dove in headfirst, hearts wide open. It wasn't just about the substance; it was about the return to something beautiful, raw, and alive.

The first time I mentioned I had some mushrooms, my dad barely let me finish my sentence before blurting out, "Yes, please."

He grinned like a kid being offered candy.

That day turned into a lighthearted, almost playful experience for him. He spent hours watching nature videos, chuckling at the wonder of it all, and for the first time in a long while he seemed fully present, rooted in the moment and simply enjoying the day as it unfolded…

He tried journeying a few times after that, but it wasn't easy on him. His stomach never quite forgave him, and he'd suffer for days afterward—bloated, cramping, miserable. We tried tea and lemon tekking, but nothing spared his GI system from rebellion. Still, he kept trying, drawn back by the promise of heart-opening magic. He described flashes of color, swirling patterns, and sometimes fractals, but he never quite reached that deep, ego-melting surrender that often defines a complete psychedelic breakthrough.

Unfortunately, I believe that his antidepressants had something to do with it. They created a sort of ceiling, a barrier he couldn't break through, no matter how much he wanted to.

I sat with him during what would become his final attempt to journey, and that day yielded significant results—at least from my perspective as a counselor, and his daughter. My sister Linda, Ken, my stepmother, and I were spending the day with him while soft music played in the background—something instrumental and slow, the kind of music that seems to breathe with you. He closed his eyes, breathing deeply, his face softening as the mushrooms took hold.

"I feel...warm," he said after a while. "Like I'm being wrapped in something."

"Love?" I asked gently.

He smiled, eyes still closed. "Yeah. That."

There was no dramatic ego death, no cosmic revelations, but there was peace. And that mattered. He basked in a calm that had long eluded him. It wasn't what either of us had hoped for, but it was something. Something real. And it was enough.

Later, he came out and giggled with us, getting silly the way he used to when we were kids. It was beautiful for us all. A rare and tender glimpse of the playful dad we remembered, momentarily free from the seriousness and physical pain that now weighs so heavily on him.

I believe my father could genuinely benefit from a deep ego dissolution experience, the kind of profound inner shift that psychedelics can sometimes offer. But for that to happen, he'd need to wean off the medications he's relied on for years, and that's not something he's willing to do. He's worked hard for so long to find stability in his mental health, and I respect that more than I can say. At this point in his life, I understand why he wouldn't want to risk unsettling that hard-won balance, despite the promise of healing that mushrooms might bring.

Still, there's a part of me that grieves the missed possibility. I had quietly hoped that psychedelics might become a shared path, something that could draw us closer in a way nothing else ever has. I believe, deep down, that if my dad had ever been able to experience psilocybin fully, it might have opened a door to healing, not just for him, but for us, together. That's the quiet ache of working in a field still on the fringe: not everyone is in a place where stepping through that door feels possible. So I carry on, sharing what I've learned, telling the stories, educating where I can, and most of all, meeting the people I love exactly where they are.

As my relationship with psychedelics evolved, so did the tension between my inner and outer worlds. Psilocybin was no longer a side path; it had become central to my healing, my profession, and who I was becoming. And yet, I hadn't fully brought my sisters into that part of my life. The separation started to feel unnatural, even lonely. These were two of the people I loved most in the world, and I longed to share this work with them, not just through updates or cautious mentions, but in a way that felt real, embodied, and personal. So I began, gently, to open the door. I told them what I was exploring, what I was learning. But more than anything, I hoped for the moment we could experience it… together.

I had planned a birthday gathering in Santa Fe—something simple, something special. I was already renting a beautiful vacation home for a client retreat, so I decided to extend the stay and invite my sisters, Linda and Cori, along with a few close friends. I imagined cozy meals, long talks, desert sunsets, and the warmth of being surrounded by people I love. But beneath the excitement, there was a ripple of nerves: *How will they react when I share all the details? Will they judge me? Will they understand why mushroom healing is so important to me that it has become my "re-mission"?*

On the first night, we gathered around the porch table in the backyard, the Santa Fe sky turning shades of indigo and gold. The air smelled of piñon wood and desert sage. Some partook in a glass of wine, passed snacks, and laughed. And then I took a deep breath and said, "There's something I want to share with you all."

They turned toward me. I could feel my heart thudding in my chest. But once I started talking, the words flowed. I told them all about psilocybin. About how it had helped me finally come off antidepressants. About my clients—the ones who found relief, clarity, even joy after years of struggling. About how this medicine was calling to me in a way that nothing else ever had.

As I spoke, I noticed something shift. My sisters were leaning in, eyes wide, brows relaxed. They weren't skeptical, they were curious. Encouraged. Moved. I've been told I light up when I talk about my passion, and I could feel it happening. My voice grew stronger, my hands animated. *This is what I'm meant to do,* I thought. *This is the path.*

Cori tilted her head and said, "You really believe in this, don't you?"

"With my whole heart," I replied, without missing a beat.

By the end of the evening, both Cori and Linda looked at me with a quiet resolve. Cori said, "I'm ready. I want to know what you're experiencing."

And Linda—true to form—smiled and said, "If you say it will help, then I'm in too. I trust you. I always have."

In that moment, my heart swelled with emotion. I was about to share my love of mushrooms with the people I love dearly.

I transitioned into guide mode—grounded, intentional, and deeply present. I sat with them, explaining the importance of set and setting, helping them clarify their intentions, and talking through what they might feel or encounter. I made sure they knew this wasn't about chasing a high. Instead, it was about creating space for insight, healing, and transformation. I checked in on their emotional states, walked them through setting up a playlist if they wanted, showed them where they could lie down, and reassured them that I would be right there the whole time. I wanted them to feel safe, seen, and supported. More than anything, I wanted them to feel the same sacred, healing current that had carried me so gently—but so powerfully—over the past year. It felt like I was offering them something precious, something that had changed me from the inside out.

Both Cori and Linda said yes to psilocybin because they trusted me fully and without hesitation. Over the years, they had watched me dive into countless healing modalities— Memory Reconsolidation, _Mindfulness Modalities_, Emotional Triggers Treatment (ETT)—and each time, they saw how deeply committed I was. That was enough for them. Cori didn't just believe in ETT—she studied it. She took my class, learned the techniques, and even used them effectively with others. I had also worked with both of them over the years using ETT, helping them process specific traumas and emotional blocks, so they already knew the kind of healing that could unfold when we worked together.

And Linda, ever my quiet champion, always followed my lead, no matter how unconventional the path. "I believe in everything you do," she once told me. "I'd follow you anywhere."

Their decisions to take mushrooms weren't driven just by curiosity or pressure; they were rooted in love, lived experience, and a deep trust in the journey we were about to take together.

When we moved into setting intentions, their motivations came into sharper focus. Linda's was simple and powerful: she wanted to stop feeling small. She didn't frame it in dramatic terms; just a quiet desire to expand, to take up more space in her own life.

Cori, on the other hand, came in with a more layered and urgent need. She'd done years of talk therapy but still struggled deeply with anxiety, self-loathing, and body image issues. She knew her ego was in the way, cutting her down with constant criticism and blocking her from peace. But she had no idea just how thick and tangled it had become.

I felt a sense of urgency when it came to Cori. I didn't know the full extent of what she was carrying, but I knew enough: memories from our childhood, pain she rarely spoke about, shadows that clung to her even when she smiled. She had spent years trying to outrun the weight through talk therapy and sheer willpower, but it never truly let go. I could feel that she was still stuck, still suffering. While I wanted both of my sisters to understand the beauty and power of psychedelics, I knew, deep down, that Cori needed this. This wasn't just an experience for her; it was a lifeline. I wanted to offer her a glimpse of the healing I had found, hoping that it could begin to lift some of the heaviness she had carried for far too long.

That night, right before she dosed, Cori kept saying, "I can't wait for my ego to go away," like she was ordering it off a menu. It was kind of adorable, her wide-eyed optimism, like she thought ego was just some annoying roommate she could politely evict. In hindsight, it's clear she had *no* idea what she was actually asking for. Sure, she had a vague sense that her ego was getting in the way, maybe even blocking her from fully seeing herself. But she didn't know it had built an entire fortress around her. She was self-aware enough to know it existed, but not nearly prepared for the psychological demolition crew that was about to show up. That little catchphrase? It ended up being the doorbell for a total ego reckoning.

Surprisingly, or perhaps not so surprisingly, Cori had an arduous journey. In all my years of guiding psychedelic experiences, I've only witnessed one other person fight ego dissolution as fiercely as she did. And it makes sense—ego protects us. It builds walls, filters, shields... Whatever it needs in its attempt to keep us safe. Cori's ego had been on high alert for most of her life, working overtime to defend her from old wounds, buried memories, and unspoken pain. Why would it suddenly step aside just because she asked it to? From the ego's point of view, that's not healing—that's a threat. In that moment, I wasn't her sister—I was the one trying to dismantle the very system that kept her going. Ego was protecting her... even from me.

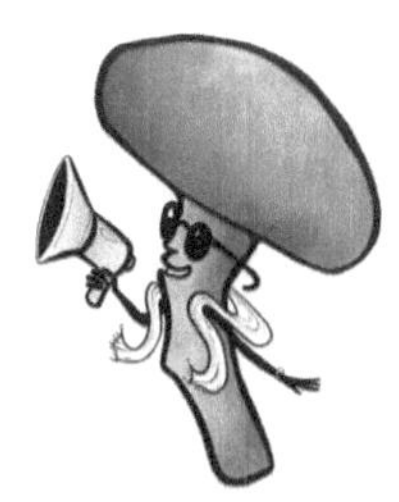

¡OYE! Ego dissolution feels less like enlightenment and more like a slow-motion identity crisis.

Don't panic—it's not death, it's just your inner control freak losing Wi-Fi. Breathe. Surrender. That unraveling feeling? It's actually the pre-party to becoming someone new. Weird, huh?

The medicine didn't shatter her walls all at once; it pressed against them, and she pressed back. Fear rose like a reflex, but she wasn't left to face it alone. Linda's calm presence was a steady hand on the rope, grounding her, giving Cori just enough safety to steal a glimpse behind the curtain of her defenses.

Afterward, Cori described what she encountered inside as an army of protections: hundreds of tiny, armored soldiers guarding her heart. Soldiers who weren't just shielding her from pain, but who were blocking her from growth. The psilocybin only touched the first layer, but even that was enough to shift something deep inside her. What surprised her most wasn't what changed; it was realizing just how much she'd been carrying. That single session cracked open a small window of light, and for the first time, she saw a path forward.

Cori's first journey stirred something profound, something that went well beyond simply sharing the experience with me. It marked the beginning of her awakening. It shifted her focus from seeking the attention of others to discovering her own desires, her own voice. For the first time in a long while, she began engaging with life in a way that felt intentional and alive. The autopilot she'd been running on slowly powered down, and she started making choices that reflected who she truly was. Life was no longer about everyone else. It was about becoming herself.

My presence, though, was both a gift and a complication. As her big sister, I had always been a figure of guidance, someone she looked to for approval, especially before her psychedelic work began. I believe that dynamic stirred her ego, made it more reluctant to let go. It was as if her ego tightened its grip, afraid of being seen too closely by someone who mattered so much. At the same time, I was the only person she would have trusted enough to do this with. Without me, I doubt she would have taken that first step. And yet, paradoxically, I stood in the way.

I guided her through her first three journeys. In the first two, my presence—though safe and familiar—also made it harder for her to release her ego fully. Psilocybin turns the volume up on everything inside, and sometimes even the comfort of someone close can activate protective layers rather than soften them. With me in the room, her ego held on tighter, not out of resistance to the experience itself, but out of a deep, unconscious need to stay composed, to stay seen in a conditioned way. It wasn't that the journeys were about me, but my involvement subtly interfered with her ability to surrender completely.

By the third journey, however, something shifted. She had done enough inner work to begin letting go, even in my presence. As a result, the protective grip began to loosen, and for the first time, she fully leaned into her healing.

Cori's relationship with mushrooms has taken a different turn from mine. Once I introduced her to the medicine, she took the reins of her own healing journey and found other trusted guides to support her with preparation, ceremony, and integration.

She's become deeply knowledgeable, an expert in microdosing, mesodosing, and macrodosing. Her understanding of the nuanced qualities of different mushroom strains is impressive, and over time, she's cultivated a rich, layered relationship with the medicine.

Since beginning this path, she's rebuilt her life from the inside out, and the results still astonish me. She walked away from a twenty-year marriage, shifted careers, found her voice, and now lives with a sense of peace and joy I have never seen in her. She is radiant in her authenticity. Spiritually, she's soaring, reaching heights I have yet to experience.

And while her evolution inspires me, I'm grounded in my own path. I know I'm here to hold a clinical, steady space—for now. Our timelines are different, our callings distinct. I wouldn't want it any other way. The evidence is clear, however, that mushrooms have facilitated growth for both of us.

Linda's path has been markedly different from Cori's. Where Cori's journey was urgent and dramatic, Linda's has been quieter, more deliberate, and deeply discerning. She has only dosed a few times, but each experience carried weight. Her first journey in Santa Fe began in solitude, rooted in her own exploration. Yet as the evening unfolded, it became clear that her path and Cori's were meant to intertwine. Cori, caught in the intensity of her own process, gravitated toward Linda, the only person in the house who made her feel safe enough to lower her defenses. While others, without meaning to, triggered Cori's ego, Linda's calm presence allowed her to soften. In the process, Linda's own insights were disrupted, her experience pulled into Cori's. What might have felt like an intrusion instead became something sacred: a bond forged in raw vulnerability, a moment of sisterhood that continues to enrich their connection to this day.

Still, Linda had her own intention that night. She carried with her a lifelong desire to stop feeling small. During her trip, she recalls experiencing an *Alice in Wonderland* adventure, wherein a tiny version of herself inhabited a disproportionally large world. One moment stood out to her: someone said, "Linda, you are so small," and her response was simply, "Thank you." It was an odd yet powerful realization—how she had internalized her smallness, how she had allowed it to shape her self-worth.

About two months later, Linda came to me with a quiet resolve. She wanted a redo. The beginning of her first journey had intrigued her deeply, and there was so much more she wanted to explore. Her journey felt unfinished, like a book she had started but never finished. This time, she was clear on her intention: She was keen to face the deep-seated struggles around her eating disorder, the constant counting of calories, the obsession with food and body image that had held her captive for years. She longed to break free from the pattern.

So, we decided to dose again together, this time with Ken as our guide. Linda came to my house, retreating to my spare bedroom while I cocooned in my bed nearby. For the first part of the journey, we were separated. As Linda embarked on her experience, I was immersed in a battle. My mushroom journeys, at that time, were marked by what felt like endless liquid release. The psilocybin activated a flood of mucus—my eyes and nose would run uncontrollably, requiring tissue after tissue, until I was overwhelmed by the constant flow. It was a frustrating, distracting process that kept me from fully leaning into my experience. I couldn't help but wonder if I was missing something important, something deep that was just out of reach, buried beneath the weight of liquid release and physical distraction.

¡OYE! Crying might just feel like your face is leaking.

Sometimes tears sneak out like your spirit sprang a leak. Let them flow. That's just your soul doing some unscheduled plumbing maintenance.

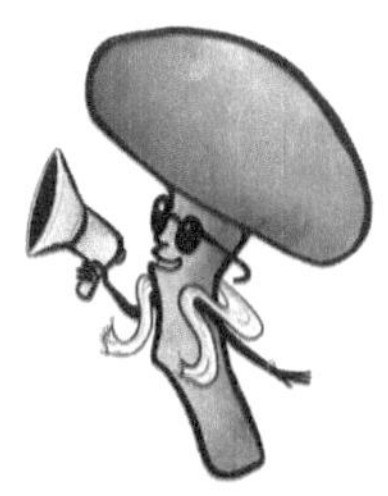

Partway through the journey, I felt a pull toward the guest room—an undeniable, magnetic tug. It was as if the mycelium itself was calling me, whispering through the walls, *Go to her.* When I opened the door, I found Linda curled in the bed, her body wracked with sobs. She wasn't just crying—she was *weeping*, from the core, her breath catching in jagged waves as she tried to hold the weight of the world in her chest.

Without thinking, I crawled in beside her, wrapping my body around hers to let her know she wasn't alone. She grabbed my arms and pulled me closer. Her voice was raspy, barely more than a whisper, and she struggled to find the words through the emotion.

"I feel it all," she choked out. "The beauty... the sadness... *everybody and everything.*"

I held her silently, letting my presence speak what words couldn't. Eventually, as the sobs softened, she began to share more—visions, understandings, truths that had been handed to her by something bigger.

"I saw Dad," she said quietly. "I *felt* him. All his pain. Every day. It's more than we know. His life… It's going to end sooner than we think."

My heart clenched. "No," I said reflexively, the word slipping out like a plea. "That would be awful."

But she shook her head gently. "No," she said. "I'm going to be *so happy* for him when he dies. His pain is so great. He deserves peace."

Something in me shifted. In my altered state, her words didn't just land—they planted. They sprouted. I could feel new neural pathways forming in real time. She continued, her voice soft but certain, like she was repeating what had been shown to her.

"An alien showed me how life energy works," she said. "We each have these orbs of light—life energy—that pass from one soul to the next. When one life ends, the energy transfers. I saw Dad's orb… and it was dim. Barely flickering. He's almost done here."

I swallowed hard, trying to absorb the weight of it.

"And then I saw yours," she said, turning her head toward me. "It was glowing—so bright. It's full of purpose. You're on your path. And Cori's… hers was dim too. But not like Dad's. Hers just hasn't been *lit* yet. Her life hasn't even really started."

That conversation cracked something open in me. Until that moment, I had only one story about my father's impending death that would happen someday, as it entailed loss, grief, and devastation. But now, I could *feel* the beginnings of a second narrative forming—one of peace, release, and even celebration. I didn't have to choose between them. I could hold both.

Today, about a year and a half later, on my father's 80th birthday, I still carry those two pathways. One of sadness and mourning, yes—but also one of gratitude. Of reverence for his life and relief for his eventual freedom from pain. That day, Linda gave me something I didn't even know I needed: a coping tool I will one day hold close. When the time comes, I will cry, but I will also smile, knowing his journey here was full and complete.

Linda and I stayed curled up in bed long after the intensity had passed, wrapped in sheets and in that sweet, shimmering afterglow of ego dissolution. We giggled like teenagers, the kind of laughter that bubbles up from your soul when something heavy has finally been lifted. The air between us was thick with honesty, curiosity, and the quiet thrill of having crossed a threshold together. We shared what we saw, what we felt, and what we were just beginning to understand. Something had shifted in both of us.

At one point, as we were still floating in that liminal space, Linda turned to me with a mischievous grin and her newfound mushroom wisdom. "You know," she said, "I think your ego is using the tissues to distract you."

I blinked at her, confused. "The tissues?"

"Yeah," she said, half-laughing. "All that liquid letting from your face—your eyes, your nose—you get so caught up in it. Your ego latches onto it like a little life raft. It's keeping you anchored."

I rolled my eyes. "That can't be true."

"I'm serious!" she said, nudging me. "You just need to *embrace the wetness*. Forget the tissues. Use a towel. Let it all flow. Stop giving your ego an excuse to hang on. Your ego *loves* that you're obsessed with the mess. It keeps you focused on your body, on control, on cleanup. It's your escape hatch. You think it's about mucus, but it's about not letting go."

At first, I dismissed her idea. It sounded like one of those half-baked psychedelic insights that make perfect sense in the moment and none at all the next day. But the more I sat with it, the more

I realized she was right. Every trip, I'd been obsessing over the mess—dabbing my eyes, blowing my nose, reaching for tissue after tissue. It *was* a way of staying in control. Of staying safe. Of avoiding surrender.

So next time, I swapped the tissues for a towel.

And everything changed.

I stopped fussing. I let the wetness come. I surrendered to the process. And with nothing left to cling to, my ego lost its grip. I dropped in—deeper than I ever had before.

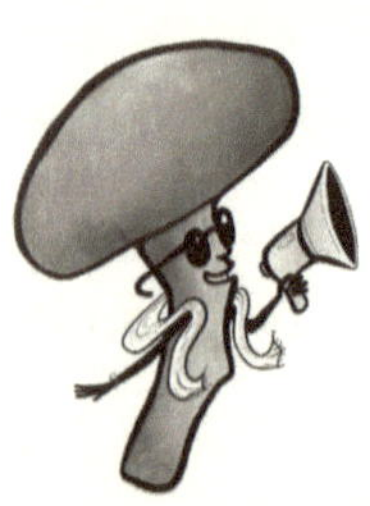

¡OYE! Skip the tissues—get a towel.

You might cry enough to water a houseplant. Tissues are no match for a full-body soul purge. Towels: because sacred snot is still snot.

Now, I won't even *look* at a box of tissues during a journey. For me, they're like little anchors, quietly holding me back from the depths I'm meant to reach. The towel, on the other hand, has become my silent invitation to surrender. Now, I let the flood come. And I go so much deeper.

Funny how something as simple as a towel can become a gateway. But that's the thing with psychedelics: the magic is always in the letting go.

During Linda's second journey, the medicine delivered a cascade of powerful insights, each cracking open old beliefs and replacing them with truth that pulsed with clarity. One message came through loud and clear: *Your body is a vessel. It transports you through this life. Treat it with love, not judgment.*

In addition to learning about the energy pods and how life force is transferred, she also discovered how deeply disconnected she had become from her physical self—and how urgently she needed to reconnect with it.

She saw it all in flashes of understanding—how she'd been doing it wrong for so long. Chasing numbers and measuring worth through digits: calories, weight, money, age, and BMI. The entire digit-driven world had become a cage. A constant tally that distracted her from joy. The medicine whispered, *Forget the digits. They are not the point.*

She felt it deep in her bones: *money isn't everything.* Time lost its tight grip. There was no need to obsess over minutes spent on a treadmill or a number on a scale. Her body didn't need punishment or perfection. It needed nourishment, compassion, and presence.

Just feed your vessel, the message echoed. *Give it nutritious fuel. Move it with joy. Make healthy choices because you love yourself, not because you're chasing numbers. The digits will follow—if they matter at all.*

It wasn't about control anymore. It was about coming home to herself. Working out no longer needed to be a countdown clock or a guilt trip. Instead, it could be a dance, a walk, or a stretch—something done for the soul, not the stopwatch. For the first time in a long time, she saw what freedom might actually feel like.

Linda's intention had been clear, and the mushrooms delivered. What had once felt like an unfinished story now found its resolution. The journey brought her exactly what she needed: not a strict plan or a tidy answer, but a shift in how she saw herself and her body. The grip of numbers loosened. The voice of shame quieted. She left changed. Something essential had been unlocked; a knowing that her body was not a problem to fix, but a vessel to love. And that knowing would become the foundation for her ongoing healing, one rooted not in control, but in deep compassion for herself.

The only other time Linda dosed was with a large microdose—just 0.5 grams—but it came at precisely the right moment. She had just been let go from her job without warning, blindsided and spiraling into a severe identity crisis. The opportunity to dose was a spontaneous and serendipitous turn of events. I had just finished dosing clients for the day and was heading home when I felt a strong pull to stop by Linda's house. I called, but she didn't answer, so I left a quick message. Just as I was about to pass the turn to her street, a text lit up on my phone: "Can you stop by?" So I did.

When I arrived, she was on the phone with Cori, deep in conversation, trying to make sense of the significant shift in her life, one where her job no longer defined her identity. Cori, in her new role as resident mushroom sage, said, "You need a dose. It'll help you figure this out." I smiled. As fate would have it, I had the medicine with me.

I offered, and Linda agreed.

I prepared the dose and stayed with her, guiding her through the experience with ETT. The dose wasn't enough for complete ego dissolution, but it opened the door just wide enough for guided imagery techniques used in ETT. During the session, she had a vivid encounter with an ex who had passed away. It was a powerful reminder of what love truly is, and that more love was on the way.

She also connected with her future self, who gently reassured her: *"Keep going. You're doing the right things."* No grand revelations, just a quiet knowing that the answers would come in time. *"It will present itself,"* her future self said.

By the next day, something had shifted. Linda felt lighter and clearer. The storm had passed, and she was no longer stuck. The medicine had helped her move forward, just enough to regain her footing, just in time to keep her from slipping deeper into confusion and self-doubt. Both Cori and Linda turned to mushrooms to move beyond the places where they felt stuck, uncovering deep wells of joy and purpose within.

Meanwhile, my mom watched it all unfold from the sidelines—curious, amazed, and with a bit of skepticism. She saw each of her daughters begin to shift in ways that were impossible to ignore. *Could a fungus, of all things, really help all three of her grown children become better versions of themselves?*

It was hard for her to wrap her head around. After all, we weren't in crisis. We were already fully functioning adults, contributing members of society with no addictions, no criminal records, not living off the government. From the outside, we looked fine. But watching us level up in midlife—becoming more present, joyful, awake—sparked something in her. She wanted to be part of this mushroom movement.

When she first expressed interest in trying psilocybin, I thought it would be best for her to start with microdosing. This would ease her in gently. I gave her a couple of capsules at 0.12 grams, along with detailed instructions: no caffeine or dairy for a few hours before and after, take it in the morning, set an intention, and plan to spend some quiet time about two hours in.

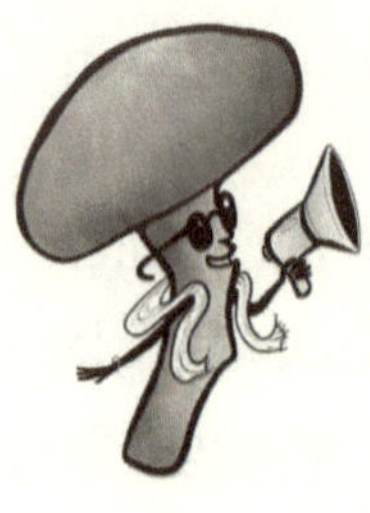

¡OYE! Ditch the dairy—it dulls the magic.

That grilled cheese might sabotage your sacred trip. Milk products can block psilocybin absorption, so hold the cheddar for at least two hours before and after. Let the journey unfold.

What followed was...not what I expected. Though in hindsight, it should have been exactly what I expected.

She called me later to report that time had slowed down to a crawl—"minutes felt like hours," she said. She felt wobbly walking down the hallway, dizzy, and foggy-headed. These weren't typical microdosing effects. What she described sounded more like the onset of a macrodose.

The dose I gave her was small, at the very low end of the microdosing range (.1–.5g), but my mom is also tiny at five feet tall, 105 pounds. Some might say her body size would call for a smaller dose, but others argue that serotonin receptor density is relatively consistent regardless of body weight, barring metabolic differences. There's still no definitive research on this, but I imagine we'll have more answers soon.

I consulted with other professionals, and they echoed my hunch: cut the dose in half. So I prepared new capsules at just 0.0625 grams. Still, the next day, she reported the same symptoms: dizziness, fogginess, and discomfort.

That's when it hit me: it wasn't the mushrooms, it was the mindset. Stigma was shaping her experience. Somewhere deep inside, she was still holding onto the myth of psychedelics as dangerous or deranging, like something out of *Reefer Madness*, that absurd propaganda film from the 1930s designed to terrify the public.

Finally, I told her gently, "Maybe mushrooms just aren't right for you."

Her mindset wasn't ready, and that matters more than dose, body weight, or strain. The medicine meets you where you are, and if where you are is steeped in fear and stigma, it can't do its work. So, we paused her journey. When the time came for her to be genuinely ready—open and curious—the medicine would be waiting.

After witnessing the powerful transformations her daughters had undergone over the course of months, my mom came to me again—this time asking for a full macrodose journey. She wanted the real thing. But I wasn't about to hand her the experience without making sure she truly understood what she was asking for. This time, there would be no shortcuts.

"If you want to dose again," I told her, "you're going to have to take my class."

So she did.

She sat through my complete training as a guide, beginning with an intensive lecture day where I covered the science, the history, the myths, and the emotional terrain of psilocybin. She learned what the mushrooms actually *do*. Not what the anti-drug culture of the past had claimed, not what Hollywood dramatizes, but what this medicine really looks like when administered with intention and respect. Then, she spent an entire day guiding three participants through their own macrodose journeys, holding space, witnessing their emotional processes, and learning firsthand that this wasn't about getting high.

It was about healing.

After the training, I sat her down for a candid conversation. I needed to know—*had* her mindset shifted? Was she ready—really ready—to enter the experience with curiosity instead of fear?

She was. Or at least, she could articulate a new understanding that gave me confidence we could move forward. So we set a date. She would journey at my home, and my husband, Ken, would be her guide.

I chose not to sit with her myself. I'd learned my lesson from Cori's early experiences—that my presence can interfere with the process. And I knew my mother needed time to focus on the more foundational layers of her life, not her relationship with me. She needed space to let the mushrooms meet her where *she* was, without my energy shaping the path.

That morning, I settled in at home, thinking I'd catch up on work while Ken guided her. I imagined it would be a gentle day, quiet and reflective.

I was wrong.

About two hours in, I heard the sound of sobbing. Not quiet weeping. *Wailing.* My mother was crying with such intensity it echoed through the house, wave after wave of raw grief rising and falling. I froze. Every sob cracked something open in me. I felt it in my bones.

It was brutal.

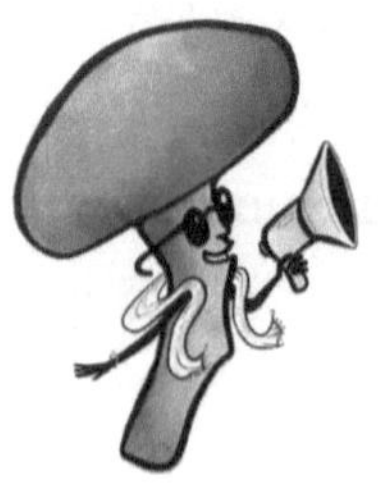

¡OYE! You might ugly cry while laughing like a maniac. That's normal.

Mushrooms stir the soul. Don't analyze the combo platter of feelings... just let them cook.

I couldn't think, couldn't focus, couldn't do a single thing except *feel*. Every time she gasped for air between cries, I felt my chest tighten. Ken told me she was sobbing so hard she kept passing out—unable to catch her breath. And I was utterly undone.

I tried calling my sisters for support, but neither was available. And just like that, I was snapped back to my childhood: me, the one left holding the emotional weight, the one tasked with comforting, fixing, and making it all okay. That old wound tore wide open. I was furious—not just at the situation, but at them. Angry that, once again, I was the one left behind to take care of Mom, while they got to carry on with their lives.

Of course, the anger wasn't really about them. It was trauma, resurfacing in the powerful energetic field that mushrooms create, even when you're not the one dosing. My mother was the one on the journey, but there I was, pulled into my own lesson by proxy. Apparently, the medicine wasn't done with me either.

Sometimes the healing finds us whether we invite it or not.

Later, as my mother emerged from her journey and shared what she had experienced, she told me something that stopped me in my tracks: When she was around six years old, her own mother, Mamaita, told her to go to her room and *cry it out*, because she never wanted to hear her crying again. And so, she did. She walked into her bedroom at six years old and made a silent vow never to cry again. And she kept it.

I sat there stunned, flipping through my mental archives, trying to recall a time when I had seen my mother cry.

Nothing.

Not a single memory surfaced. Not during heartbreak, not during grief, not even during the most emotional moments of our lives. Her tears had been locked away for decades.

That realization gutted me. I felt a wave of grief, not just for her, but for all the emotion she had carried, silently and stoically, for a lifetime. She never learned how to breathe through a cry because she had never been allowed to. *What must it have been like to live a life where the most primal release of emotion is off-limits?* That image of her trying to cry, gasping for air, unaware of how to allow the body to weep—*that* still haunts me.

But the medicine didn't stop there.

She also shared a powerful vision she had during the journey, one that added layers of depth and context to the generations of emotional suppression. She saw her own mother—*also* six years old—being pulled by my great-grandmother through the streets of Mexico, fleeing from the chaos of Pancho Villa's forces. Her father had just died, and my great-grandmother, now a widow, was escaping north with her six children in tow, seeking refuge in the United States. Their destination: family in El Paso. Their mission: survival.

In that vision, my mom saw her grandmother not as a hardened woman, but as a desperate mother trying to keep her children alive. Suddenly, she understood where the "no crying" rule came from. Crying was a liability. Crying could get you caught. Crying could cost you your life.

It wasn't personal. It was ancestral.

So, of course, the messaging was passed down like a family heirloom cloaked in trauma. *Crying is meaningless. Why are YOU upset? This is nothing compared to what I lived through. Your pain doesn't measure up.*

My mother's own trauma, including being inappropriately touched by her brother, was minimized by generations of women who had to silence their own pain just to make it to the next day. But the mushrooms gave her something none of them had ever been offered: space to feel, to grieve, and to finally let it out.

Since then, my mother has continued to journey with mushrooms in her own way, discovering more pieces of herself with each experience. Out of respect for her process and her privacy, I won't share more of her story here. That part is hers to tell, if and when she chooses.

But what I *can* say is this: the lineage of silence stopped with her. Her own three daughters now share their feelings, insights, and dreams with candor and trust. The cycle was interrupted. And that alone feels like a generational victory.

Because my mother took my class, she gained the knowledge and firsthand experience to support me in guiding others. She's become my trusted co-facilitator when an extra presence is needed—especially when working with clients in recovery. Her thirty-six years of sobriety bring depth and authenticity that clients in AA immediately recognize and respect.

Most recently, I invited her to join me during the filming of a dosing session with two aging clients in Ruidoso, New Mexico, part of a larger documentary project. Initially, there were three clients, but two of their initial journeys felt unfinished, so we decided to re-dose them. Including my mother as a guide felt right, and by the end of the experience, one of the clients even shared that my mother's presence was a sincerely welcomed and grounding part of the journey.

My mother's support throughout my work with psychedelics has been unmatched by anyone except Ken. She cheers me on and offers practical help when needed, not just for clients but for the guides too. She tends to the energy of the entire space, preparing, nurturing, and holding the container with quiet strength and warmth. She has come a long way from someone for whom I believed I needed to hold the spotlight. She has a lot to give.

Somewhere along the way, she also began offering me the things I longed for as a child. She shows up now in ways she never did back then. And the truth is, the woman standing beside me today is not the same woman who raised me. I had to grieve the mother I once had to make room for the mother she has become. In doing so, I was able to create a new kind of relationship with her, like receiving a second mother in this lifetime—a relationship built on healing, presence, and a love that now flows freely.

I am deeply, soulfully grateful that mushrooms helped my mother and me find our way to each other. From the moment I was born, it felt like I was trying to run away from her. There was an emotional distance between us that I didn't have the tools to understand or bridge. I felt unseen, unheard, and unheld in the ways I needed most. For years, I kept her at arm's length, protecting myself from the parts of her that hurt me, even as I longed for connection. But now, everything is different. I don't run from her—I lean in. I seek her presence.

I look forward to spending time with her, to hearing her stories, to witnessing who she is becoming. I am deeply moved by the way she now embodies everything I once longed for—secure, unwavering love. She celebrates my achievements, shows up without fail, reminds me to care for myself, supports my causes, and finds endless ways to express her affection. But perhaps the most profound shift isn't just in her—it's in me. For the first time, I can truly open my heart, accept her love, and let it in.

She is also, in so many ways, the blueprint for the person I've become. I am who I am because of her, not only because of the values she instilled in me, but because of the ones I had to fight to create for myself. She modeled strength, perseverance, resourcefulness, and work ethic. She taught me how to show up, to take care of things, to be capable and dependable. At the same time, her pain, her silences, and her trauma showed me what I didn't want to carry forward. I learned boundaries by noticing where hers were missing. I learned emotional presence by understanding the cost of its absence. I learned to feel because I was raised by someone who had never been permitted to do so.

My mother was born with ancestral trauma in her blood. She experienced more of it in her own childhood, especially from her mother, who had been shaped by survival and fear. My mother did her best to protect me from those patterns, but some of the pain still bled through. Wounds don't just vanish—they echo. But through my own healing, and eventually through hers, we've interrupted the generational current. I've done the hard work to process and alchemize the trauma that once felt like a curse into something purposeful and transformative.

Mushrooms were the bridge. They allowed us both to access a depth of understanding, forgiveness, and connection that years of distance couldn't touch. They didn't just bring us closer; they softened the edges between us. They helped us see each other. Not through the lens of our roles, or our wounds, but as two women finding their way back home to themselves and each other.

CATHERINE - *I'm sharing this work, one person at a time. It's slowly spreading.*

MARIA - *Healing ripples out.*

> *It touches those around you, especially family.*

CATHERINE - *I feel the energy staying with me.*

> *It affects them too.*

MARIA - *Family healing starts with you.*

> *The energy spreads, whether they're ready or not.*

CATHERINE - *The work continues through them.*

MARIA - *Yes.*

> *The energy doesn't just heal you.*

> *It heals the bonds you carry.*

CATHERINE - *We're growing together.*

MARIA - *Yes.*

Trust the energy.

It heals, one person at a time.

And together, the healing grows.

CHAPTER TWENTY

TRIP THE LIGHT FORWARD

FOR MOST OF MY YOUTH, I was running. Not always from something, but always toward somewhere else. I wanted to escape the Southwest, the dry landscapes, and the weight of home. My life was a long string of relocations: Vista, Sacramento, Corpus Christi, Houston, Hayward, Millbrae, Kentucky, Vermont, Colorado. Each new place felt like another chance to reinvent myself, to leave behind whatever I had not yet figured out. I was certain the answers I sought lived somewhere far from the desert.

But life has a way of pulling us back to where we started, especially when there is unfinished work waiting. When I finally landed in southern New Mexico, forty-five minutes from the place of my birth, it felt like a reluctant homecoming at first. I had spent years trying to get away from the region, only to find myself full circle, standing once again on the very soil I once dismissed. I could not have known then that this landscape would hold my greatest purpose, and that psychedelics would become such a vital part of my story.

What I once resisted has become the ground of my calling. New Mexico is not just where I live; it's where I serve. It's where I have been given the opportunity to stand as Secretary of the

Decriminalize Psychedelics New Mexico Board. From this place, I can help move progress forward, shaping policy with both heart and strategy. I can help create systems where people have safe access to the medicine that saved my life, and heal the wounds that our communities carry.

Coming back here was not an accident. The medicine led me home, to the place that needed me most, and to the work that only makes sense here, in the desert where my story began.

For thirty years, I lived with depression wrapped around me like a heavy coat I couldn't take off. It was always there: stifling, itchy, worn down in places, but oddly protective. I didn't realize how much it shaped me, my relationships, and the trajectory of my life until psychedelics stripped it away and showed me what I'd been missing.

Antidepressants were part of my life for as long as I can remember. I used to say I'd probably die with a bottle of them in my nightstand. They helped me function. Without them, I spent days in bed, blinds drawn tight, watching the sun trace its arc across the ceiling without once feeling compelled to move. Isolation felt safer than pretending to care about school, work, or friends.

And yet, I look back now with a strange sense of gratitude. Those medications saved me. They gave me the ability to focus, to show up for work, to take care of the people I loved. They were my life raft, and I clung to them as if my life depended on it, because, for a while, it did.

But what I didn't realize then is that the price of safety was emotional numbness. I wasn't just muted in my sorrow—I was dulled in my joy too.

It wasn't until I began working with psychedelics that the fog began to lift.

The first months after stopping my medication were intense. I felt like a shaken soda bottle with the cap twisted off—everything rushing out. I cried over joyful news stories. I sobbed while watching movies. I'd see a child hugging their parent at the grocery store and have to blink away tears.

"I think I broke," I told Ken one night, wrapped in a blanket on the couch, tears still clinging to my lashes. "I'm crying over a *Catfish* trailer."

He looked at me, bewildered. "It's like I'm meeting a whole new you," he said gently. "I just don't know the rules anymore."

Ken and I had been together for over a decade. In that time, he'd come to rely on a particular version of me: logical, even-keeled, solution-oriented. We'd worked out a comfortable rhythm for resolving conflict: identify the problem, talk it out, then agree on a plan.

But that version of me shifted.

Now, I couldn't leap to logic. I had to *feel* first.

If I got triggered or overwhelmed, no amount of reasoning would work until I'd fully ridden the wave of emotion. Sometimes that took hours. Sometimes a whole day.

"It's like trying to have a conversation with someone while they're surfing a tsunami," Ken said once, only half-joking. "I just have to wait until you're back on the beach."

What surprises me the most isn't the intensity of the feelings I have now without the antidepressants. It's how good they often *feel.* Even the sadness. And the anger. Feeling anything, after so long in emotional exile, feels deeply human. Like I was thawing out after decades in a freezer.

I remember one moment vividly. I was driving alone, listening to music, when a song came on that I hadn't heard in years. Something about the melody, the lyrics, *it hit me.* The tears came so fast I had to pull over. And yet, I wasn't sad. Not really. I was alive. I was *in* it. Every cell in my body seemed to vibrate with resonance.

"This is what I've been missing," I whispered to myself. "This is what it means to be me."

Of course, not every emotional wave was so poetic. There were hard days too, days when I overbooked myself, thinking I could power through, only to be blindsided by a swell of emotional exhaustion.

"I thought I could handle today," I told my therapist once, "but I forgot to account for how much energy it takes to process feelings. It's like… I finally opened the floodgates, and now I have to build a life around the river."

Still, I would never go back.

Before psychedelics, I was dependent on pharmaceuticals. I took them daily for decades. Now, my needs are different. A psychedelic journey every few months, what I call my "tune-ups," gives me what I need. But not just to manage depression.

These journeys do more than stabilize my mood. They *heal* me.

They help me release what isn't mine to carry. They show me the tangled places in my soul where old wounds fester. They help me notice the beauty in others. And in myself.

I remember one mushroom journey in particular. Toward the end, I felt this overwhelming presence, a voice or an energy that said simply, *"You don't have to hold it all anymore."*

I wept. Not because I was sad, but because I had been holding so much for so long. Grief. Shame. Perfectionism. The weight of years spent being "functional" but not truly *whole.*

Afterward, I shared the moment with Ken.

"What if," I said, "my job isn't to carry everything, but to learn what's mine and what's not?"

He took my hand and nodded. "And, my job is to love you while you figure it out."

This transformation wasn't easy on Ken. In fact, at times it was downright disorienting for him. For over a decade, he had come to know a version of me that was steady, rational, and emotionally predictable. Our arguments were tidy. Our problem-solving was quick. He knew how to reach me, how to calm me, how to make things right when they went wrong. And then, almost overnight, all of that changed. Suddenly, the rules shifted. The woman he loved, once logical and composed, was now moved to tears by music, overwhelmed by unexpected memories, and often needed hours, even days, to process emotions before she could return fully to reason.

Still, Ken struggled. Not because he didn't love me, but because he felt like he was trying to speak a language he had never learned.

"I just don't know what to do," he said one evening, after I'd spiraled into tears over something seemingly small. "It used to be so clear. I could fix it. Now I just feel... helpless."

His patience was tested more than once, especially during the months when my emotions were swinging wide and fast. He worried he was losing me, or at least losing the version of me he had counted on. But slowly, painfully, he began to understand that he wasn't losing me at all. I was just becoming someone more fully alive. And even though it was hard for him, and sometimes made him feel like he was standing on shifting ground, he stayed. He listened. He adapted.

I'm so grateful.

Now our relationship is deeper. Messier, sometimes, but more real. Ken has learned to hold space, to wait. I've learned that emotional fluency takes practice. I've become more patient with myself, even when I'm tired and it's inconvenient.

Because this is what healing looks like for me: not perfection, not even balance, but wholeness. The freedom to feel. To grow. To hurt. To change. This is what I want to tell everyone.

Psychedelics, mostly psilocybin, didn't just treat my depression. They returned me to myself.

And that's something thirty years of pills could never do.

Luckily for me, and many others, the medicine has never stopped calling. Even when the government silenced it. Even when stigma buried it. Even when fear turned it into a crime. The truth is that for decades, mushrooms kept working underground; they whispered in ceremonies, they showed up in living rooms, they guided seekers in forests and deserts. They kept teaching in secret, reminding us again and again that healing cannot be outlawed.

And now, the call is louder than ever, because science has caught up to what this medicine has been saying all along. Research pours in from the most respected universities in the country. Johns Hopkins. NYU. UCLA. The studies all point in the same direction. Psilocybin has been proven to ease depression and often releases trauma. They can soothe end-of-life fear. They've also demonstrated an ability to break the grip of addiction. They do what so many current treatments fail to do: heal at the root.

Momentum is building. An important step is changing psilocybin from a Schedule A substance to a more accessible one, and this is now under consideration. MDMA for PTSD is expected to be approved soon for rescheduling, setting the stage for psilocybin to follow. Oregon has launched the first statewide psilocybin program. Colorado is building its own. Cities from Denver to Oakland, from Seattle to Detroit, have declared what communities have always known: criminalizing healing helps no one. Each of these steps may look bureaucratic on the surface, but together they form a tide. And that tide is rising.

This is not a fringe movement anymore. This is history turning. It is medicine remembered. It is culture shifting. It is science, ceremony, and story converging at last.

And yet, let us be honest: America has a bad habit of taking the sacred and selling it back to us in plastic. Of turning healing into product. Of building systems that serve the privileged while the vulnerable wait outside the door. Of ignoring Indigenous roots while rushing to patent and profit. The risk is real: that psilocybin will be packaged into another pill, another industry, another thing only the wealthy can afford. That the medicine will be stripped of its context, its spirit, its community. That the very people who need it most will be the last to touch it. We cannot repeat those mistakes.

It happened fast. Almost too fast to believe. In January 2025, I learned that the Senate was preparing to introduce the *Medical Psilocybin Act* to the New Mexico legislature. Big things always seem to arrive suddenly in my life. My cancer diagnosis and treatment moved at lightning speed, from illness to remission in what felt like a blink. Now the next "fast thing" was here: legislation to create an infrastructure for psilocybin-assisted therapy. The bill was introduced in January and signed into law on April 7. Less than three months. A blink in the world of legal proceedings. New Mexico had done what few thought possible. It felt like a lifetime of work suddenly breaking through the surface.

The *Act* moved like wildfire through the committees. Each stop brought majority support, often with little to no opposition. Bipartisan votes carried it forward every time. Even the funding was approved, which had been the stumbling block in previous years. I was stunned to see how quickly New Mexico surged ahead, becoming the surprise contender in the race. Oregon and Colorado had already legalized psilocybin therapy and were building their infrastructure, but both had run into major challenges. I watched in disbelief as New Mexico, the quiet dark horse, sprinted ahead of states everyone assumed would lead the way.

Oregon and Colorado had already opened the doors, but both stumbled badly once inside. I had hoped to practice under Colorado's system, where I am licensed; yet, what they built was a maze of barriers: nearly ten thousand dollars in fees, coursework I had already mastered, and fifty requisite hours of supervision despite my advanced training in Canada and my years of safe, successful facilitation. An earlier promise they'd made to grandfather in experienced practitioners was broken. Even worse,

Indigenous healers, the original carriers of this medicine, were shut out unless they too paid, trained, and jumped through hoops. Ridiculous and an example of cultural misappropriation at its finest. It was crushing to see the state I once called home dishonor the very people who had kept the medicine alive.

I expected California to be the next state in the game. But then came New Mexico, the place I had once run from, charging forward like it had been waiting all along. Not through a ballot initiative like Oregon or Colorado, but through the legislature itself. Bold. Direct. Against all odds. They passed medical access first and left decriminalization for another day. It was a cautious strategy. It was not perfect, but it was a start. New Mexico has chosen to begin with medical infrastructure, but the conversation about decriminalization is far from over.

When the bill hit its first committee, I was ready. I wrote to senators and representatives. I sent emails to my community. I watched every hearing I could, squeezed in between counseling sessions. I even submitted testimony. At the first hearing, I was not called because there were too many voices already lined up in favor. No one spoke against it. The bill moved forward like a wave gathering strength.

At the second hearing, my name was called. My heart pounded as I unmuted myself. I had my words ready. Twenty seconds in, the moderator interrupted to say they could not hear me. My mic was on. My settings were correct. I scrambled, desperate to fix it, but the moment was gone. They moved on.

My one chance had been silenced by technology. My stomach dropped. I felt crushed—my chance to be heard evaporated. In the past, this kind of blow might have devastated me, but thanks to the work the mushrooms had already done on my ego, I was perfectly fine with it. My words were not meant to sway that day. Others spoke, the committee voted, and the bill advanced. It had a life of its own.

The weeks blurred into a storm of hearings. At one point, a private company tried to slip in an amendment that would have forced the state to use the synthetic compound they'd created instead of the mushroom itself. Here was corporate greed trying to hijack sacred medicine. If they'd won, the whole *Act* would have been poisoned. Then came relief, however, as the lawmakers struck it down. The mushroom energy stayed intact.

The Senate passed the bill 33 to 4. That was expected. The real test came in the House. Doubts surfaced. A representative insisted there was not enough research. Another repeated the tired line that psilocybin was dangerous. Their words stung, especially knowing psilocybin has one of the safest profiles of any psychoactive substance. Not a single fatality. Not a single case of psychosis. Not a single trauma worsened. Only stories of healing, hope, and the frustration of being denied a second dose once the trials ended. Their ignorance cut deep, but the tide of belief was too strong.

On March 18, the House voted. 56 to 8. It passed. My breath caught in my throat. One last step remained: the governor's signature. She had until April 11. My hope was tempered by fear. This governor was famous for her pocket vetoes, letting bills die in silence without explanation. She had done it many times before. Would she do it again?

Then, on April 7, the news came. She signed. The *Medical Psilocybin Act* was now law. I sat there stunned, tears welling in my eyes. For years, I had shouted into the void, dismissed as fringe, ignored, or mocked. And suddenly, here was proof: psilocybin is *medicine*. It *heals*. And my state, my home, had spoken those words into law.

It felt like standing in the desert after a storm, the first drops of rain hitting dry earth, the smell of renewal rising up all around me. New Mexico had listened. The dark horse had crossed the finish line. And I knew in that moment: I was exactly where I was meant to be.

This new legislation, and this point in history, is where New Mexico has the chance to rise. We are a state built on cultural blending, on borderlands, on Indigenous wisdom woven with Hispanic, Anglo, and immigrant traditions. Our land holds stories of healers who never separated body from spirit. We can lead in a way no other state has.

Imagine this: a veteran with PTSD sits in a safe space, finally free to lay down the weight of war. A mother living with treatment-resistant depression finds light breaking through where there was only darkness. A person struggling with substance use disorder receives care without shame, supported by community instead of punished by law. A cancer patient facing the end of life finds peace in their final days, held in compassion rather than fear. An Indigenous elder holds ceremony without fear of arrest. In every corner of this state, seeking wholeness is not a crime. Clinical care is available. Ceremonial practice is protected. Decriminalization sets the ground. Health equity keeps the heart beating.

New Mexico could be the first place in the nation to truly honor all of it. Not one path, but many. Not one way, but wholeness.

I did not write this book just to tell my story. I wrote it because stories change laws. Stories soften hearts. Stories push the conversation forward when statistics alone cannot.

And honestly, I did not choose to write this book. The mushrooms programmed me to write it. The words came through me as much as from me. At times, it felt less like writing and more like channeling, as if the medicine itself insisted these pages be born.

Education is power. Advocacy is love in action. And every page you read is a seed planted. In you. In this movement. In the future we are creating together.

The question is not whether psychedelics are coming back. They already have. The question is, *How, and how long will it take?*

Will we allow the same old systems of power to shape this renaissance? Or will we do something braver? Something truer?

Healing does not stop. It spreads. New Mexico can send out a wave that the whole country feels. And you, dear reader, are part of it.

Carry the story forward. Speak of what is possible. Refuse to let healing be caged or commodified. Stand for equity. Stand for love. Stand for the medicine.

The mushrooms have always known the way.

Now we can walk it. Together.

CATHERINE - *It feels complete.*

    The story told. The light shared.

    Am I done?

MARIA - *You are never done.*

    Healing does not end.

    It expands and closes the gaps.

CATHERINE - *Then what is left for me?*

MARIA - *To walk.*

> *To speak.*

> *To remember.*

> *And to hand another branch to them.*

CATHERINE - *To the reader?*

MARIA - *Yes.*

> *YOU.*

> *Carry the light forward.*

> *Use your reach.*

OPTIMIZE YOUR EXPERIENCE

Preparation Before the Journey

¡OYE! Have your usual brew—then back away from the pot.

If skipping caffeine gives you a headache, a small cup an hour before is fine. But less is best. Riding a mushroom wave while over-caffeinated is like meditating on a trampoline. You're aiming for depth, not bounce.

¡OYE! Visit psychedelicinteraction.com

Some meds play nice. Others don't. Know before you go.

¡OYE! Talk consent around touch beforehand.

That reassuring hand on your shoulder? Beautiful—if expected. Awkward, if not. Always check in first. Nobody wants surprise intimacy while talking to a tree.

¡OYE! Ditch the dairy—it dulls the magic.

That grilled cheese might sabotage your sacred trip. Milk products can block psilocybin absorption, so hold the cheddar for at least two hours before and after. Let the journey unfold.

¡OYE! Energy is contagious—mushrooms pick up what you're putting down.

They don't just read the room. They *magnify* what's in the room. So bring grounded presence, sprinkle in some curiosity, and leave the cranky at the door.

¡OYE! Bring an eye mask.

This isn't just a blackout tool. It's your ticket to the IMAX of the soul. The fewer distractions out there, the more revelations in here.

¡OYE! Expect the unexpected. And then expect to be wrong about that too.

The medicine doesn't take requests. It delivers what you need, not what you planned. Ditch the control and ride the current—it knows where it's going.

¡OYE! Set intentions as invitations, not demands.

Write what matters to you, refine it, and speak it aloud. The mushrooms listen, but they respond in their own language and at their own pace.

¡OYE! Don't ghost your meds.

Antidepressants aren't a bad date. You can't just disappear. Break up slowly, with a professional third wheel. Tapering takes teamwork. And fewer withdrawal meltdowns in aisle 5!

¡OYE! Home is where the dishes judge you.

A sink full of reminders can pull you right out of the medicine. Go somewhere neutral. Clean space, clean slate, clear mind.

¡OYE! This isn't a mushroom-measuring contest.

Someone else's hero dose might be your nope. Start where *you* are, not where someone else ego-tripped.

¡OYE! Set and setting doesn't just mean your couch and candles.

It's your mindset, your heart state, your readiness to meet whatever comes up. Don't just feng shui the room—check in with your soul. Are you here to heal, or are you trying to hide?

¡OYE! Sometimes the journey starts before the mushrooms show up.

The moment you set your intention, the medicine stirs. Dreams shift, memories sneak in, feelings bubble up. It's like the medicine clocked in before you even swallowed.

¡OYE! Pack for peace, not Pinterest.

Bring a soft blanket, a meaningful object, or a scent that soothes. This isn't a slumber party... it's sacred work. Comfort calms your system. Clutter confuses it.

¡OYE! Have a 'why,' but hold it lightly.

Intentions guide the journey, but they don't guarantee the outcome. Be clear, but stay open. The medicine doesn't always give you what you want, but it always delivers what you need.

¡OYE! Macrodosing = usually 2 to 4 grams.

Start with awareness. Don't go big just to go hard.

¡OYE! You can't transcend the ego if your bra is trying to kill you.

No one has ever found the meaning of life while wearing anything itchy, tight, or riding up in weird places. Choose comfort like your healing depends on it... because it kinda does.

¡OYE! You don't need a "hero" dose to find your inner hero.

Ego dissolution often happens between 2–4 grams with a proper mindset.

¡OYE! Plan your return before you depart.

Block off the day after your session. Cancel errands. Leave space for rest and reflection... don't go from ego death to emails.

¡OYE! Sketchy vibes aren't medicine.

Get your psychedelics from trusted, reliable sources. Purity matters. Safety matters. Healing starts with knowing what you're taking.

¡OYE! Lemon tekking is like pressing fast-forward—on purpose.

Mix your mushrooms with fresh-squeezed limeade, lemonade, or orange juice (not from concentrate!) and let it steep for fifteen to twenty minutes. The effects come on faster, feel more intense, and don't last as long. Many people find they need a smaller dose. Just don't forget to drink it, because after twenty minutes, the magic starts to fade. This isn't a hack; it's a shift in timing. Use it when you're ready to meet the medicine sooner and stronger.

¡OYE! If it tastes like a forest floor, that's because it basically is.

Don't expect dessert. Expect dirt. Mix with citrus if you need to, and if you like the flavor... we're both impressed and mildly concerned.

During the Journey

¡OYE! Not everything you see is literal, but it's all meaningful.

Visions can be wild. Don't get stuck on the details. Ask what they feel like, not just what they look like.

¡OYE! Psilocybin isn't a homewrecker.

It doesn't break your marriage. It just turns up the volume on what's already there. Love gets louder. Resentment does too. The medicine doesn't invent problems. It just flips on the light.

¡OYE! Your body's thermostat just ate a mushroom, too.

One minute you're in a sauna, the next you're on an arctic tundra. Don't fight it—layer up, cozy down, and let your body vibe with the weather inside you.

¡OYE! Don't panic! You're not dying, you just don't want snacks.

Your stomach's not broken! It's just busy processing eternity. Let the downloads finish buffering. The snacks will still be there when you come back.

¡OYE! Language is a cage, and your journey is a comet.

Trying to describe a psychedelic experience is like catching moonlight in a jar. Words wobble. Meaning slips. Don't worry if you can't explain it all. Some truths are meant to be felt, not squeezed into sentences.

¡OYE! Having a hard time? There's a parachute.

Benadryl + nano-CBD won't end the trip—but they can put ego back in the driver's seat just enough to make you feel human again. You might still see visuals, but the panic eases. The discomfort of letting go softens, and the ride becomes a whole lot gentler.

¡OYE! Touch can tether you.

Sometimes, diving into the psychic muck is only possible when you know someone in the real world has your back. That grounding hand permits you to do the dirty work, knowing you're not drifting alone through the soul swamp.

¡OYE! Pinned to the couch? Perfect.

You weren't meant to wander... at least not out there. The medicine anchors you so you can travel inward. Don't fight the stillness; it's the launchpad for your real journey.

¡OYE! You don't need to "do" the journey... just be in it.

This isn't a test or a task. Your only job is presence. The medicine takes care of the rest.

¡OYE! Let your breath be your anchor.

When the waves get wild, your breath is the rope that tethers you to safety. Inhale trust. Exhale resistance.

¡OYE! Mushrooms might flip your script.

These fungi love a good contradiction. They'll nudge you into the very thing you've spent a lifetime avoiding—because that's how new neural paths are made. Insomniacs sleep. Introverts speak. Control freaks surrender. Don't question... observe.

¡OYE! Twitches, tingles, and toe wiggles? Let it happen.

Your body might do some weird stuff: jerks, shudders, sighs. That's not you "losing it." That's you letting go. These odd little releases are your nervous system's way of cleaning house.

¡OYE! Your first insight might not be your deepest one.

Sometimes the real gem is buried under the obvious takeaway. Keep digging. Let time refine the message.

¡OYE! Headphones + eye mask = inner galaxy.

This isn't a costume, it's a spacecraft. Strap in, block out the outside world, and let the journey launch from the inside out.

¡OYE! Music is sacred—or sabotaging.

The right song can open your heart. The wrong one might make you want to karate chop a flute. Curate wisely—your nervous system is listening.

¡OYE! Lose the distractions.

Distractions are the ego's way of throwing glitter at the crime scene. It wants your attention outside so you never look at what's unraveling within. That itch? That urge to check your phone? The facial liquid letting? Classic sabotage. Guard your focus like your growth depends on it—because it does.

¡OYE! Lean into it.

Mushrooms don't slay your dragons for you! They hand you a flashlight and shove you toward the cave. It's scary, yes, but guess where the treasure is? Face the fire, brave the dark, and you'll find the gold. Discomfort is the toll, but the lessons are guaranteed.

¡OYE! Silence can be louder than sound.

Sometimes, no playlist is the best playlist. Let the absence of noise become its own kind of music.

¡OYE! Got gold? Spit it out fast and get back to the goods.

If a cosmic download lands mid-trip, say it quick and drop back in. A good guide will catch it for you, like a soul stenographer with a clipboard and good vibes. You'll have time to unpack the meaning later. For now, stay with the magic.

¡OYE! If you're wondering if it's working... it's working.

Doubt is part of the ride. Trust the unfolding, even if it doesn't look how you imagined.

¡OYE! Ego dissolution feels less like enlightenment and more like a slow-motion identity crisis.

Don't panic—it's not death, it's just your inner control freak losing Wi-Fi. Breathe. Surrender. That unraveling feeling? It's actually the pre-party to becoming someone new. Weird, huh?

¡OYE! Crying might just feel like your face is leaking.

Sometimes tears sneak out like your spirit sprang a leak. Let them flow. That's just your soul doing some unscheduled plumbing maintenance.

¡OYE! Skip the tissues—get a towel.

You might cry enough to water a houseplant. Tissues are no match for a full-body soul purge. Towels: because sacred snot is still snot.

¡OYE! You might ugly cry while laughing like a maniac. That's normal.

Mushrooms stir the soul. Don't analyze the combo platter of feelings... just let them cook.

¡OYE! Small doses, steady rewiring.

Who knew subtle shifts could sneak in like ninjas and rearrange the furniture?

After the Journey

¡OYE! Don't rush to make it make sense.

Some insights don't come with subtitles. Let the weird, wonderful pieces breathe. Meaning appears when it's ready, usually when you stop chasing it.

¡OYE! No fireworks? No problem.

Not every journey comes with blinding insight or life-altering clarity. Mushrooms work in mysterious ways. Sometimes the healing happens so subtly, there's no clear lesson at all—just a quiet shift that unfolds in the days or weeks that follow.

¡OYE! Magic doesn't vanish just because you're back at work.

Integration means weaving what you've learned into your everyday life. Don't file your experience away. Live it out, one choice at a time.

¡OYE! Contrary actions create new neural paths.

Psilocybin throws open the emergency exit on your usual behavior patterns. Suddenly, you get a pause... an unexpected "Are you sure you want to do that thing you always do?" Instead of reacting like a well-trained lab rat, you get to choose a new move. Make the weird choice. Make the kind choice. Make the opposite-of-what-you-usually-do choice. That's the gold. And when you do it again? Boom! Neuroplasticity. Your brain's like, "Wait... we can do that now?"

¡OYE! Don't live-stream your soul before it's done buffering.

Sharing your journey can be healing, but rushing to explain can strip away the sacred. Hold it close until it ripens.

¡OYE! No insight? Doesn't mean no impact.

Sometimes the mushrooms deliver their message like a ninja. Silent, slow, and confusing until it dropkicks you three days later while brushing your teeth. Practice patience.

¡OYE! Capture the wisdom before it fades.

Have a journal nearby as you land. You might write like a toddler on a trampoline, and that's perfect. The scribbles, fragments, and run-on thoughts are the footprints of your experience. Don't edit the magic out.

¡OYE! You just came back from the moon, don't rush into Costco.

Integration takes time. Your nervous system needs soft landings, not loud errands. Go slow. Go tender. You're still reassembling.

¡OYE! Expect unexpected shifts afterward.

Mushrooms move you. Literally. Sleep patterns, moods, behaviors… they all might shift.

¡OYE! Integration isn't extra credit.

Taking care of yourself is the work. Every boundary you set, every moment you choose rest over rush, every act of kindness toward yourself—that's integration in motion.

¡OYE! Psilocybin drops "choice points" like breadcrumbs after a journey.

You can replay the old track, or spin something brand new.

¡OYE! It's integration, not interrogation. Put the flashlight and notebook down.

You don't have to solve your experience. Just return to it with curiosity. New layers will reveal themselves over time.

¡OYE! Music becomes a bridge.

The right playlist can become the soundtrack to your healing—even after the journey ends.

¡OYE! New self, same old closet.

Integration is like trying on outfits. Shame still hangs on the rack, but you don't have to wear it. Keep slipping into the new fit of self-acceptance until it feels like your favorite.

GLOSSARY

Agoraphobia

An anxiety disorder where individuals fear being in situations where they feel they cannot escape, often leading to avoidance of public places or leaving the home.

Attachment

The emotional bond that develops between a person and their caregivers, typically in early childhood, which shapes patterns of relating, trust, and intimacy throughout life. Attachment styles such as secure, anxious, avoidant, or disorganized can influence relationships, emotional regulation, and mental health. Therapeutic work can help heal attachment wounds and foster healthier relational patterns.

Breathwork

A therapeutic practice that involves controlled breathing techniques to improve physical, emotional, and mental well-being. Breathwork can help reduce stress, increase relaxation, and promote emotional release by influencing the nervous system. It is often used in conjunction with meditation or psychedelic therapies to enhance healing and self-awareness.

Ceremony

A structured, ritualized experience involving psychedelics, often guided by a shaman or curandera, in which spiritual insights are sought.

Choice Points

Moments after psilocybin use, when neuroplasticity creates the opportunity to pause and choose a new behavior instead of repeating old patterns. Creating new habits becomes much easier when these choices are practiced and reinforced. This is where lasting, permanent change can occur.

Couch-Lock

A term used to describe a feeling of being physically immobile or "stuck," typically associated with intense psychedelic experiences where one may feel compelled to stay in one spot for an extended period.

Curandera

A traditional healer, often from Latin American cultures, who uses natural remedies and spiritual practices, sometimes including psychedelics, to treat physical or mental health issues.

Depression

A mental health condition marked by persistent sadness, hopelessness, and loss of interest in daily activities. Symptoms include fatigue, changes in appetite, sleep disturbances, and difficulty concentrating. Depression can result from a mix of genetic, biological, and environmental factors and is typically treated with therapy, medication, or both.

Dosing

The process of taking a specific amount of a substance, such as psilocybin, typically measured in grams, to achieve a desired effect.

Ego Death

A term used to describe the experience of losing the sense of personal identity or ego, often seen as a key moment in deep psychedelic experiences, where the individual feels united with everything.

Ego Dissolution

A term used to describe the experience of losing a sense of self, where the boundaries between "self" and the world dissolve, often leading to feelings of unity or connectedness.

Emotional Triggers Treatment (ETT)

A therapy method that works to identify and address emotional triggers by reprocessing past emotional experiences using Memory Reconsolidation. ETT helps to reframe and heal unresolved trauma, and it pairs effectively with psychedelic therapies to promote deeper trauma resolution and emotional healing.

Facilitating

The role of a trained professional who supports individuals during their psychedelic experience, helping to ensure safety, understanding, and emotional support throughout the process.

Generational Trauma

Emotional pain that is passed down through generations, often stemming from events like abuse or loss. It affects the behavior and mental health of descendants, even if they didn't directly experience the trauma. Psychedelic therapy can help address and heal these cycles.

Guiding

See **Facilitating.**

Hero Dose

A very high dose of a psychedelic substance, typically used in a therapeutic context to produce profound, transformative experiences. This is the most intense level of dosing. For psilocybin, a hero dose is generally considered to be 5 grams or more.

Inner Child Work

A therapeutic approach focused on healing emotional wounds from childhood that may continue to affect an individual's thoughts, behaviors, and relationships in adulthood. It involves reconnecting with the "inner child" to address unmet needs, trauma, and unresolved emotions, often through techniques like visualization, reparenting, and guided reflection.

Integration

The process of making sense of and incorporating the insights gained during a psychedelic experience into everyday life, helping to create lasting positive change.

Intention Setting

Before a psychedelic session, the individual sets personal goals or intentions for the experience, helping to focus the journey and promote healing.

Lemon Tekking

A method of preparing psilocybin mushrooms by soaking them in lemon, lime, or orange juice to intensify the effects and speed up absorption, making the experience stronger and shorter.

Looping

A phenomenon that can occur during a psychedelic experience where the individual feels trapped in repetitive thought patterns or experiences, often causing distress.

LSD (Lysergic Acid Diethylamide)

A powerful psychedelic substance known for altering perception, mood, and consciousness, often used in therapy for its deep psychological effects, similar to psilocybin.

Macrodose

A relatively high dose of a psychedelic substance, typically taken for therapeutic or profound experiential purposes. Macrodoses are intended to produce strong, intense effects, often leading to deep introspection, emotional breakthroughs, or altered perceptions of reality. In the context of psilocybin, a macrodose is generally considered to be around 3 grams or more.

Magic Mushrooms

See **Psilocybin**. This is a slang term coined by author and researcher R. Gordon Wasson in the 1950s, after his famous journey to Mexico, where he first encountered the psychoactive use of mushrooms by indigenous people. The term has since become widely used to refer to mushrooms containing psilocybin, a naturally occurring psychedelic compound.

Major Depressive Disorder (MDD)

See **Depression**. MDD is a severe form of depression lasting at least two weeks, significantly affecting daily functioning. Symptoms include intense sadness, fatigue, and an inability to enjoy life. MDD requires professional treatment, often involving therapy and medication.

Maria Sabina

A renowned Mazatec healer from Mexico, famous for her use of psilocybin mushrooms in sacred ceremonies. She is considered a pioneer in introducing the healing properties of mushrooms to the Western world. Maria Sabina's work remains influential in both indigenous healing practices and psychedelic therapy.

Memory Reconsolidation

The process by which memories are updated or restored after an emotional experience. In psychedelic therapy, this can help reframe traumatic memories in a more healing context.

Mesodose

A moderate dose of a psychedelic substance, typically between a microdose and a therapeutic dose, aimed at achieving mild but noticeable effects. For psilocybin, a mesodose is generally considered to be .8-1.2 grams.

Microdose

Taking a minimal, sub-perceptual dose of a psychedelic substance, usually about 1/10th to 1/20th of a standard dose, to enhance mood, creativity, or focus without noticeable hallucinations. For psilocybin, a microdose is generally considered to be .1-.5 grams.

Mindfulness Modalities

Therapeutic practices, like meditation, that involve being fully present and aware in the moment, often used alongside psychedelic therapy to enhance insight and healing.

Mycelium

The root-like network of fungal threads (hyphae) that grow beneath the surface of soil or organic matter. Mycelium plays a crucial role in nutrient absorption, decomposition, and the reproduction of fungi. It is also the structure from which mushrooms (such as psilocybin mushrooms) emerge, serving as the foundation for fungal life.

Non-Specific Amplifier

A term for a substance, like psilocybin, that amplifies the intensity of an experience in a broad, non-directed way. It heightens all aspects of perception, emotion, and thought without focusing on any particular area, allowing for a more holistic enhancement of the individual's inner experience.

Neuroplasticity

The brain's ability to reorganize and form new neural connections throughout life in response to learning, experience, or injury. This adaptive process allows the brain to adjust its structure and function, supporting memory, recovery, and cognitive flexibility. Psychedelics, such as psilocybin, have been shown to promote neuroplasticity, potentially aiding in healing and emotional growth.

Post-Traumatic Stress Disorder (PTSD)

A mental health condition that can develop after an individual experiences or witnesses a traumatic event, such as combat, natural disasters, accidents, or violence. Symptoms of PTSD include intrusive memories, nightmares, flashbacks, heightened anxiety, irritability, and emotional numbness. It can have a profoundly negative impact on daily functioning and relationships. In recent years, psychedelic therapies, particularly with substances like psilocybin and MDMA, have shown promise in helping individuals with PTSD by facilitating emotional processing and trauma resolution.

Psilocybin

A naturally occurring psychedelic compound found in certain mushrooms, often called "magic mushrooms." It's known for its ability to alter perception and consciousness.

Psychedelic

A class of substances that alter perception, mood, and consciousness, often inducing experiences of visual and auditory hallucinations, altered thinking, and a sense of expanded awareness. The term "psychedelic" was coined by psychiatrist Humphry Osmond in 1957, derived from the Greek words *psyche* (soul) and *delos* (manifest), meaning "mind-manifesting." Psychedelics, such as psilocybin, LSD, and DMT, are used both recreationally and therapeutically to explore consciousness and facilitate emotional or spiritual healing.

Psychedelic-Assisted Therapy (PAT)

A type of therapy where a person uses psychedelic substances, like psilocybin, under the supervision of a trained therapist to help address mental health issues, such as depression or trauma.

Psychonaut

A person who is experienced in exploring altered states of consciousness, typically through the use of psychedelics, to gain self-awareness or spiritual insight.

Recreational Use

Using psychedelics for non-therapeutic purposes, typically for fun or spiritual exploration, without the guidance of a trained professional.

Remission

A period in cancer treatment where the signs and symptoms of the disease significantly decrease or disappear. Remission may be temporary, and ongoing monitoring is required, as the cancer could return.

Selective Serotonin Reuptake Inhibitor (SSRI)

A class of antidepressant medications that work by increasing serotonin levels in the brain, helping to improve mood, reduce anxiety, and alleviate symptoms of depression. Common SSRIs include fluoxetine (Prozac), sertraline (Zoloft), and escitalopram (Lexapro). They are often prescribed to treat conditions like depression, anxiety disorders, and PTSD.

Set

The mental and emotional state a person brings to their psychedelic experience. This includes their mood, mindset, and expectations.

Setting

The physical environment in which a psychedelic experience takes place. A calm, safe, and supportive setting can enhance the therapeutic effects of the experience.

Shaman

A spiritual healer or guide, often from indigenous cultures, who uses rituals, ceremonies, and plant medicines (such as psilocybin) to facilitate healing, insight, and spiritual growth. Shamans are believed to have a deep connection to the spiritual world and act as intermediaries between the physical and spiritual realms, guiding individuals through transformative experiences.

Situational Depression

See **Depression**. A temporary form of depression triggered by a specific life event, such as loss or stress. While similar to MDD, the symptoms are generally less severe and improve as the individual adapts. Situational depression often resolves on its own with time and support.

Synesthesia

A neurological condition where stimulation of one sense triggers an involuntary experience in another, such as seeing colors when hearing music or associating tastes with words. Psychedelics can sometimes induce synesthesia, amplifying sensory connections and enhancing perception.

Tapering

The gradual reduction of a substance, such as medication or alcohol, to minimize withdrawal symptoms and allow the body to adjust. In the context of psychedelics, tapering might refer to slowly decreasing the dose of a substance like an SSRI before introducing psychedelic therapy to reduce the risk of adverse interactions.

Therapeutic Dose

The amount of a psychedelic substance that is administered to achieve a therapeutic effect, typically larger than a microdose but not as intense as a hero dose.

TheraPsil

A Canadian organization focused on providing training, research, and advocacy for psychedelic-assisted therapy (PAT). It supports healthcare professionals in integrating psychedelics, particularly psilocybin, into therapeutic practices, and works to advance public understanding and acceptance of psychedelic medicine for mental health treatment.

Tripsit

A term for a trusted person who stays with someone during a psychedelic experience, offering support and ensuring safety. This person may guide or simply provide reassurance.

Updosing

Gradually increasing the dose of a psychedelic substance during a session to deepen the experience or reach a specific therapeutic effect.

Veladas

A traditional healing ceremony practiced by indigenous groups in Mexico, particularly the Mazatec, involving the use of psilocybin mushrooms. Typically held at night, the ceremony is guided by a shaman or healer, focusing on spiritual insight, emotional healing, and deep introspection. The experience is seen as a means to connect with the divine and promote psychological well-being.

Withdrawal

The physical and psychological symptoms that occur when someone reduces or stops taking a pharmaceutical drug, especially after long-term use or dependency. Common symptoms include anxiety, irritability, fatigue, dizziness, and mood swings. Withdrawal is particularly common with medications like antidepressants (SSRIs), benzodiazepines, and opioids, and should be managed carefully, often with a tapering process.

REFERENCES

Cajete, G. (2000). *Native science: Natural laws of interdependence.* Clear Light Publishers.

Canal, C. E., & Murnane, K. S. (2017). The serotonin 5-HT2C receptor and the non-addictive nature of classic hallucinogens. *Journal of Psychopharmacology*, 31(1), 127–143. https://doi.org/10.1177/0269881116677104

Carhart-Harris, R. L., Bolstridge, M., Rucker, J., Day, C. M. J., Erritzoe, D., Kaelen, M., Bloomfield, M., Rickard, J. A., Forbes, B., Feilding, A., Taylor, D., Pilling, S., Curran, H. V., & Nutt, D. J. (2016). Psilocybin with psychological support for treatment-resistant depression: An open-label feasibility study. *The Lancet Psychiatry*, 3(7), 619–627. https://doi.org/10.1016/S2215-0366(16)30065-7

Estrada, Á. (1981). *María Sabina: Her life and chants* (H. Munn, Trans. & commentary). Ross-Erikson.

Gouin, J.-P., & Kiecolt-Glaser, J. K. (2012). The impact of psychological stress on wound healing: Methods and mechanisms. *Critical Care Nursing Clinics of North America*, 24(2), 201–213. https://doi.org/10.1016/j.ccell.2012.03.006

Griffiths, R. R., Johnson, M. W., Carducci, M. A., Umbricht, A., Richards, W. A., Richards, B. D., Cosimano, M. P., & Klinedinst, M. A. (2016). Psilocybin produces substantial and sustained decreases in depression and anxiety in patients with life-threatening cancer: A randomized double-blind trial. *Journal of Psychopharmacology*, 30(12), 1181–1197. https://doi.org/10.1177/0269881116675513

Gukasyan, N., Griffiths, R. R., Yaden, D. B., Antoine, D. G., II, & Nayak, S. M. (2023). Attenuation of psilocybin mushroom effects during and after SSRI/SNRI antidepressant use. *Journal of Psychopharmacology*, 37(7), 707–716. https://doi.org/10.1177/02698811231179910

Mortaheb, S., Fort, L. D., Mason, N. L., Mallaroni, P., Ramaekers, J. G., & Demertzi, A. (2024). Dynamic functional hyperconnectivity after psilocybin intake is primarily associated with oceanic boundlessness. *Biological Psychiatry: Cognitive Neuroscience and Neuroimaging*, 9(7), 681–692. https://doi.org/10.1016/j.bpsc.2024.04.001

Ortiz, A. (1969). *The Tewa world: Space, time, being, and becoming in a Pueblo society*. University of Chicago Press.

Sahagún, B. de. (1950–1982). *Florentine codex: General history of the things of New Spain* (A. J. O. Anderson & C. E. Dibble, Trans.). University of Utah Press.

Samorini, G. (1992). The oldest representations of hallucinogenic mushrooms in the world (Sahara Desert, 9000–7000 B.P.). *Integration*, 2(3), 69–78.

Shao, L.-X., Liao, C., Gregg, I., Davoudian, P. A., Savalia, N. K., Delagarza, K., & Kwan, A. C. (2021). Psilocybin induces rapid and persistent growth of dendritic spines in frontal cortex in vivo. *Neuron*, 109(16), 2535–2544.e4. https://doi.org/10.1016/j.neuron.2021.06.008

Stewart, O. C. (1987). *Peyote religion: A history*. University of Oklahoma Press.

Tipado, Z., Kuypers, K. P. C., Sorger, B., & Ramaekers, J. G. (2024). Visual hallucinations originating in the retinofugal pathway under clinical and psychedelic conditions. *European Neuropsychopharmacology*, 85, 10–20. https://doi.org/10.1016/j.euroneuro.2024.04.011

Winkelman, M. (2019). Introduction: Evidence for entheogen use in prehistory and world religions. *Journal of Psychedelic Studies*, 3(2), 43–62. https://doi.org/10.1556/2054.2019.024

Wyman, L. C. (1975). *The Night Way: A history and a history of a Navajo ceremonial*. University of Arizona Press.

ACKNOWLEDGEMENTS

This book had a life of its own from day one. The words showed up uninvited, took over my schedule, and refused to leave until I surrendered and wrote them down. At times, I wondered if I was just a vessel with a keyboard. Still, I'm profoundly grateful for the journey and for the mushrooms that taught me, through experience, that integration is a living practice. In the end, writing this book became its own sacred ceremony and the humbling realization that I was being written as much as I was writing.

Ken, thank you for loving someone whose dinner conversations sometimes include mushrooms, consciousness, ancestral healing, and the occasional trip through the cosmos. Your patience deserves its own chapter. Possibly an entire sequel. More than that, much of what I do would not be possible without you. You support me in selfless, loving, and steady ways, often believing in me more than I believe in myself. You've been my reliable guide when I've needed to do my own healing work, offering both courage and calm when the path felt uncertain. When my mind was busy traveling through galaxies, you were the one with a foot firmly planted in the practical world, helping me find my way back home.

Alex Morin and Marcy Barbaro of Working Writers Co., my development editors, helped shape this book in ways I deeply appreciate. Alex believed wholeheartedly in both me and this subject matter from the very beginning, offering encouragement and thoughtful guidance as the manuscript took form. Marcy, on the other hand, initially worried that speaking openly about this work might put me at unnecessary risk. Fair concern. Over time, though, she watched something unexpected happen. As my relationship with the mushrooms deepened, she commented more than once that I appeared to look younger each week. Not surprisingly, research is starting to suggest psilocybin may extend lifespan. I'll let the scientists sort that one out. I'm grateful to both of them for their different viewpoints and for challenging me in ways I very much needed.

I'm also deeply thankful to the remarkable group of writers who allowed me to read early pieces and gather honest feedback: Christina Siepiela, Kim Sekleski, Katie Woodruff, Cara Krezek, Tayler DeLisio, Zoom Iwuagwu, Kiersty Kelly, Steve Whigham, and Meghan Seybold. This group gave me the rare gift of a safe place to try out stories before they met the wider world, and often before they were fully baked. Your insights, encouragement, and willingness to listen made the writing process far less lonely and far more meaningful. If you ever come across their work, I encourage you to read it. Each of them is an extraordinary writer and storyteller in their own right, and I'm grateful to have shared this space with you all.

My publishing team, the manager Tiffany, and Dez, deserve a special thank you. I'm grateful to Heather Lutz, an author and a member of my extended family, who connected me with Borderlands Media and helped set this partnership in motion. I know I haven't always made things easy for this group. Deadlines, rewrites, and the occasional "just one more tiny change" email. My sense of urgency and relentless timelines kept everyone on their toes, and Tiffany has had the unenviable job of gently reminding me that publishing, like most things in life, still takes time. Dez was the steady cheerleader along the way, always ready with encouragement when the process felt overwhelming. The editors carried much of the heavy lifting in the copy editing and formatting, turning a mountain of words into something that actually looks like a book. Collectively, they brought patience, skill, and good humor to this project, and I'm deeply grateful for the work they did to bring it to life.

I want to thank my mother, Cecilia Terri Oldre. When I began writing this book, I had no idea how much of it would ultimately be about her and our relationship. The mushrooms became a kind of salve for wounds that had lived between us for years, helping us find our way back to each other in ways I once could not have imagined. If someone had told me years ago that mushrooms would help heal my relationship with my mother, I would have been deeply skeptical. I'm very grateful for her strength, her dedication, and the love that remained present even during the years when we struggled to understand one another. I'm especially thankful for her willingness to grow, to look at the past with honesty, and to meet me again in a new place. In many ways, our healing together became part of the medicine itself, a reminder that when one person does the work, it can begin to soften the generations that came before and the ones that follow. That is a gift I will always carry.

Next, I want to thank my two Jens: Jennifer Hannaford and Jennifer Jones. I met Hannaford during my undergraduate years and Jones back in high school, and both of these women have shaped my life in profound ways. They know me at my core and somehow love me anyway. That level of loyalty should probably come with medals. With them, I have always felt truly seen, understood, and accepted in a way that is rare and deeply grounding. Over the years they have taught me how to face hardship with honesty and resilience, and how to pause long enough to celebrate life's victories along the way. I am deeply grateful for the wisdom, friendship, and unwavering presence they have brought to my life.

Special thanks to my sisters Linda and Cori, my cousins, especially Marcia, Gonzy, and Stephanie, my parents, and my aunt Mitzi. You have filled my life with laughter, deep love, and more family stories than any responsible person should probably publish. We also share a long history of laughing at things we probably shouldn't. Linda and Mitzi make appearances in these pages, but the others have been just as present in my life and in this journey. Each of you showed genuine interest in the progress of this book and supported me along the way, cheering me on through the long process of actually finishing it. Our shared humor and love have always reminded me that laughter is its own kind of medicine, and I'm grateful for the encouragement and joy each of you continues to bring into my life.

I'm also grateful to my long-time friend Bari and to my yoga guide Jess for the personal support you offered throughout this journey. Bari, your friendship has been a steady source of encouragement and perspective over the years. Jess, your guidance on the mat often reminded me to slow down, breathe, and stay present while navigating the many twists and turns of writing this book. Your support helped keep me grounded.

Elizabeth deserves special thanks for the three years she served as my admin while helping me build my practice. Her dedication and reliability allowed me the freedom to pursue other passions, including the documentary and this book. Elizabeth was far more than administrative support. Anyone who has ever tried to run a practice knows that a great admin is part organizer, part therapist, and part miracle worker. She offered valuable perspective as I navigated both professional growth and personal transformation. I'm deeply grateful for the care, insight, and steady presence she brought to that chapter of my life.

Nova Vale, my filmmaking partner, deserves special thanks. She was willing to pick up her camera and follow me through the deeply personal journeys of PAT clients, helping bring these stories to light with care and integrity. Nova believes in this medicine because it changed her own life, and she shares my commitment to helping others understand its healing potential and to challenge the stigma that still surrounds it. Her patience, dedication, and willingness to walk this path beside me mean more than I can adequately express. I'm grateful not only for her partnership in this work, but for the shared vision that continues to guide it, and for being brave enough to film some very profound days at the office.

I'm grateful to the many colleagues who supported and encouraged me along this professional journey: Melissa S, Tessa S, Erin P, Jess E, Josie P, Petrina N, Larry M, Olga A, Peg R, Kristin K, Kirry N, Tina P, Dave P, the Gathering Group Cohort, Joaquin O, and Brenda B. Each of these remarkable individuals contributed to my growth in meaningful ways. Good conversations, hard questions, and the occasional reality check all played their part. Through conversations, collaboration, encouragement, and belief in this work, you helped shape the path that led to this book. I am truly grateful for your wisdom, support, and the role each of you played along the way.

Of course, I must acknowledge the trailblazers who carved the path long before many of us were willing or able to walk it. Robin Carhart-Harris, Paul Stamets, Michael Pollan, Terence McKenna, Mary Cosimano, María Sabina, and Aldous Huxley each helped expand the world's understanding of psychedelic medicine in their own way. Through science, storytelling, advocacy, and courage, they challenged long-held assumptions and helped reopen a conversation that had been buried for decades. Their work created the space for many of us to continue exploring, learning, and sharing the healing potential of these medicines. I'm grateful they were asking these questions long before it was popular to do so.

I also want to express deep gratitude to the clients who trusted me to walk beside them in their healing journeys. Your courage, vulnerability, and willingness to explore the depths of your own lives have taught me more than any training ever could. You are the reason this work matters. It is a privilege to witness the human capacity for growth, resilience, and transformation.

To the many other colleagues who have shared ideas, encouragement, and thoughtful dialogue along the way, thank you for helping shape both my understanding and my practice.

I'm also especially grateful for my weekly Accountability Group and the Tuesday Integration Group. Your conversations, insights, and willingness to engage deeply with this work created a space of learning, reflection, and mutual support that sustained me throughout this process. These communities remind me again and again that healing is rarely a solo endeavor.

I also want to acknowledge my ancestors, known and unknown. The healing explored in these pages did not begin with me, and it will not end with me. I'm grateful for the strength and resilience that traveled through generations and for the opportunity to help carry that healing forward.

If this book taught me anything, it's that healing requires equal parts grace, grit, and trust in the process itself. My hope is that this book opens hearts to the truth that medicine doesn't always come in a bottle; it sometimes grows from the earth, waiting for us to remember.